# Behavioral Medicine: Work, Stress and Health

# NATO ASI Series

## Advanced Science Institutes Series

*A Series presenting the results of activities sponsored by the NATO Science Committee, which aims at the dissemination of advanced scientific and technological knowledge, with a view to strengthening links between scientific communities.*

The Series is published by an international board of publishers in conjunction with the NATO Scientific Affairs Division

| | | |
|---|---|---|
| A | Life Sciences | Plenum Publishing Corporation |
| B | Physics | London and New York |
| | | |
| C | Mathematical and Physical Sciences | D. Reidel Publishing Company Dordrecht and Boston |
| | | |
| D | Behavioural and Social Sciences | Martinus Nijhoff Publishers Dordrecht/Boston/Lancaster |
| E | Applied Sciences | |
| | | |
| F | Computer and Systems Sciences | Springer-Verlag Berlin/Heidelberg/New York |
| G | Ecological Sciences | |

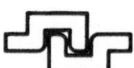

Series D: Behavioural and Social Sciences – No. 19

# Behavioral Medicine: Work, Stress and Health

edited by

## W. Doyle Gentry, PhD

Psychological Associates of Lynchburg
Lynchburg, VA 24502, USA

Formerly:
Department of Behavioral
Medicine & Psychiatry
University of Virginia, USA

## Herbert Benson, MD

Department of Medicine
Harvard Medical School and
Beth Israel Hospital, USA

## Charles J. de Wolff

Director, Workgroup on Psychology
of Work and Organization
University of Nijmegen, The Netherlands

1985 **Martinus Nijhoff Publishers**
Dordrecht / Boston / Lancaster
Published in cooperation with NATO Scientific Affairs Division

Proceedings of the NATO Advanced Study Institute on Behavioral Medicine: Work, Stress and Health, Castera-Verduzan, France, August 1-16, 1981

**Library of Congress Cataloging in Publication Data**

NATO Advanced Study Institute on Behavioral Medicine:
  Work, Stress, and Health (1981 : Castera-Verduzan,
  France)
  Behavioral medicine--work, stress, and health.

  (NATO ASI series. Series D, Behavioral and
social sciences ; no. 19)
  "Proceedings of the NATO Advanced Study Institute
on Behavioural Medicine: Work, Stress, and Health,
Castera-Verduzan, France, August 1-16, 1981"--T.p.
verso.
  "Published in cooperation with NATO Scientific
Affairs Division."
  Includes bibliographies and index.
  1. Coronary heart disease--Psychosomatic aspects--
Congresses. 2. Occupational diseases--Psychosomatic
aspects--Congresses. 3. Stress (Psychology)--
Congresses. 4. Medicine and psychology--Congresses.
I. Gentry, W. Doyle (William Doyle), 1943-
II. Benson, Herbert, 1935-      . III. Wolff,
Charles J. de (Charles Johannes) IV. North Atlantic
Treaty Organization. Scientific Affairs Division.
V. Title. VI. Series. [DNLM: 1. Behavioral Medicine--
congresses. 2. Cardiovascular Diseases--psychology--
congresses. 3. Mental Health Services--congresses.
4. Occupational Diseases--psychology--congresses.
5. Occupational Health Services--congresses. 6. Stress,
Psychological--congresses. WA 495 N279b 1981]
RC685.C6N36  1981        616.07'1          85-28368


ISBN-13: 978-94-010-8792-6    e-ISBN-13: 978-94-009-5179-2
DOI: 10.1007/978-94-009-5179-2


Distributors for the United States and Canada: Kluwer Boston, Inc., 190 Old Derby Street, Hingham, MA 02043, USA

Distributors for the UK and Ireland: Kluwer Academic Publishers, MTP Press Ltd, Falcon House, Queen Square, Lancaster LA1 1RN, UK

Distributors for all other countries: Kluwer Academic Publishers Group, Distribution Center, P.O. Box 322, 3300 AH Dordrecht, The Netherlands

Softcover reprint of the hardcover 1st edition 1985

To

Marilyn Hall

in recognition of and appreciation
for her unselfish and untiring
efforts throughout all phases of
the BONAS ASI, including publication
of this volume...

# PREFACE

This volume contains the entire proceedings of a
North Atlantic Treaty Organization (NATO) Advanced
Study Institute held on August 2-15, 1981 in Castera-
Verduzan, France. The ASI was entitled "Behavioral
Medicine: Work, Stress, and Health." Its major theme
was that health risk attributable to work stress is
defined in terms of a balance between those factors
which influence an individual's susceptibility and his/
her resistance to illness. At the level of the individual
employee, susceptibility factors include psychological
(e.g., Type A behavior pattern) as well as social (e.g.,
blue vs. white collar workers) variables. At an organizational level, they may include company size, level
of employment (e.g., middle-management), and type/extent
of demands placed on workers. Resistance factors,
currently viewed only at the individual level, include:
social support, anger expression, and hardiness, the
latter a personality trait found in highly stressed
executives who remain healthy.

Previous attempts to ameliorate work stress so as
to reduce illness morbidity in employees have focused
on teaching workers to relax under stress, alter stress-
producing Type A characteristics, and ventilate pent-up
anger resulting from day-to-day frustrations at work,
all of which clearly alter physiological function and
account for a high incidence of stress-related illness
(e.g., coronary heart disease, hypertension) in industrialized societies. Such efforts have met with modest
success and warrant further study/application. Efforts
at organizational intervention, as opposed to those aimed
at individual workers, are less evident.

This type of "behavioral medicine" approach to understanding the complexities of work stress and its impact
on health of employees goes beyond the single-discipline
understanding of psychological, sociological, or medical
facets of same and offers a framework for integrating
data obtained from all bio-behavioral fields of study.

It also highlights (a) the need for additional study of "resistance resources" both at the individual and systems level and (b) a shift toward a "balance sheet approach" to effective stress management. The latter is important, e.g., in allowing one to plan for increased social support or anger expression among employees, since early studies show that altering stress factors at the individual level can be difficult because of non-compliance/resistance problems.

New research findings, in addition to those summarized in this volume, presented at the ASI indicated that: (1) under-utilization at work (too few demands) can result in chronic boredom and affect worker health status much the same as over-load; (2) failure to cope with unpredictable stress (e.g., economic instability due to unemployment) results in increased incidence of depression among workers and their dependents; (3) national policies resulting in restriction of high-responsibility jobs to certain race/social class groups can influence disease (e.g., CHD) rates among these same groups; (4) employee "resource inadequacy" and "role ambiguity" are more influential in explaining employee health than are "role conflict" or "overload"; and, (5) cultural factors to some extent modify stress-strain relationships at work.

We are grateful to the 60 faculty and student participants who attended the ASI from 12 NATO and 5 non-NATO countries. It was their enthusiastic sharing of diverse professional expertise and life experience that ensured the educational success of the Institute.

We also wish to express our appreciation to Dr. Tilo Kester for his advice and assistance as regards preparation of the NATO-ASI grant application and selection of Institute site, to Dr. M. di Lullo and Mr. Robert Chabbal for their invaluable assistance in implementing the grant, to all members of the NATO Science Committee, and to Maryse Lagarde, secretary to the Association Scientifique Culturelle et Educative de Bonas, who was so helpful as regards day-to-day administrative matters throughout the two-week Institute.

We are also grateful to Harvard Medical School, Boston, Massachusetts, USA, for accepting the NATO award in our behalf.

    We especially wish to thank our hosts, Professor
Jean-Claude and Mme Simon, whose intellect, charm, and
gracious French hospitality added immeasurably to our
scientific proceedings.  The Chateau de BONAS, set amid
rolling green hils in a region of France famous for its
Armagnac and its excellent cuisine, provided, we believe,
the perfect ecological niche for an international,
interdisciplinary conference; our memories of it shall
not soon fade!

    Finally, we wish to thank Mrs. Henny Hoogervorst,
of Martinus Nijhoff Publishers, for her unfailing patience
in seeing this volume through to completion.  Without
her help, this book would not have been published.


                            The Editors

TABLE OF CONTENTS

XII

# BEHAVIORAL MEDICINE: A MANDATE FOR INTEGRATED RESEARCH

W. Doyle Gentry

Department of Behavioral Medicine
and Psychiatry
University of Virginia
Charlottesville, Virginia (USA)

## 1  INTRODUCTION

The now historic Yale Conference on Behavioral Medicine (1) was held at Yale University on February 4-6, 1977. At this Conference, a group of leading biomedical and behavioral/social science researchers from the USA met and defined the concept of <u>behavioral medicine</u> as follows:

> ... the field concerned with the development
> of behavioral science knowledge and techniques
> relevant to the understanding of physical
> health and illness and the application of this
> knowledge and these techniques to prevention,
> diagnosis, treatment and rehabilitation.

Shortly thereafter, this same group of researchers met at a similar conference held at the Institute of Medicine (USA) and sponsored by the National Academy of Sciences. Here, they (2) further elucidated the concept to more explicitly highlight the issue of <u>integration of thought and technology</u>; the amended definition was as follows:

> ... the interdisciplinary field concerned
> with the development and integration of
> behavioral and biomedical science knowledge
> and techniques relevant to health and ill-
> ness and the application of this knowledge

and these techniques to prevention, diagnosis, treatment and rehabilitation.

The essence of the behavioral medicine research
model is presented in Figure 1. That is, the basic
idea is to examine the complexities of stress and disease (e.g., coronary heart disease) across a broad
range of biobehavioral disciplines, rather than simply
focusing on relationships or empirical findings provided
by a single discipline in terms of its particular tools,
theories, and dogma. As others have noted, behavioral
medicine represents "a pooling of talent and diverse
perspectives" (3), a type of "holistic problem-solving"
(4), a "conceptual crucible" (5), and finally a syn-
thetic "systems theory" model for understanding important
links between stress and disease in humans (6).

It is the Yale definition of behavioral medicine
that has thus far spawned the new JOURNAL OF BEHAVIORAL
MEDICINE (7), the Academy of Behavioral Medicine Research
in the USA, a new mechanism for peer review funding of
research and training grants (8) in the National Institutes of Health (USA), and recent volumes such as that
be Weiss, Herd, & Fox (9) and/or Gentry (10).

While behavioral medicine to date is hardly more
than "an integrative ideal" (11) or "point of departure"
(12) for future research efforts that draw on several
disciplines simultaneously, it is indeed an idea whose
time has come (12-14). The reasons for this include:

- the fact that biomedical and social/behavioral
  science researchers operating along "single
  discipline" lines have failed to explain in any
  all-or-nothing way why some people become ill
  under stress and others do not

- the general maturity of research in the social
  and behavioral sciences, as well as advances in
  behavioral epidemiology (13), in recent years

- the rapid growth of medical or health psychology
  (14), which has added a dimension of applied
  clinical science previously lacking in so-called
  psychosomatic medicine (15)

Whether or not it will realize its initial impetus
(16) is at this point somewhat in doubt. There are
those who reject the concept in favor of the term "bio-

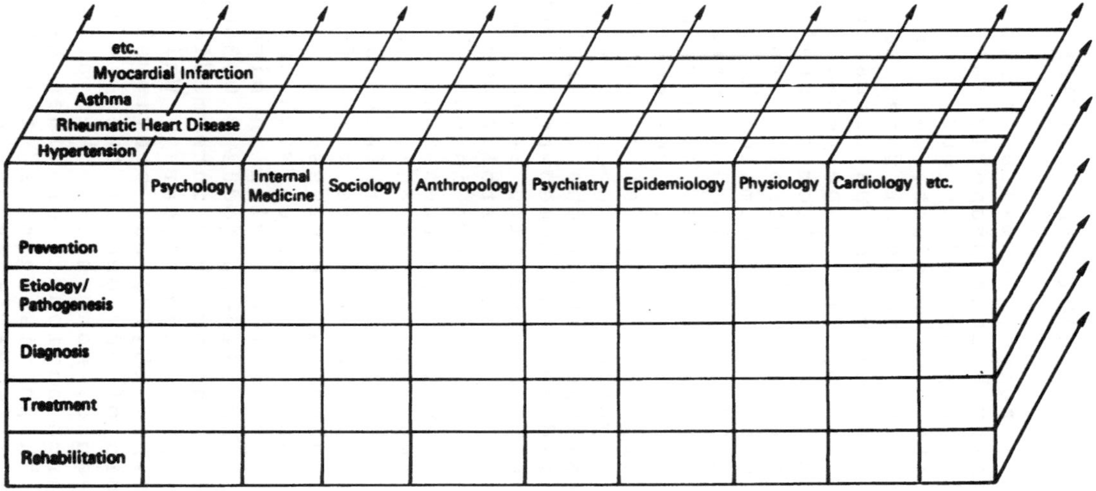

Figure 1. Matrix of Problems in Behavioral Medicine (1).

psychosocial" (17) and there are those who believe it
will misdirect the future growth of research either in
the behavioral sciences or medicine (18). Still and
yet, its proponents seem to far outweigh its detractors!

## 2  EXAMPLES OF BEHAVIORAL MEDICINE AT WORK

At this point, it may be helpful to illustrate the
type of research that properly falls under this rubric.
One example is provided by our own research group (17).
In this particular project, we were attempting to examine
the interactive effects of race, sex, socioecological
stress, and anger-coping patterns on mean blood pressure
and risk for essential hypertension.  In doing so, we
obtained relevant data from a total of 1,006 adults residing in the city of Detroit.  Roughly half of the
sample were male, half female; half were white, half
black; and, half lived in high stress neighborhoods
(low education and income, high crime and divorce rates),
half in low stress areas.  Respondents were also classified as "anger in" vs. "anger out" based on their response to 5 hypothetical anger-provoking situations,
including alleged reactions to an angry boss, policeman,
spouse, children, and homeowner.  Our results suggested
that race and anger-coping style were the significant
determinants of mean diastolic and systolic blood pressure
whereas, all four factors independently affected one's
risk for essential hypertension.  Also of note was the
fact that the etiologic contribution of each factor
added to that of the other factors such that the group
at least risk for HBP were white females who lived in
low stress areas and expressed their anger openly (odds
= 0.0658), while the group with the greatest risk for
HBP were black males living in high stress areas who kept
their anger bottled-up (odds = 0.3860).  Groups with 1,
2, or 3 risk factors had intermediate odds of developing
HBP during their adult years.  While single discipline
studies (e.g., 18,19) had previously isolated the risk
relationship of any one of these 4 factors to elevated
blood pressure, none had looked at them in combination.
Such research obviously provides useful information for
targeting "high risk groups" for this dread disease!  It
also, perhaps more importantly from the behavioral standpoint, provides us with some fairly objective guideline
as to the potential impact of altering behavior (in this
case anger-coping styles) on risk for HBP and subsequent
CHD morbidity.  For example, black males residing in high
stress areas who were classified as "anger in" had a 14%

greater risk of essential hypertension than did their black, male, high stress area, "anger out" counterparts.

A second good example of behavioral medicine research is provided by James et al. (20). They looked at the interactive effects of education and an attitude of environmental mastery (referred to as John Henryism - i.e., belief that persons can control the stress level(s) in their day-to-day environment through hard work and determination) on blood pressure in black American males, a group (as noted above) with a high risk for hypertensive disease. They noted that education and John Henryism interact such that the men with high JH levels and high education are at less risk for HBP (lower mean blood pressure) than their high JH, low education colleagues. They argue that education may be the key to understanding the differential risk for HBP in this instance, i.e., those men with low education were stressed by their attempts to work hard and control their environment, while those with higher education levels could expect to have more control over routine day-to-day stressors and thus be more at ease (relaxed) and thereby less prone to chronic uncertainty and strenuous active coping - both of which they note set one up for elevated blood pressure. Again, previous research had looked at the singular impact of such variables rather than their interactive influence.

Third, there is a very nice study by Kobasa, Maddi, and Puccetti (21) that examines the interactive effects of hardiness (see chapter by Kobasa this Volume) and regular physical exercise in buffering individuals from stress-induced illness. In their study of 137 male business executives, they found that persons who were both hardy (flexible, committed, and in control) and who engaged in nonsport exercise regularly had one-sixth as much self-reported illness as did their non-hardy, non-exercise counterparts. Again, executives who either were hardy or exercised regularly were intermediate in their illness scores. Such research importantly argues for the combined protective effects of personality and behavioral (non-personality) variables in mediating stress-illness relationships, and also points to "high risk" target groups in the work setting.

Finally, in a conceptual rather than empirical paper, Margolis et al. (22) present "an ecological approach" to understanding the emergence of Type A (coronary-prone) behavior (see chapter by Kornitzer this Volume), it link to CHD, and intervention strategies for altering same at

primary, secondary, and tertiary prevention levels. They
argue that Type A behavior can be considered at several
levels of analysis: intrapersonal, interpersonal, institutional, and cultural. For example, at the <u>intrapersonal</u>
level, they propose that Type As (a) have higher performance standards than Type Bs and (b) tend to make attribu-
tions of achievement to effort rather than ability and to
expect future outcomes to be the result of increased or
intense effort rather than ability. On the <u>interpersonal</u>
level, they suggest that (a) Type As tend to select competitive rather than cooperative situations, (b) Type As
will have weaker and less reciprocal social networks
than Type Bs, and (c) Type A behavior will be more evident
in males vs. females because of differential sex role
socialization practices inherent in the society. At the
<u>institutional</u> level, they argue that Type A behavior will
vary as a function of the reward system(s) within the
institution; at the <u>cultural</u> level, Type A behavior will
be seen more in groups where industrialization has des-
troyed social cohesion and where the locus of responsibility has shifted from the larger social group to the
level of the individual. With regard to intervention,
they propose that: (a) multi-level intervention will be
more successful than single-level intervention because
(b) interventions directed at only one level will be unsuccessful because of influences from other levels. As
Roskies (see chapter this Volume) describes, efforts at
altering Type A behavior have thus far <u>only</u> been directed
at the intrapersonal level! In short, the study of Type
A behavior is not the sole province of any single discipline or sub-discipline (e.g., psychology); rather, it can
only be fully understood within the "behavioral medicine"
context of simultaneous, integrated contributions from
sociology, social epidemiology, psychology (social, personality, clinical, developmental), anthropology, history,
etc., as mandated by the matrix model shown earlier (see
Figure 1).

## 3  BALANCE AND COUNTERBALANCE: ROLE OF MEDIATING FACTORS IN BEHAVIORAL MEDICINE RESEARCH

As we have noted elsewhere, health/illness whether
viewed at the individual or group level can no longer be
defined in simplistic, unidimensional terms, i.e., as a
function of exposure to some known or suspected stressor
(23,24). Rather, researchers (and clinicians alike)
must consider the interplay between what we prefer to
call <u>susceptibility</u> factors (those that increased one's

risk for illness) and <u>resistance</u> factors (those which
reduce one's risk). Figure 2 illustrates this model of
balance or counterbalance. While relationships between
susceptibility factors and health/illness, both in and
outside the work setting, have been studied in some
detail over the last several decades, those between
resistance factors and illness are few in number and
essentially date back only 5-10 years to the writings of
Cassel (25), Cobb (26), and Wolf (27). We believe it
is important to keep in mind the fact that susceptibility
and resistance are not simply "two sides of the same
coin," i.e., one is defined as the presence/absence of
the other. On the contrary, we believe that each category of variables functions in an interdependent, or
independent manner in its relationship(s) with the others.
As we try to convey in Figure 3, an individual can
evidence a <u>high health risk</u> if he/she has a dispropor-
tionate loading of susceptibility versus resistance. On
the other hand (see Figure 4), other individuals can be
seen as having <u>little or no health risk</u>, despite such
things as Type A behavior or a high dose of critical
life events (see chapter by Theorell this Volume), if
they have ample resistance resources at their disposal.

Again, the idea here is integration and interaction,
both at the conceptual and statistical level(s).


4   GOALS AND ORGANIZATION OF THE BONAS ASI

This NATO Advanced Study Institute on "Behavioral
Medicine: Work, Stress, and Health" is a natural outgrowth
of the behavioral medicine movement. It is an integrated,
interdisciplinary Institute, not dominated by any single
theoretical approach, disciplinary dogma, experimental
or statistical approach, etc. In fact, it three co-
directors represent rather divergent professional backgrounds and research interests, ranging from clinical/
industrial medicine (Benson) through clinical/medical
psychology (Gentry) to industrial/organizational psychology
(de Wolff). The proceedings too are broad-ranging, while
at the same time focusing on the topic of mutual interest,
that being a more precise understanding of health risk
resulting from stress in the workplace. As such, this
volume includes contributions from epidemiologists,
sociologists, psychologists, physicians, as well as
persons working in- and outside the work setting. While
one will see immediately that much of the focus is on
the level of the individual (employee), this we would

8

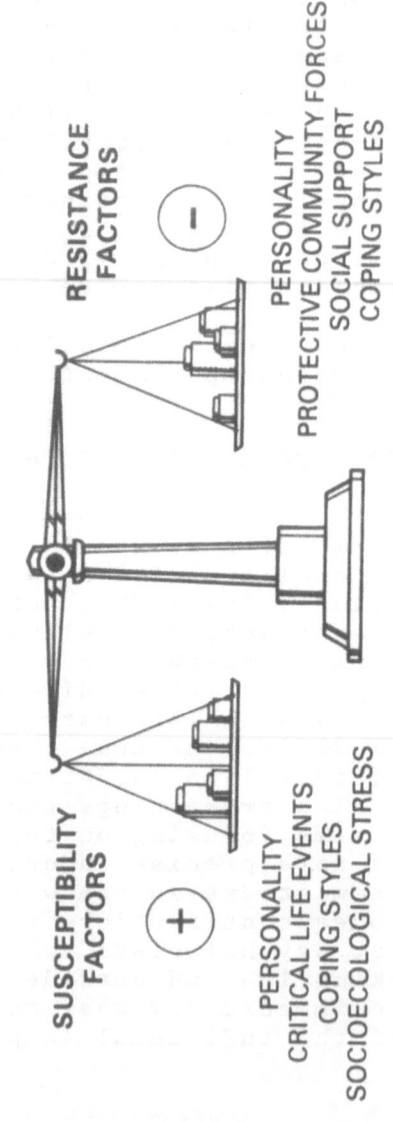

Figure 2. Model of Health Risk (23).

9

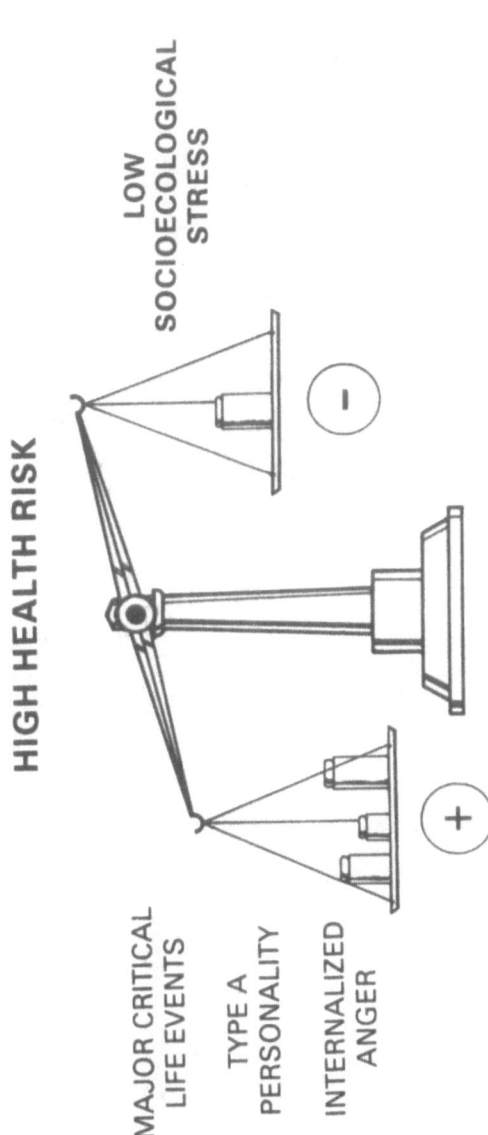

Figure 3.   High Health Risk (23).

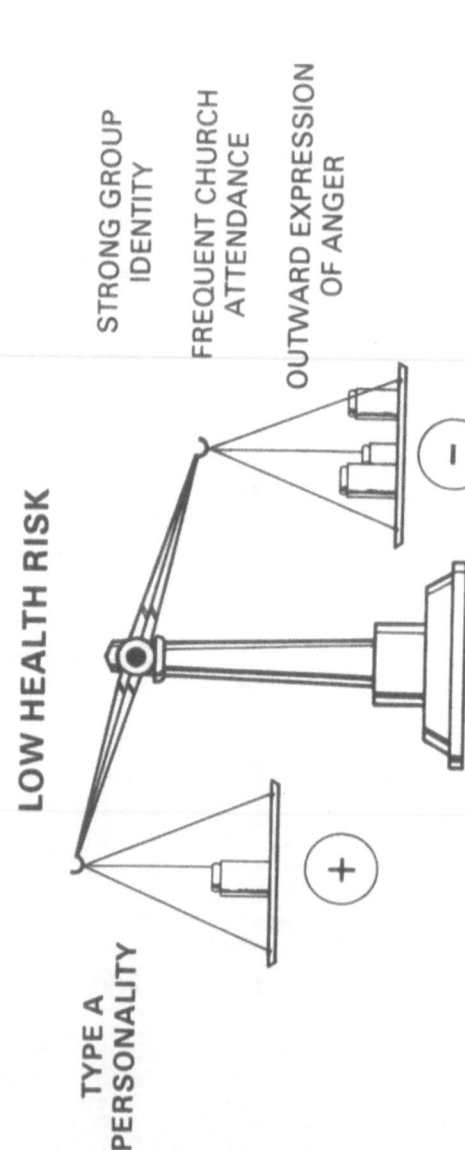

Figure 4. Low Health Risk (23).

suggest is more a reflection of the present <u>state-of-the-art</u> than any bias on our part. It represents, as does behavioral medicine per se, a "point of departure" and not "the final word" (1). It also represents, we believe, the first step toward deriving the "high-need, high-yield" equation postulated by Collings (see chapter this Volume) as being so necessary for cost-effective preventive intervention in the workplace; again, referring to the ecological model of Margolis et al. (22), we believe that both <u>need</u> and <u>yield</u> will be determined by factors operating at several levels (including those at the individual and organizational), as well as be factors which both contribute to (susceptibility) and detract from (resistance) one's ultimate health risk.

## REFERENCES

1    Schwartz, G.E. and S.M. Weiss. Yale Conference on Behavioral Medicine: A Proposed Definition and Statement of Goals. Journal of Behavioral Medicine 1 (1978) 3-12.
2.   Schwartz, G.E. and S.M. Weiss. Behavioral Medicine Revisited: An Amended Definition. Journal of Behavioral Medicine 1 (1978) 249-252.
3.   Weiss, S.M. and G.E. Schwartz. Behavioral Medicine: The Biobehavioral Perspective. In R.S. Surwit, R.B. Williams, A. Steptoe, and R. Biersner (Eds.) Behavioral Treatment of Disease. (New York, Plenum, 1982).
4.   Gentry, W.D. What is Behavioral Medicine? In J.R. Eiser (Ed.) Social Psychology and Behavioral Medicine. (New York, Wiley, 1982).
5.   Weiss, S.M. and G.E.Schwartz. Behavioral Medicine: The Biobehavioral Perspective. In R.S. Surwit, R.B. Williams, A. Steptoe, and R. Biersner (Eds.) Behavioral Treatment of Disease. (New York, Plenum, 1982).
6.   Schwartz, G.E. Behavioral Medicine and Systems Theory: A New Synthesis. National Forum 60 (1980) 25-30.
7.   Gentry, W.D. Developing a New Journal in the Area of Medicine: An Editorial Perspective. National Forum 60 (1980) 33-35.
8.   Weiss, S.M. and J.L. Shields. The National Institutes of Health and Behavioral Medicine. National Forum 60 (1980) 30-32.
9.   Weiss, S.M., J.A. Herd, and B.H. Fox (Eds.) Perspectives on Behavioral Medicine. (New York, Academic, 1981).

10. Gentry, W.D. (Ed.) Handbook of Behavioral Medicine. (New York, Guilford, 1984).

11. Eiser, J.R. (Ed.) Social Psychology and Behavioral Medicine. (New York, Wiley, 1982).

12. Agras, W.S. Behavioral Medicine in the 1980s: Non-random Connections. Journal of Consulting and Clinical Psychology 50 (1982) 797-803.

13. Blanchard, E.B. Behavioral Medicine: A Perspective. In R.B. Williams and W.D. Gentry (Eds.) Behavioral Approaches to Medical Treatment. (Cambridge, Mass., Ballinger, 1977).

14. Weiss, S.M. Behavioral Medicine: An Idea. In J.R. McNamara (Ed.) Behavioral Approaches to Medicine. (New York, Plenum, 1979).

15. Schwartz, G.E. and S.M. Weiss. What is Behavioral Medicine? Psychosomatic Medicine 39 (1977) 377-381.

16. Eiser, J.R. Behavioral Medicine: What Kind of Medicine? What kind of Behavior? Journal of the Royal Society of Medicine 76 (1983) 629-632.

17. Gentry, W.D. et al. Habitual Anger-Coping Styles: I. Effect on Mean Blood Pressure and Risk for Essential Hypertension. Psychosomatic Medicine 44 (1982) 195-202.

18. James, S.A. and Kleinbaum, D.G. Socioecologic Stress and Hypertension Related Mortality Rates in North Carolina. American Journal of Public Health 66 (1976) 354-358.

19. Fries, E.D. Age, Race, Sex, and Other Indices of Risk in Hypertension. American Journal of Medicine 55 (1973) 275-280.

20. James, S.A., S.A. Harnett, and W.D. Kalsbeek. John Henryism and Blood Pressure Differences Among Black Men. Journal of Behavioral Medicine 6 (1983) 259-278.

21. Kobasa, S.C., S.R. Maddi, and M.C. Puccetti. Personality and Exercise as Buffers in the Stress-Illness Relationship. Journal of Behavioral Medicine 5 (1982) 391-404.

22. Margolis, L.H., et al. Type A Behavior: An Ecological Approach. Journal of Behavioral Medicine 6 (1983) 245-258.

23. Chesney, A.P. and W.D. Gentry. Psychosocial Factors Mediating Health Risk: A Balanced Perspective. Preventive Medicine (1983) in press.

24. Gentry, W.D. and S.C. Kobasa. Social and Psychological Resources Mediating Stress-Illness Relationships in Humans. In W.D. Gentry (Ed.) Handbook of Behavioral Medicine. (New York, Guilford, 1984).

25. Cassel, J. The Contribution of the Social Environment
    to Host Resistance. American Journal of Epidemiology
    104 (1976) 107-123.
26. Cobb, S. Social Support as a Moderator of Life Stress.
    Psychosomatic Medicine 38 (1976) 300-314.
27. Wolf, S. Protective Social Forces That Counterbalance
    Stress. Journal of the South Carolina Medical
    Association Supplement, February (1976) 57-59.

# STRESS, HEALTH, AND THE RELAXATION RESPONSE

Herbert Benson

Department of Medicine
Harvard Medical School
Boston, Massachusetts

The relaxation response is believed to be an integrated hypothalamic response which results in generalized decreased sympathetic nervous system activity (11). This response, termed the "trophotropic response," was first described by Hess in the cat (24). Electrical stimulation of hypothalamic areas results in hypo- or adynamia of skeletal musculature, decreased blood pressure, decreased respiratory rate, and pupil constriction. Hess states, "Let us repeat at this point that we are actually dealing with a protective mechanism against overstress belonging to the trophotropic-endophylactic system and promoting restorative processes. We emphasize that these adynamic effects are opposed to ergotropic reactions which are oriented toward increased oxidative metabolism and utilization of energy" (24). The "ergotropic" reactions of Hess correspond to the "emergency reaction" first described by Cannon, popularly referred to as the fight or flight response and also called the "defense reaction" by others (1, 25).

To better understand the relaxation response (the trophotropic response), a discussion of its counterpart, the fight or flight response (the ergotropic response) is appropriate. The fight or flight response is mediated by the sympathetic nervous system. When a specific hypothalamic area is electrically stimulated, dilation of the pupils, increased blood pressure, increased respiratory rate, and heightened motor excitability are consistently produced. Cannon reasoned that this integrated response prepared the animal for "fight or flight" when faced with a threatening environmental situation. Man also responds to threatening environmental conditions or to environmental situations which require behavioral adjustment by a coordinated physiologic response which mimics that of the increased sympathetic nervous system activity of the fight or flight response (22).

The relaxation response in man consists of changes opposite to those of the fight or flight response (2, 64-66). During the practice of one well-investigated technique called Transcendental Meditation, the major elements of the relaxation response occur: decreases in oxygen consumption, carbon dioxide elimination, heart rate, respiratory rate, minute ventilation, and arterial blood lactate. Systolic, diastolic and mean blood pressures remain unchanged compared to control levels. Rectal temperature also remains unchanged while skin resistance markedly increases and skeletal muscle blood flow slightly increases (34). The electroencephalogram demonstrates an increase in the intensity of slow alpha waves and occasional theta wave activity. Muscle tonus decreases (29, 38). These changes are consistent with generalized decreased sympathetic nervous system activity and are distinctly different from the physiologic changes noted during quiet sitting or sleep. The changes occur simultaneously and are consistent with those noted by Hess (24).

## 1 THE TECHNIQUE OF ELICITING THE RELAXATION RESPONSE

Four basic elements are usually necessary to elicit the relaxation response in man:

### 1.1 Mental Device

There should be a constant stimulus, e.g., a sound word, or phrase repeated silently or audibly, or fixed gazing at an object. The purpose of these procedures is to shift from logical, externally-oriented thought.

### 1.2 Passive Attitude

If distracting thoughts do occur during the repetition or gazing, they should be disregarded and one's attention should be redirected to the technique. One should not worry about how well he is performing the technique.

### 1.3 Decreased Muscle Tonus

The subject should be in a comfortable posture so that minimal muscular work is required.

### 1.4 Quiet Environment

A quiet environment with decreased environmental stimuli should be chosen. Most techniques instruct the practitioner to

close his eyes. A place of worship is often suitable, as is a
quiet room.


2 HISTORICAL SUBJECTIVE WRITINGS SUPPORTING EXISTENCE OF THE
  RELAXATION RESPONSE

Techniques have existed for centuries, usually within a
religious context, which allow an individual to experience the
relaxation response. For example, in the West a fourteenth-
century Christian treatise entitled The Cloud of Unknowing
discusses how to attain an altered state of consciousness which
is required to attain alleged union with God (51). The anonymous
author states that this goal cannot be reached in the ordinary
levels of human consciousness, but rather by use of "lower" levels.
These levels are reached by eliminating all distractions and
physical activity, all worldly things including all thoughts.
As a means of "...beating down thought," the use of a single-
syllable word, such as "god" or "love," should be repeated.

> Choose whichever one you prefer, or, if you like, choose
> another that suits your taste, provided that it is of one
> syllable. And clasp this word tightly in your heart so
> that it never leaves it no matter what may happen.
> This word shall be your shield and your spear...
> With this word you shall strike down thoughts of
> every kind and drive them beneath the cloud of
> forgetting. After that, if any thoughts should
> press upon you...answer him with this word only
> and with no other words. (pp. 76-77)

There will be moments when "every created thing may suddenly and
completely be forgotten. But immediately after each stirring,
because of the corruption of the flesh, it (the soul) drops
down again to some thought or some deed" (p. 68). An important
instruction for success is "...do not by another means work in
it with your mind or with your imagination" (p. 69)

Another Christian work, The Third Spiritual Alphabet,
written in the tenth century by Fray Francisco de Osuna (46),
deals with an altered state of consciousness. He wrote that
"Contemplation requires us to blind ourselves to all that is
not God" (p. viii), and that one should be deaf and dumb to all
else and must "...quit all obstacles, keeping your eyes bent on
the ground..." (pp. 293-294). The method can be either a short,
self-composed prayer, repeated over and over, or simply saying
"no" to thoughts when they occur. This exercise should be
performed for one hour in the morning and evening and should be
taught by a qualified teacher. Fray Francisco wrote that such
an exercise would help in all endeavors, making us more efficient

in our tasks and the tasks more enjoyable. All men, especially
the busy, secular as well as religious, should be taught this
meditation for it is a refuge to which one can retreat when faced
with stressful situations.

The famous fifteenth-century Christian mystics Saints John
and Terese described the major steps required to achieve the
mystical state (4, 54), which include ignoring distractions,
usually by repetitive prayer.

Christian meditation and mysticism was well developed
within the Byzantine church and known as Hesychasm (43). This
method of repetitive prayer was described in the fourteenth
century at Mount Athos in Greece by Gregory of Sinai and is
called "The Prayer of the Heart" or "The Prayer of Jesus." It
dates back to the beginnings of the Christian era. The prayer
itself was called secret meditation and was transmitted from older
to younger monks through an initiation rite. Emphasis was placed
on having a skilled instructor. The method of prayer recommended
by these monks was:

> Sit down alone and in silence. Lower your head,
> shut your eyes, breathe out gently, and imagine
> yourself looking into your own heart. Carry your
> mind, i.e., your thoughts, from your head to your
> heart. As you breathe out, say 'Lord Jesus Christ,
> have mercy on me.' Say it moving your lips gently,
> or simply say it in your mind. Try to put all other
> thoughts aside. Be calm, be patient and repeat the
> process very frequently (19, p. 10).

To reach such a state, a tranquil environment is necessary.
"It may happen that a man who has been busy all day gives himself
to prayer for an hour...so that during that time the thoughts
of his earthly preoccupations are forgotten (53, p. 87).

In Judaism, similar practices leading to this altered
state of consciousness date back to the time of the second temple
in the second century B.C. and are found in one of the earliest
forms of Jewish mysticism, Merkabalism (56). In this practice
of meditation, the subject sat with his head between his knees,
whispered hymns and songs, and repeated a name of a magic seal.
In the thirteenth century A.D., the works of Rabbi Abulafia
were published and his ideas became a major part of Jewish
Kabbalistic mysticism (56). Rabbi Abulafia felt that the normal
life of the soul is kept within limits by our sensory perceptions
and emotions, and since these perceptions and emotions are
concerned with the finite, the soul's life is finite. Man
therefore needs a higher form of perception, which instead of
blocking the soul's deeper regions, opens them up. An "absolute"

object upon which to meditate is required. Rabbi Abulafia found this in the Hebrew alphabet. He developed a mystical system of contemplating the letters of God's name. Bokser (14) describes Rabbi Abulafia's prayer:

> ...immersed in prayer and meditation, uttering the divine name with special modulations of the voice and with special gestures, he induced in himself a state of ecstasy in which he believed the soul had shed its material bonds, and, unimpeded, returned to its divine source. (p. 9)

The purpose of this prayer and methodical meditation is to experience a new state of consciousness, described as harmonious movement of pure thought, which has severed all relation to the senses. This is compared by Scholem to music and yoga. Scholem (56) feels that Rabbi Abulafia's

> ...teachings represent but a Judaized version of that ancient spiritual technique which has found its classical expression in the practices of the Indian mystics who follow the system known as Yoga. To cite only one instance out of many, an important part of Abulafia's system is played by the technique of breathing; now this technique has found its highest development in the Indian Yoga, where it is commonly regarded as the most important instrument of mental discipline. Again, Abulafia lays down certain rules of body posture, certain corresponding combinations of consonants and vowels, and certain forms of recitation, and in particular some passages of his book, "The Light of the Intellect", give the impression of a Judaized treatise on Yoga. The similarity even extends to some aspects of the doctrine of ecstatic vision, as preceded and brought about by these practices (p. 139).

The basic elements which elicit the relaxation response in certain practices of Christianity and Judaism are also found in Islamic mysticism or Sufism (62). Sufism developed as a reaction against the external rationalization of Islam and made use of intuitive and emotional faculties which are claimed to be dormant until they are utilized through training under the guidance of a teacher. The method of employing these faculties is known as Dhikr. It is a means of excluding distractions and of drawing nearer to God by the constant repetition of His name, either silently or aloud, and by rhythmic breathing. Music, musical poems, and dance are also employed in the ritual of Dhikr, for it was noticed that they could help induce states of ecstasy. Originally, Dhikr was only practiced by the members of

the society who made a deliberate choice to redirect their lives
to God as the preliminary step in the surrender of the will.  Upon
initiation to his order, the initiate received the wird, a secret,
holy sound.  The old Masters felt that the true encounter with
God could not be attained by all, for most men are born deaf to
mystical sensitivity.  However, by the twelfth century, this
attitude had changed.  It was realized that this ecstasy could be
induced in the ordinary man in a relatively short time by rhythmic
exercises involving posture, control of breath, coordinated
movements, and oral repetitions (62).

In the Western world, the relaxation response elicited by
religious practices was not part of the routine practice of
religions, but rather was within the mystical tradition.  In the
East, however, meditation which elicited the relaxation response
was developed much earlier and became a major element in religion
and in everyday life.  Writings from Indian scriptures, the
Upanishads, dated sixth century B.C., note that individuals
might attain "...a unified state with the Brahman (the Diety) by
means of restraint of breath, withdrawal of senses, meditation,
concentration, contemplation and absorption" (45).

There are a multitude of Eastern religions and ways of life,
including Zen and Yoga with their many variants, which can elicit
the relaxation response.  They employ mental and physical methods
including the repetition of a word or sound, the exclusion of
meaningful thoughts, a quiet environment,  and a comfortable
position, and they stress the importance of a trained teacher.
One of the meditative practices of Zen Buddhism, Zazen, employs a
yoga-like technique of the coupling of respiration and counting to
ten, i.e., one on inhaling, two on exhaling, and so on, to ten.
With time, one stops counting and simply "follows the breath"
(32) in order to achieve a state of no thought, no feeling, to be
completely in nothing (28).

Shintoism and Taoism are important religions of Japan and
China.  In Shintoism, one method of prayer consists of sitting
quietly,  inspiring through the nose, holding inspiration for a
short time, and expiring through the mouth, with eyes directed
toward a mirror at their level.  Throughout the exercise, the
priest repeats ten numbers, or sacred words, pronounced according
to the traditional religious teachings (23).  Fujisawa (20, p. 23)
noted, "It is interesting that this grand ritual characteristic
of Shintoism is doubtlessly the same process as Yoga..."  Taoism,
one of the traditional religions of China, employs, in addition
to methods similar to Shinto, concentration on nothingness to
achieve absolute tranquility (16).

Similar meditational practices are found in practically
every culture of man.  Shamanism is a form of mysticism associated

with feelings of ecstasy and is practied in conjunction with tribal
religions in North and South America, Indonesia, Oceania, Africa,
Siberia, and Japan. Each shaman has a song or chant to bring
on trances, usually entering into solitude to do so. Music,
especially the drum, plays an important part in Shamanistic
trances (31).

Many less traditional religious practices are prevalent
in the United States. One aim of these practices is achievement
of an altered state of consciousness which is induced by technique
similar to those that elicit the relaxation response. Subub,
Nichiren Sho Shu, Hare Krishna, Scientology, Black Muslimism,
Meher Baba, and the Association for Research and Enlightenment
are but a few of these (42).

In addition to techniques which elicit the relaxation
response within a religious context, secular techniques also
exist. One method often used is gazing upon an object and keeping
attention focused upon that object to the exclusion of all else
(35, 63). Others, the so-called nature mystics, have been able
to elicit the relaxation response by immersing themselves in
quiet, often in the quiet of nature. Wordsworth believed "...that
when his mind was freed from preoccupation with disturbing
objects, petty care, 'little enmities and low desires,' that he
could then reach a condition of equilibrium, which he describes
as a 'wise passiveness' or 'a happy stillness of the mind'..."
(57, p. 61). Wordsworth believed that anyone could deliberately
induce this condition in himself by a kind of relaxation of the
will. Thoreau made many references to such feelings attained
by sitting for hours alone with nature. Indeed, Thoreau compares
himself to a Yogi (55). William James describes similar experiences may be found in Johnson's Watcher on the Hills (31).

## 3  OBJECTIVE DATA SUPPORTING THE WIDESPREAD EXISTENCE OF THE RELAXATION RESPONSE

Physiologic changes occur during the practice of various
techniques which elicit the relaxation response. These consist,
in part, of decreased oxygen consumption, respiratory rate, heart
rate, and muscle tension. Increases are noted in skin resistance
and EEG alpha wave activity.

Autogenic training is a technique of medical therapy which
is said to elicit the trophotropic response of Hess or the
relaxation response. Autogenic therapy is defined as "...a self-
induced modification of corticodiencephalic interrelationships"
which enables the lower brain centers to activate "trophotropic
activity" (38). The method of autogenic training is based on six
psychophysiologic exercises devised by a German neurologist,

22

H. H. Shultz, which are practiced several times a day until the subject is able to voluntarily shift to a wakeful low-arousal (trophotropic) state. The "Standard Exercises" are practiced in a quiet environment, in a horizontal position, and with closed eyes (38). Exercise 1 focuses on the feeling of heaviness in the limbs, and Exercise 2 on the cultivation of the sensation of warmth in the limbs. Exercise 3 deals with cardiac regulation, while Exercise 4 consists of passive concentration on breathing. In Exercise 5, the subject cultivates the sensation of warmth in his upper abdomen, and Exercise 6 is the cultivation of feelings of coolness in the forehead. Exercises 1 through 4 most effectively elicit the trophotropic response, while Exercises 5 and 6 are reported to have different effects (38). The subject's attitude toward the exercise must not be intense and compulsive, but rather of a quiet, "let it happen," nature. This is referred to as passive   concentration and is deemed absolutely essential (39).

Progressive relaxation (29) is a technique which seeks to achieve increased discriminative control over skeletal muscle until a subject is able to induce very low levels of tonus in the major muscle groups. Jacobson, who devised the technique, states that anxiety and muscular relaxation produce opposite physiologic states, and therefore cannot exist together. Progressive relaxation is practiced in supine position in a quiet room; a passive attitude is essential because mental images induce slight, measurable tensions in muscles, especially those of the eyes and face. The subject is taught to recognize even slight contractions of his muscles so that he can avoid them and achieve the deepest degree of relaxation possible.

Hypnosis is an artificially induced state characterized by increased suggestability. A subject is judged to be in the hypnotic state if he manifests a high level of response to test suggestions such as muscle rigidity, amnesia, hallucination, anesthesia, and post-hypnotic suggestion, which are used in standard scales such as that of Weitzenhoffer and Hilgard (68). The hypnotic induction procedure usually includes suggestion (autosuggestion for self-hypnosis) of relaxation and drowsiness, closed eyes, and a recumbent or semisupine position (6).

Procedures for self- and hetero-hypnotic induction and for the elicitation of the relaxation response appear to be similar. Further, before experiencing hypnotic phenomena, either during a traditional or an active induction, a physiological state exists which is comparable to the relaxation response. This state is characterized, in part, by decreased heart rate, respiratory rate, and blood pressure. After the physiological changes of the relaxation response occur, the individual proceeds to experience other exclusively hypnotic phenomena, such as perceptual distortions, age regression, posthypnotic suggestion, and amnesia (10).

Yoga has been an important part of Indian culture for thousands of years. It is claimed to be the culmination of the efforts of ancient Hindu thinkers to "give man the fullest possible control over his mind" (26). Yoga consists of practices and physical techniques usually performed in a quiet environment, and it has many variant forms. Yoga began as Raja Yoga, which sought "union with the absolute" by meditation. Later, there was an emphasis on physical methods in attempts to achieve an altered state of consciousness. This form is termed Hatha Yoga. It has developed into a physical culture and is claimed to prevent and cure certain diseases. Essential to the practice of Hatha Yoga are appropriate posture and control of respiration (52). The most common posture helps the spine stay erect without strain and is claimed to enhance concentration. The respiratory training promotes control of duration of inspiration and expiration, and the pause between breaths, so that one eventually achieves voluntary control of respiration. Bagchi and Wenger (5), in studies of Yoga practitioners, reported that Yoga could produce a 70% increase in skin resistance, decreased heart rate, and EEG alpha wave activity. Yet others have described decreased oxygen consumption (3, 59) and decreased respiratory rate (44). These observations led them to suggest that Yoga is "deep relaxation of a certain aspect of the autonomic nervous system without drowsiness or sleep."

Transcendental Meditation is a form of Yoga. The technique, as taught by Maharishi Mahesh Yogi, comes from the Vedic tradition of India. Instruction is given individually, and the technique is allegedly easily learned at the first instruction session. It is said to require no physical or mental control. The individual is taught a systematic method of repeating a word or sound, the manta, without attempting to concentrate specifically on it.

Zen is very much like Yoga, from which it developed, and is associated with the Buddhist religion (44). In Zen meditation, the subject is said to achieve a "controlled psychophysiologic decrease of the cerebral excitatory state" by a crossed-leg posture, closed eyes, regulation of respiration, and concentration on the Koan (an alogical problem, e.g., What is the sound of one hand clapping?), or by prayer and chanting. Respiration is adjusted by taking several slow deep breaths, then inspiring briefly and forcelessly, and expiring long and forcefully, with subsequent natural breathing. Any sensory perceptions or mental images are allowed to appear and leave passively. A quiet, comfortable environment is essential. Experienced Zen meditators elicit the relaxation response more efficiently than novices (59).

Incorporating the four elements common to a multitude of historical techniques, a simple noncultic technique was developed in our laboratory (7). Use of the technique results in the same physiologic changes that our laboratory first noted using Transcendental Meditation as a model. The instructions for this technique are the following:

1. Sit quietly in a comfortable position and close your eyes.
2. Deeply relax all your muscles, beginning at your feet and progressing up to your face. Keep them deeply relaxed.
3. Breathe through your nose. Become aware of your breathing. As you breathe out, say the word one silently to yourself. For example, breathe in...out, one; in...out, one; etc. Continue for 20 minutes. You may open your eyes to check the time, but do not use an alarm. When you finish, sit quietly for several minutes at first with closed eyes and later with open eyes.
4. Do not worry about whether you are successful in achieving a deep level of relaxation. Maintain a passive attitude and permit relaxation to occur at its own pace. Expect other thoughts. When these distracting thoughts occur, ignore them by thinking, "Oh well" and continue repeating "one." With practice, the response should come with little effort. Practice the technique once or twice daily, but not within two hours after any meal, since the digestive processes seem to interfere with the subjective changes.

## 4  CLINICAL USEFULNESS OF THE RELAXATION RESPONSE

The continual stresses of contemporary living have led to the excessive elicitation of the fight-or-flight response (22). Within the constructs of our society, the behavioral features of this response, running or fighting, are often inappropriate. Indeed, the excessive and inappropriate arousal of the fight-or-flight response with its corresponding sympathetic nervous system activation may have a role in the pathogenesis and exacerbation of several disorders. Regular elicitation of the relaxation response may be of preventive and therapeutic value in diseases in which increased sympathetic nervous system activity is implicated.

Several longitudinal investigations have demonstrated that the regular elicitation of the relaxation response lowers blood pressure in both pharmacologically treated and untreated hypertensive patients (12, 13, 17, 47, 48, 58). In an early investigation done by our laboratory, would-be initiates of Transcendental Meditation who were also hypertensive, volunteered

to participate in the study (12, 13). Baseline measurements
of blood pressure were taken weekly for approximately six weeks,
after which the subjects were taught to bring forth the relaxation
response through the practice of Transcendental Meditation. Of
the 36 patients included in the study, 22 received no medication
during the investigation and 14 remained on unaltered antihypertensive medications during both the control and experimental
periods. In the 22 nonmedicated subjects, control blood pressures
averaging 146.5 mm Hg systolic and 94.6 mm Hg diastolic decreased
significantly to 139.5 mm Hg systolic and 90.8 mm Hg diastolic
after the regular elicitation of the relaxation response through
the practice of Transcendental Meditation. In the 14 patients
who maintained constant antihypertensive medications, mean control
blood pressures of 145.6 mm Hg systolic and 91.9 mm Hg diastolic
dropped significantly to 135.0 mm Hg systolic and 87.0 mm Hg
diastolic post-intervention.

Several other researchers report similar findings. Datey
and co-workers (17) noted decreases in both systolic and diastolic
blood pressures in 47 hypertensive patients who evoked the
relaxation response through the practice of another Yogic
technique, called Shavasan. In this study, subjects served as
their own controls. Information regarding the length of the
pre-intervention control period and the number of control blood
pressure measurements made, however, was not reported.

In two well-controlled longitudinal investigations, Patel
(47, 48) combined Yogic relaxation with biofeedback techniques in
the treatment of 20 patients with hypertension. The average
systolic blood pressure in these subjects was reduced by $20.4\pm$
11.4 mm Hg, while mean diastolic pressure was reduced by $14.2\pm$
7.5 mm Hg. A hypertensive control group matched for age and sex
was employed. Length of testing sessions, number of attendances,
and the procedure for measuring the blood pressure of the control
group were identical to those of the treatment group. Control
patients were not given instruction in the relaxation technique,
however, but simply were asked to rest on a couch. No significant
changes in blood pressure occurred in the control group.

Further substantiation of the usefulness of the relaxation
response in the treatment of hypertension has come from Stone
and DeLeo (58), who obtained significant decreases in systolic
and diastolic blood pressures using a Buddhist meditation exercise.
The control group, which received no psychotherapeutic intervention,
was matched for blood pressure, age, and race, and exhibited
virtually no change in systolic and diastolic pressures.

A more recent example of the clinical usefulness of the
relaxation response is that of reducing the number of premature
ventricular contractions (PVCs) (9). Participating in a study

were 11 nonmedicated ambulatory patients who had proven ischemic heart disease for at least one year's duration, with documented relatively stable PVCs. Frequent PVCs are correlated with an increased mortality in such patients (18, 61). The frequency of the PVCs was measured over 48 consecutive hours, after which the subject was taught to elicit the relaxation response by using the noncultic technique described above. After four weeks of regularly practicing the relaxation technique and recording their frequency of practice, the patients returned to repeat the two days of monitoring.

A reduced frequency PVCs was observed in 8 of the 11 patients. Before intervention, the PVCs per hour per patient for the total group had averaged 151.5 for the entire monitoring session. Four weeks after the intervention was instituted, the average PVCs per hour per patient dropped to 131.7. The reduction of PVCs was even more marked during sleep. Initially, the number of PVCs per hour per patient during sleeping hours averaged 125.5, while after four weeks of regular elicitation of the relaxation response, the PVCs during sleep decreased to 87.9. When the PVCs were expressed per 1,000 heartbeats per patient for the entire group, there was a significant decrease during sleeping hours from 29.0 to 21.1.

The results suggest that the regular elicitation of the relaxation response with its hypothesized decreased sympathetic nervous system activity may have been the mechanism by which PVCs were reduced. This finding is consistent with that of Lown and his co-workers (36), who, in a recent case study, reported that a patient was able to abolish his arrhythmias by meditation. These results were attributed to lessened sympthetic tone (37), although others (67) implicate increased parasympathetic activity as a mechanism for the reduction of the PVCs.

## 5 USEFULNESS IN PREVENTION AND AT THE WORK SITE

An experiment conducted at the corporate offices of a manufacturing firm investigated the effects of daily relaxation breaks on five self-reported measures of health, performance, and well-being (49). For 12 weeks, 126 volunteers filled out daily records and reported bi-weekly for additional measurements. After four weeks of baseline monitoring, they were divided randomly into three groups: Group A was taught a technique for producing the relaxation response; Group B was instructed to sit quietly; Group C received no instructions. Groups A and B were asked to take two 15-minute relaxation breaks daily. After an eight-week experimental period, the greatest mean improvements on every index occurred in Group A; the least improvements occurred in Group C. Group B was intermediate. Difference between the

the mean changes in Groups A vs. C reached statistical significance
on four of five indices: Symptoms, Illness Days, Performance,
and Sociability-Satisfaction. Improvements on a Happiness-
Unhappiness Index were not significantly different among the three
groups. The relationship between amount of change and rate of
practicing the relaxation response was different for the different
indices. While less than three practice periods per week produced
little change on any index, two daily sessions appeared to be more
practice than was necessary for many individuals to achieve
positive changes. Somatic symptoms and performance responded with
less practice of the relaxation response than did behavioral
symptoms and measures of well-being.

During the baseline period, mean systolic blood pressures
were 119.7, 118.4 and 114.2 mm Hg for Groups A, B and C
respectively; mean diastolic pressures were 78.7, 76.8 and 75.7
(50). Between the first and last measurements, mean changes in
systolic blood pressure were -11.6, -6.5 and +0.4 mm Hg in Groups
A, B and C; mean diastolic blood pressure decreased by 7.9, 3.1
and 0.3 mm Hg. Between the four-week baseline period and last
four weeks of the experimental period, mean systolic blood
pressure decreased by 6.7, 2.6 and 0.5 mm Hg; while mean diastolic
blood pressure and diastolic blood pressure, mean changes in
Group A were significantly greater than those in Group B (p = 0.05)
and in Group C (p = 0.001). The same pattern of changes among
the three groups was exhibited by both sexes, all ages, and at
all initial levels of blood pressure. However, in general, within
Group A, the higher the initial blood pressure, the greater the
decrease. Thus, blood pressure within the "normal" range was
significantly lowered after regular elicitation of the relaxation
response. This lowered blood pressure might ultimately prevent
the development of subsequent hypertension.


6  RECENT FINDINGS

Although the physiologic changes of the relaxation response
are consistent with decreased sympathetic nervous system activity,
the direct measurement of plasma norepinephrine during its
elicitation did not reveal significant decreases in the concentration of this hormone (41). Indeed, some have found increased
levels of plasma norepinephrine in subjects who regularly elicit
the relaxation response (33).

Recent physiologic data resolve this apparent paradox of
unchanged or increased plasma norepinephrine levels associated
with the elicitation of the relaxation response (27). Sympathetic
nervous system reactivity was assessed in 10 experimental and 9
control subjects who were exposed to graded orthostatic and
isometric stress on monthly hospital visits. Between visits,

experimental subjects practiced a technique that elicited the
relaxation response, whereas control subjects sat quietly for
an equivalent time. Heart rate and blood pressure reactions
to the graded stresses did not differ between visits in either
group. However, in the experimental group, the levels of plasma
norepinephrine corresponding to graded stresses were significantly
augmented after the elicitation of the relaxation response. No
changes in plasma norepinephrine levels were noted in the control
group. After completion of this phase, these results were then
replicated in the control group in a crossover experiment. That
is, heart rate and blood pressure responses were unchanged, but
plasma norepinephrine levels were significantly higher after this
group crossed over and elicited the relaxation response. Hence,
the repeated elicitation of the relaxation response resulted in
greater sympathetic nervous system reactivity that was not reflected
in larger heart rate and blood pressure responses. These observations are most consistent with reduced norepinephrine end-organ
responsivity.


## 7 CONCLUSIONS

Although emphasis has been placed on the processes by which
mind and behavioral processes lead to disease states, we should
be aware of the beneficial, healthful aspects of other thought
processes. Specific behaviors and thought patterns elicit the
innate physiologic changes termed the relaxation response. The
relaxation response appears to be a valuable adjunct to our
current therapies, and it may also be useful as a preventive
measure, e.g., in mediating stress at the work site. This
response can be elicited by nonreligious or noncultic techniques
or by other methods, which a practitioner may prefer. A religious
person, for example, may select meditative prayer as the most
appropriate method for bringing forth the relaxation response. The
freedom to choose a technique that conforms to one's own personal
beliefs should enhance compliance. Elicitation of the relaxation
response is a simple and natural phenomenon; it does not require
complex equipment for monitoring of physiologic events or involve
the expense and side effects of drugs.

REFERENCES

1. Abrahams, V.C., et al. Active Muscle Vasodilatation by
       Stimulation of the Brain Stem: Its Significance in
       the Defense Reaction. Journal of Physiology 154 (1960)
       491.

2. Allison, J. Respiration Changes During Transcendental Meditation. Lancet 1 (1970) 833–834.
3. Anand, B.K., et al.  Studies on Shri Ramananda Yogi During His Stay in an Air-Tight Box.  Indian Journal of Medical Research 49 (1961) 82–89,
4. Anonymous: A Benedictine of Stanbrook Abbey.  Mediaeval Mystic Tradition and Saint John of the Cross (London, Burns and Oates, 1954).
5. Bagchi, B.K. and M.A. Wenger.  Electrophysiological Correlations of Some Yoga Exercises.  Electroencephalography and Clinical Neurophysiology 7 (1957) 132–149.
6. Barber, T.X.  Physiological Effects of Hypnosis and Suggestion, in Biofeedback and Self-Control 1970 (New York, Aldine-Atherton, 1971).
7. Beary, J.F., and H. Benson.  A Simple Psychophysiologic Technique Which Elicits the Hypometablic Changes of the Relaxation Response, Psychosomatic Medicine 36 (1974) 115–120.
8. Benson, H.  The Relaxation Response. (New York, William Morrow, 1975).
9. Benson, H., S. Alexander, and C.L. Feldman.  Decreased Premature Ventricular Contractions through Use of the Relaxation Response in Patients with Stable Ischemic Disease. Lancet 2 (1975) 380–382.
10. Benson, H., P.A. Arns, and J.W. Hoffman.  The Relaxation Response and Hypnosis.  International Journal of Clinical Experimental Hypnosis 29 (1981) 259–270.
11. Benson, H., J.F. Beary, and M.P. Carol.  The Relaxation Response.  Psychiatry 37 (1974) 37–46.
12. Benson, H., B.A. Rosner, B.R. Marzetta, et al.  Decreased Blood Pressure in Borderline Hypertensive Subjects Who Practiced Meditation.  Journal of Chronic Disease 27 (1974a) 163–169.
13. Benson, H., B.A. Rosner, B.R. Marzetta.  Decreased Blood Pressure in Pharmacologically Treated Hypertensive Patients Who Regularly Elicited the Relaxation Response. Lancet 1 (1974b) 289–291.
14. Bokser, R.B.Z.  From the World of the Cabbalah. (Philosophical Library, 1954).
15. Cannon, W.B.  The Emergency Function of the Adrenal Medulla in Pain and the Major Emotions, American Journal of Physiology 33 (1941) 356.
16. Chang, Chung-Yuan.  Creativity and Taoism.  (New York, Julian Press, 1963).
17. Datey, K.K., S.N. Deshmukh, C.P. Dalvi, et al.  "Shavasan": A Yogic Exercise in the Management of Hypertension. Angiology 20 (1969) 325–333.
18. Desai, D., P.I. Hershberg, and S. Alexander.  Clinical Significance of Ventricular Premature Beats in an Out-Patient Population.  Chest 64 (1973) 564.

19. French, R.M. The Way of a Pilgrim. (New York, Seabury Press, 1968).
20. Fujisawa, C. Zen and Shinto (Philosophical Library, 1959).
21. Gellhorn, E. Principles of Autonomic-Somatic Interactions. (University of Minnesota Press, 1967).
22. Gutmann, M.C. and H. Benson. Interaction of Environmental Factors and Systemic Arterial Blood Pressure: A Review. Medicine 50 (1971) 543-553.
23. Herbert, J. Shinto: At the Fountain-head of Japan. (London, Allen and Unwin, 1967).
24. Hess, W.R. Functional Organization of the Diencephalon. (Grune and Stratton, 1957).
25. Hess, W.R. and M. Brugger. Das Subkortikale Zentrum der Affektiven Abwehrreaktion, Helv. Physiol. Acta 1 (1943) 33-52.
26. Hoenig, J. Medical Research on Yoga. Confin. Psychiatr. 11 (1968) 69-89.
27. Hoffman, J.W., P.A. Arns, et al. Altered Sympathetic Nervous System.Reactivity with the Relaxation Response. Clinical Research 29 (1981) 207A.
28. Ishiguro, H. The Scientific Truth of Zen (Tokyo, Zenrigaku Society, 1964).
29. Jacobson, E. Progressive Relaxation (University of Chicago Press, 1938).
30. James, W. Letters (Atlantic Monthly Press, 1920).
31. Johnson, R.C. Watcher on the Hills (Harper, 1959).
32. Johnston, W. Christian Zen (Harper & Row, 1971).
33. Lang, R., K. Dehof, K.A. Meurer and W. Kaufmann. Sympathetic Activity and Transcendental Meditation, Journal of Neural Transmission 44 (1979) 117-135.
34. Levander, V.L., et al. Increased Forearm Blood Flow during a Wakeful Hypometabolic State. Federation Proceedings 31 (1972) 405.
35. Lowell, P. The Soul of the Far East. (Houghton-Mifflin, 1892).
36. Lown, B., J.V. Temte, P. Reich, et al. Basis for Recurring Ventricular Fibrillation in the Absence of Coronary Heart Disease and Its Management. New England Journal of Medicine 294 (1976) 623-629.
37. Lown, B., M. Tykocinski, A. Garfein, et al. Sleep and Ventricular Premature Beats. Circulation 48 (1973) 691.
38. Luthe, W. (Ed.) Autogenic Therapy (Vols. 1-5) (Grune & Stratton, 1969).
39. Luthe, W. Autogenic Therapy: Exerpts on Applications to Cardiovascular Disorders and Hypercholesterolemia. In Biofeedback and Self-Control 1971 (New York, Aldine-Atherton, 1972).
40. Maharishi Mahesh Yogi. The Science of Being and Art of Living (London, International SRM Publishers, 1966).

41. Michaels, R.R., M.J. Haber, D.S. McCann. Evaluation of Transcendental Meditation as a Method of Reducing Stress. Science 192 (1976) 1242-1244.
42. Needleman, J. The New Religions (Doubleday, 1970).
43. Norwich, J.J. and R. Sitwell. Mount Athos (Harper & Row, 1966).
44. Onda, A. Autogenic Training and Zen. In W. Luthe (Ed.) Autogenic Training (Grune & Stratton, 1965).
45. Organ, T.W. The Hindu Quest for the Perfection of Man. (Athens, Ohio, Ohio University Press, 1970).
46. Osuna, Fray Francisco de. The Third Spiritual Alphabet. (London, Benziger, 1931).
47. Patel, C.H. Yoga and Biofeedback in the Management of Hypertension. Lancet 2 (1973) 1053-1055.
48. Patel, C.H. Twelve-Month Follow-Up of Yoga and Biofeedback in the Management of Hypertension. Lancet 1 (1975) 62-64.
49. Peters, R.K. H. Benson, and D. Porter. Dailey Relaxation Response Breaks in a Working Population. I. Effects on Self-reported Measures of Health Performance, and Well-Being. American Journal of Public Health 67 (1977a) 946-953.
50. Peters, R.K., H. Benson, J.M. Peters. Dailey Relaxation Response Breaks in a Working Population. II. Effects on Blood Pressure. American Journal of Public Health 67 (1977b) 954-959.
51. Progoff, I. The Cloud of Unknowing (New York, Julian Press, 1969).
52. Ramamurthi, B. Yoga: An Explanation and Probable Neurophysiology. Journal of the Indian Medical Association 48 (1967) 167-170.
53. Ross, F.H. Shinto, The Way of Japan (Beacon Press, 1965).
54. Saint Terese of Avila. The Way of Perfection A. R. Waller (Ed.) (London, J.M. Dent, 1901).
55. Sanborn, F.B. Familiar Letters of Henry David Thoreau (Houghton-Mifflin, 1894).
56. Scholem, G.G. Jewish Mysticism (Schocken Books, 1967).
57. Spurgeon, C.F.E. Mysticism in English Literature (Port Washington, Kennikat Press, 1970).
58. Stone, R.A. and J. DeLeo. Psychotherapeutic Control of Hypertension. New England Journal of Medicine 294 (1976) 80-84.
59. Sugi, Y. and K. Akutsu. Studies on Respiration and Energy-Metabolism during Sitting in Zazen. Research Journal of Physical Education 12 (1968) 190-206.
60. Thoreau, H.D. Walden. (Princeton University Press, 1971).
61. Tominaga, S., H. Blackburn and the Coronary Drug Project Research Group. Prognostic Importance of Premature Beats Following Myocardial Infarction. JAMA 223 (1973) 1116.
62. Trimingham, J.S. Sufi Orders in Islam. (Oxford, Clarendon, 1971).

63.Underhill, E.  Mysticism. (London, Methuen, 1957).
64.Wallace, R.K.  Physiological Effects of Transcendental Medi-
     tation.  Science 167 (1970) 1751-1754.
65.Wallace, R.K. and H. Benson.  The Physiology of Meditation.
     Scientific American 226 (1972) 85-90.
66.Wallace, R.K. H. Benson, and A.F. Wilson.  A Wakeful Hypo-
     metabolic State.  American Journal of Physiology.
     221 (1971) 795-799.
67.Weiss, T., G.W. Lattin and K. Engelman.  Vagally mediated
     suppression of premature ventricular contractions in man.
     American Heart Journal 89 (1975) 700.
68.Weitzenhoffer, A.M. and E. Hilgard.  Stanford Hypnotic
     Suggestibility Scale. (Palo Alto, Consulting Psychologist
     Press, 1959).

STRESS AND STRAIN IN THE WORK ENVIRONMENT: DOES IT LEAD
TO ILLNESS?

Charles J. de Wolff

Workgroup on Psychology of Work
and Organization
University of Nijmegen
Nijmegen, the Netherlands

1   INTRODUCTION

This paper discusses the relationship between
stressors and strains in the work setting.  Common wisdom
has it that work makes people sick.  Workers themselves
may attest to same.  But, until recently, in the social
sciences, a precise understanding of such relationships
has be non-existent.  Industrial and organizational
psychologists have concentrated on non-illness dependent
variables, e.g., performance, satisfaction and motivation.
Health and illness are lesser known concepts.  For
example, the handbook of Dunnette (1), widely seen as a
milestone in the field, does not even mention these terms
in its subject index.

In the past two decades, though, there have been
some pioneers of research on stress in organizations,
most notably researchers at the Institute of Social,
Research, Ann Arbor, Michigan (USA), e.g., Kahn (2) and
French and Caplan (3).

In the latter half of the 1970s, the interest in
stress-strain relationships in the work setting has increased considerably.  There are now several stress
research centers in the USA and Europe, producing findings
which are being published in journals and books.

Put together, the emerging findings offer a rather
confusing picture.  In an excellent article, Kasl (4)
reviews many of these studies, pointing out a number of

methodological flaws and questioning the nature of evidence linking stressors to illness.

In the present paper, we will discuss the relationship between stressors and strains, drawing upon results
from studies carried out by the Stress Research Group at
Nijmegen University. We will discuss a number of
methodological problems and point out some consequences
of the way research has been conducted to date. We will
also draw some tentative conclusions about how stressors
lead to strain(s).

One of the most striking characteristics of stress
research is that the scientists involved in it come from
very different backgrounds. Not only psychologists and
sociologists are interested in this area, but also
physiologists, physicians and endocrinologists. And,
within these main disciplines, there are sub-disciplines
(e.g., clinical psychology, experimental and social
psychology) each approaching the subject matter in different ways. The kind of problems researchers face
obliges them to cross traditional boundaries and to
enter into other domains, i.e., cross-fertilization.
Although this may involve certain risks on the part of
the investigator(s), it also presents some exciting
challenges! It forces all of us to reconsider many
questions. The present author has experienced his discussions with representatives from other disciplines as
a most stimulating and refreshing activity. In this
paper, we will try to stay in our own territory (i.e.,
industrial and organizational psychology), yet offer
concepts and empirical findings that will be of interest
to researchers from other parent disciplines.

2   THE STRESS RESEARCH GROUP - NIJMEGEN UNIVERSITY

In this paper, we will make use of studies from the
Stress Research Group at Nijmegen University. This
group was established in the Department of Industrial
and Organizational Psychology at Catholic University,
Nijmegen, in 1976. The group has a small permanent staff,
who have concerned themselves with research on relationships between work and various indices of mental and
physical health. We have asked specific questions such
as "What factors in the work environment cause strain?,"
"What processes lead from stressors to strains?," "What
is the influence of individual differences and other
enabling conditions upon these processes?," and "What
interventions are possible and how can these be introduced

into the organization?"

Until now, our research group has concentrated mainly on field studies of occupational groups (e.g., middle managers, personnel officers, head nurses), adopting for the most part an explorative, partly model-testing approach. In these studies, "role sets" were studied (2); not only were members of the relevant occupational group studied (interviewed), but also members of the organizations with whom they interacted frequently and who influenced their behavior. By doing so, we tried to get a more complete picture of the nature of stress-stress relationships, hoping to correct somewhat the subjective views offered by individual respondents. In addition, we used a questionnaire so that we could obtain comparable data across all study groups. Most recently, we have started a longitudinal study of 2,500 employees of small and middle-sized companies in one region of the Netherlands.

Throughout our research, we have used the stress model developed at the Institute of Social Research, Ann Arbor (2,3). This model specifies a process. The objective environment induces certain stressors in the individual employee, which in turn lead to responses on their part (strain), and then to disease (5). The relationships are modified by the properties of individuals (genetic, demographic, personality) and by interpersonal relationships. On the basis of this model, Caplan (6) developed a questionnaire, which was adapted and translated into Dutch. It was tried out on different samples, and a number of studies were carried out to explore its psychometric properties. The results of these studies have been published in two manuals, one technical and one for test administration (7,8). This questionnaire now has a modular form and is being used in all of our research projects. Taking into account the small number of items per variable, the psychometric properties are quite satisfactory.

3   THE MAGNITUDE OF PSYCHOSOCIAL STRAIN(S)

It is assumed that stressors lead to strains. In a recent study for the Dutch Government (9), we collected data on absenteeism, work disability, heart disease, neoplasmata, suicide, medical care usage, blood pressure, and cholesterol levels. Among other things, we noted that absenteeism has grown steadily in the Netherlands during the past two decades. We also noted that mortality

and morbidity for CHD and neoplasmata increased, particularly for younger age groups. To summarize: We noted
that: the general level of psychosocial strain was
disturbingly high; it was on the increase; lower socio-
economic classes suffer from strain the most; the
increase in mental disorders seems especially elevated;
and, mental disorders occur much more frequently in
the young.

## 4  PSYCHOSOCIAL STRESSORS

Most experts agree that the changes in health as
described above cannot be explained entirely on medical
grounds, but should be seen as the result of psychosocial
stressors. In the Netherlands, the available medical
service system is excellent and compares favorably to
other countries in the world. Also, a substantial part
of the Dutch national economy is spent on improving
this system; thus, there is no apparent deterioration in
services being delivered. Data from other European
countries have been published recently in a report prepared by a group of experts for the European Foundation
for the Improvement of Living and Working Conditions (10).

It is not claimed that changes in health status
(strain) can be attributed entirely to stressors. It
is, of course, possible that other factors exert some
influence. Those, however, will not be considered here.

What are the psychosocial factors that lead to
strain and illness in the work environment? The literature cites almost an infinite number. A sampling of
these include: work overload, role ambiguity, role
conflict, job future uncertainty, lack of participation.
Others have to do with adjustments to critical life
events, e.g., death of a partner, unemployment, rape,
etc. Still others refer to stressful environments, e.g.,
noise. It is likely that cultural and economic factors
are also involved, e.g., educational programs, rates of
unemployment, etc.

## 5  RELATIONSHIP BETWEEN STRESSORS AND STRAINS

The fact that there is a great deal of literature
on stressors and strains does not mean that we precisely
understand the relationship between the two.

Most studies have concentrated on cross-sectional
data. We did likewise, although recently we started on

some longitudinal studies. A first step, then, is to compute correlation coefficients. In our field, this approach is widely used and accepted. To summarize our findings, it appears that there are significant relationships between stressors and psychological strains (e.g., work satisfaction, anxiety, depression, psychosomatic complaints, etc.). Many of these relationships are in the magnitude of .30 to .40. Those between stressors and behavioral and physiological strains (e.g., smoking, blood pressure, cholesterol level, etc.) are much lower and usually non-significant. In our studies, we have not used data about frank illnesses (e.g., CHD) because of their low frequencies.

If one takes into account moderator variables, the results look more impressive. In that case, there are significant relationships between stressors and both behavioral and physiological strains. The moderator variables we examined include: A/B typology, rigidity, age, and social support.

In our studies, the differences between occupational groups are striking. We have computed correlations for total groups, but also for homogeneous subgroups (e.g., middle managers). In the latter case, there are clear differences in the magnitude(s) of correlations between stressor-strain variables. We have asked ourselves whether the differences should be attributed to chance, but have become more and more convinced that they are systematic in nature. In our middle-management study, we had four groups representing different levels in the organization (i.e., operators, first-line supervisors, middle managers, and managers). It is striking that in some cases we found significant correlations for higher levels and non-significant ones for lower levels, and visa versa. Table 1 gives an example.

These results suggest that one should not compute correlations for heterogeneous groups, but rather concentrate on homogeneous subgroups of specific interest. Furthermore, there are substantial differences between mean scores, which can be seen from both t-tests and ANOVA studies. There are clear differences related to occupational group and to level in the organization. In the middle-management study, for example, we found that the higher levels report a greater work load, more responsibility for other people, role conflicts, role ambiguity, little support from colleagues, psychological complaints, and little self-actualization. Also, the

Table 1.   Correlations Between Stressors and
           Strains for 4 Occupational Groups
           Representing Different Levels in the
           Organization.


           Stressor:   Lack of Participation
           Strain:     Work             Self-Esteem
                   Dissatisfaction         (low)

Occupational Groups

| | Work Dissatisfaction | Self-Esteem (low) |
|---|---|---|
| Higher Management | .05 | .08 |
| Middle Management | .17 | .18 * |
| First Line Supervisor | .33** | .28** |
| Operators | .29** | .19 * |

Note:   * significant at .05 level
       ** significant at .01 level

higher levels report more lack of participation, future
uncertainty, work dissatisfaction and absenteeism.

    Differences between organizations are substantial
too and studies show them to be related to size.  In
medium-size organizations (500-2,000 employees), we
found that for a number of occupational groups, the
levels of stressors and strains were much higher than
in very big organizations (greater than 10,000 workers).
This is also true for physiological strains.  In the
medium-size organizations, diastolic blood pressure
was 10 mm Hg higher.  This is confirmed in other studies
(11,12).  ANOVA studies on the same data show that
"organization" is a very significant factor in explaining differences between scores (13,14).

    In other studies, path analysis was used.  These
studies were able to demonstrate clear relationships
between different kinds of variables, including physiological variables.  Here also, there are clear differences between occupational groups.  Van Dijkhuizen (15)
presents some of these results (see Figure 1); although,
strictly speaking, these are not path analyses since
he uses eta's rather than the required product-moment
correlation coefficients.

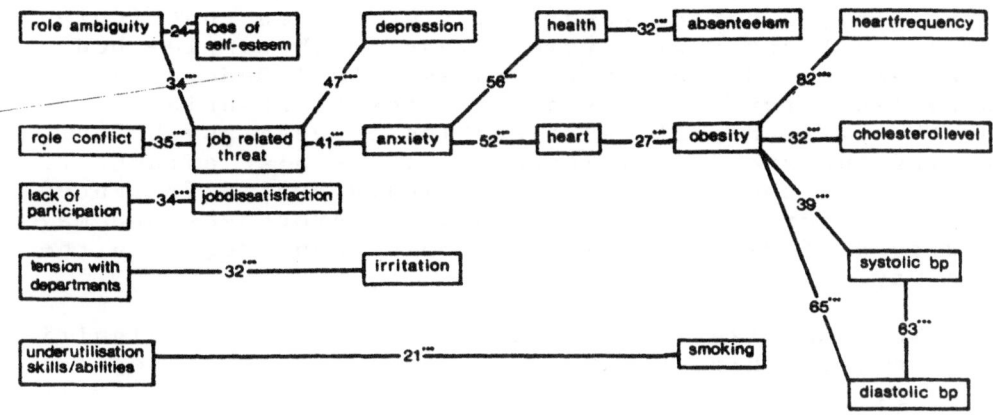

Figure 1. Path analysis based on data from middle management study (15).

Experimental studies appear to be the most adequate means for proving that there are causal relationships between stressors and strains, but they entail serious ethical problems. One may not expose any random sample to stressors in order to compare the results with those of a control group. Occasionally, there are opportunities for quasi-experiments, for example when a factory shuts down. Even then, it is difficult to conduct a study, because under such circumstances organizations usually are not very cooperative or willing to let researchers carry out their measurements. In the literature there is, however, one case reported by Gore (16). She concentrated on the influence of social support and was able to demonstrate that individuals who had been unemployed for a long time, but who reported high levels of support, displayed fewer strains than those reporting low levels of support. This effect was demonstrated for depression, health problems and cholesterol levels.

There are, however, many laboratory studies, especially on endocrinological and physiological variables, but almost all of them fall outside the domain of industrial psychology. Frankenhaueser (17) did some interesting studies in which work variables were included

which are of relevance here. She demonstrated, for
example, that control of working speed has important
consequences for endocrinological processes. For the
validation of the French and Caplan (3) model, and
especially for its latter part where psychological
variables are related to physiological ones, endocrinological and physiological studies are important.
Selye (18), a noted endocrinologist, noted that individuals confronted with threat react with complex body
defenses and adaptation processes. As I understand it,
these laboratory studies now provide substantial evidence
for the existence of relationships between psychological
strains and specific illnesses. It is also evident from
a number of these studies, that individual differences
have an important influence on these processes and may
lead to different states. No two persons react in the
same way to stressors.

To summarize: Correlation studies reveal significant relationships between stressors and psychological
strains, while correlations with behavioral and physiological strains are non-significant. Moderator variables
are important; taking them into account, relationships
with behavioral/physiological outcome(s) turn out to
be significant. There are considerable differences
between mean scores related to "organization" (including
size) and occupational group (level in the organizational
hierarchy). Experimental studies are difficult to
carry out, although there is at least one example where
relationships with a physiological variable can be demonstrated. Physiological and endocrinological studies
support a theory relating stressors to physiological
strains and frank illness. Individual differences are
important.

What may be concluded from this overview? Some
argue that, considering the correlational studies, the
scientific proof is insufficient. And, even if there
were a significant correlation, there is no proof for
causality, i.e., strains might cause stressors! It is
said that the correlations between stressors and strains
could indeed be attributed to an overlap in the contents
of measurement instruments (4).

It is possible to explain the lack of correlation
between stressors and physiological strains in other
ways. Selye (18) notes that strains have much to do
with wearing out, what today is often referred to as
burnout. Thus, physiological strains could well be the

result of a long process. In that case, the time variable will be of great importance. Maybe, some strains can only be demonstrated after long exposure to stressors. But then cross-sectional studies will not be adequate; such effects can be measured only in longitudinal studies. Incidentally, a recent longitudinal study (12) shows that role ambiguity is related to behavioral and physiological strains. Our studies indicate that individual differences (e.g., A/B typology and rigidity), conditions such as social support, and occupational differences are all very important. This has serious implications for the design of studies. One should be careful using heterogeneous samples; homogeneous samples are preferred. Also, designs should include moderator variables. Finally, it could be worthwhile to look for cumulative effects of stressors and not only stressors in the work setting per se, but also of family life and elsewhere.

Thus, the methodology most commonly used in industrial/organizational psychological studies may not be that adequate at this point. Simple correlation studies might fail to prove that there are existing relationships between stressors and illnesses. If so, negative findings should be attributed to the methods employed. There exists an obvious need for longitudinal studies, so that time effects can be taken into account. Also, the effects of individual variables and conditions should receive more attention.

All the results, taken together, strongly suggest a relationship between psychosocial variables and illnesses. In this respect, the fact that there are no competing theories, and certainly none fitting the combined results, is of importance too. In their chapter on work and health, Katz and Kahn (5) state that "No one could claim that a mature theory (of work and health) yet exists, much less that its components have been subjected to empirical test." To a considerable extent, this is still true. But so far, results from studies have made it clear that stressors do have a significant influence on health and thus provide the elements for a theory. To construct an adequate theory, other types of studies are needed, particularly longitudinal ones, that take into account both differences between occupational groups and organizations and moderator variables. Such a theory should concentrate on processes in which stressors lead to strains that in turn lead to other strains.

REFERENCES

1. Dunnette, M.D. (Ed.) Handbook of Industrial and Organizational Psychology. (Chicago, Rand McNally, 1976).
2. Kahn, R.L. et al. Organizational Stress: Studies in Role Conflict and Ambiguity. (New York, Wiley, 1964).
3. French, J.R.P. and R.D. Caplan. Organizational Stress and Individual Strain. In A.J. Marrow (Ed.) The Failure of Success. (New York, Amacon, 1973).
4. Kasl, S.V. Epidemiological Contribution to the Study of Work Stress. In C.L. Cooper and R.L. Payne (Eds.) Stress at Work. (New York, Wiley, 1978).
5. Katz, D. and R.L. Kahn. The Social Psychology of Organizations, 2 Edition. (New York, Wiley, 1978).
6. Caplan, R.D. et al. Job Demands and Worker Health: Main Effects and Occupational Differences. Washington D.C., U.S. Government Printing Office, 1975).
7. van Bastelaer, A. and W. van Beers. Vragenlijst Organisatie-Stress, Testhandleiding deel 2: Konstruktie en Normering. (Nijmegen, Katholieke Universiteit, publ. 24, 1980).
8. Reiche, M. and N. van Dijkhuizen. Vragenlijst Organisatie-Stress. Testhandleiding deel 1, Testafname. (Nijmegen, Katholieke Universiteit, publ. 23, 1980).
9. de Wolff, C.J. et al. Werk en Gezondheid. (Nijmegen, Report prepared for WRR, 1981).
10. Lawrence, W.G. et al. Physical and Psychological Stress at Work. (Dublin, European Foundation for the Improvement of Living and Working Conditions, 1981).
11. Reiche, M. and N. van Dijkhuizen. Bedrijfsgrootte, Hierarchie en Persoonlijkheid, Beinvloeden zij het Ervaren van Stressoren en Strains? Gedrag 7 (1979) 58-75.
12. van Bastelaer, A. and W. van Beers. Stress and Some Public Background Variables: An Analysis of Variance on Replicated Data. (1981) Unpublished paper.
13. van Bastelaer, A. Onderzoek Naar Stress Bij Personeelsfunktionarissen. (1980) Unpublished paper.
14. Reiche, M. Stress Aan Het Werk. (Nijmegen, Katholieke Universiteit, 1981).
15. van Dijkhuizen, N. From Stressors to Strains. (Lisse, Swets and Zeitlinger, 1980).
16. Gore, S. The Influence of Social Support in Ameliorating the Consequences of Job Loss. Doctoral

Dissertation, University of Pennsylvania, 1973.
17. Frankenhaueser, M. Psychobiological Effects of Life
    Stress. In S. Levine and H. Ursin (Eds.) Coping
    and Health. (New York, Plenum, 1980).
18. Selye, H. The Stress of Life. (New York, McGraw-
    Hill, 1956).

# PSYCHOSOCIAL CORONARY RISK CONSTELLATIONS IN THE WORK SETTING

Johannes Siegrist

Department of Medical Sociology
University of Marburg
Marburg, West Germany

## 1 INTRODUCTION

This paper examines three basic issues in the field of relationships between workload and cardiovascular disease (CVD). As a starting point, an obviously paradoxical finding in contemporary social epidemiology is discussed: on the one hand, coronary-prone behavior (CPB) has been linked, although with a rather low specificity, to the incidence of CVD, and especially ischemic heart disease (IHD), as an independent risk factor. It has also been demonstrated that CPB is prevalent among higher economic or educational groups. On the other hand, the incidence of IHD is especially high among lower socio-economic groups, even if one controls for somatic risk factors. How can we explain these discrepant findings? Our answer will suggest that one should differentiate dimensions of stressful experiences between white-collar and blue-collar occupations. In the case of white collars, and this is the first issue raised here, the role of CPB in certain types of occupations has to be specified on a conceptual as well as on an empirical level. There is good reason to conceive of CPB in terms of an interactional phenomenon, being elicited and reinforced by specific characteristics of the work setting, and being changed over time as a function of exposure.

Workload in the blue-collar world is a second issue. We will show that stressful experiences are of a different nature here, calling for a broader analysis which includes non-mental influences in the work setting as well as socio-emotional conditions outside the working place.

After having demonstrated differences of psychosocial risks between the two groups, we ask about possible underlying mechanisms on a psychoendocrinological level, introducing the concept of active distress. In discussing this third issue, we also present recent evidence on more specific links between stress-induced arousal, neurohormonal imbalance and precursors of cardiovascular pathology. It is thought that conceptual developments which go beyond simple correlations of, say, CPB and heart disease, or workload and heart disease, could contribute to coping with some of the current weaknesses in the field. It is along these lines that empirical results from research done by our institute during the last five years are presented, and that some practical conclusions will be suggested.

As mentioned, socio-epidemiologic findings are somewhat paradoxical. It is well established that CPB (1,2,3) is associated "with an increased risk of clinically apparent CHD in employed, middle-aged U.S. citizens. This increased risk is over and above that imposed by age, systolic blood pressure, serum cholesterol, and smoking, and appears to be of the same order of magnitude as the relative risk associated with any of these factors." (4)

Several studies, however, have shown that incidence of IHD (CHD) is significantly higher among blue-collar or lower educational groups after controlling for main somatic risk factors. Rose and Marmot, for example, demonstrate a ratio of 3.6 between highest and lowest occupational groups in a large sample of civil servants, analyzing coronary mortality (5). Koskenvuo et al. find an increased mortality of CHD in unskilled workers (6). This has been documented independently by Holme (7). The risk of sudden cardiac death (SCD) after first myocardial infarction (MI) has been linked with low educational level in a very careful study which revealed that after controlling for type of documented arrhythmia, SCD is over three times as high in the low education group as compared to the better educated one (8). It does not seem that CPB contributes much to this excess mortality. In the contrary, CPB has been reported to be more prevalent in white-collar occupations (9-11). The basic evidence for a correlation between CPB and heart disease comes "from a male sample which is only 10% blue collar, with most of the remainder in middle and upper levels of managerial and technic-scientific work" (12). Consistent with this result are data from the Framingham heart study which recently reported an association between CPB and CHD among white-collar but not blue-collar workers (13).

Is it possible to explain this finding by measurement bias? It may be that applied questionnaires, mainly the Jenkins Activity Survey and Framingham Type A scales, are better

adjusted to patterns of attitudes and linguistic codes of middle-
class populations. But it seems rather unlikely that the
structured interview developed by Rosenman et al. (14) with
its emphasis on speech and motor characteristics and on response
style is biased with regard to social or occupational status.
Thus, another explanation may be more appropriate. It has been
suggested that in higher social classes several protective
mechanisms such as social support or a healthier lifestyle may
lead to the fact that CPB becomes the main leading psychosocial
coronary stressor, whereas, heavy socio-environmental burden
such as workload, including mental and physical stressors,
increased social instability, interpersonal conflicts and lack
of social support are especially prevalent among lower class
working groups (15,16). The following data present some evidence
for this hypothetical explanation. First, it is shown on a large-
scale basis with administative data on about 22,000 men undergoing rehabilitation after first MI in West Germany that specific
occupations can be identified which are overrepresented as
compared to total population in this age and sex group in either
occupational sector. White-collar occupations at risk seem to be
associated with characteristics of mental workload, calling for
more intense analysis of work demands and personal coping styles,
whereas blue-collar occupations at risk seem to be associated
with multiple physical and mental stressors. This general
finding is elaborated in analyses based on a retrospective case-
control study on 380 male patients with clinically defined
first MI and a healthy control group matched on the basis of
age, sex, and occupational status with the sample half. Data
presented from this study elucidate a more specific relationship
between demands of a particular work setting and CPB as a relevant
coping style in white-collar groups. In this context, we also
present data from a follow-up study of this MI-population showing
a marked intraindividual change in the degree of CPB which can
be linked to exposure to work and social problems. Finally,
information on blue-collar work settings is given, including
general living conditions outside the work place as well, such
as critical life events and lack of social stability.


2 MATERIALS AND METHODS OF THE STUDIES

Results are based on two types of studies. The first one
is a reanalysis of administrative data on occupational
characteristics of 22,689 West German men aged 35 to 64 years
who experienced and survived their first MI in 1977 and 1978
and who underwent a rehabilitation program. As there is a high
rate of using, in this age and sex group, these programs offered
by social security, a very high percentage of all survivors could
be included in this sample. Distribution of frequency of
occupations (on the basis of an official classification made out

of 86 groups) in this sample was compared to distribution of
frequency of the total male working population in this age
group in West Germany. Differences between observed and expected
rates were checked, and statistical significance of o/e rates
was established. This work has been conducted as a doctoral
dissertation by U. Bolm in our Institute (17, 18).

The second study reported here is a medical-sociological
analysis of 380 male patients, aged from 30 to 55, with
clinically proven first MI, participating in a rehabilitation
program, and of a control group of 190 healthy males, matched
with the sample half of the MI patients on the basis of age
and occupational status. All MI patients were contacted once
more 18 months later by means of a questionnaire focusing on
occupational, medical, and psychosocial rehabilitation. Thirteen
patients died of a second infarction. Seventy percent valid
answers could be obtained (N = 258).

As a principal investigator, I could rely on crucial help
from and intense cooperation with my co-workers, K. Dittman,
K. Rittner and I. Weber. Results of this study have been
published in German (19), and only partially in English
(20-22). A larger part of results reported here has not yet
been published.

A retrospective study can be justified only, first, if it
starts from and attempts to differentiate knowledge accumulated
by previous prospective studies, second, if it, by utilizing
additional measures, guarantees that biases in data collections
due to retrospective interpretations are controlled as far as
possible, third, if the criterium variable is specified as
exactly as possible, leading to a high homogeneity of the sample,
and finally, if the comparative criteria regarding a control
group are adhered to as closely as possible.

We have shown elsewhere how we tried to fulfill all these
conditons (19). Controls, however, were not individually
assigned to the sample half of the MI patients, but matched as
groups with regard to occupational status and age. As controls
were slightly younger, we had to adjust the sample half to the
age distribution of the control group. No systematic differences
between the original and the younger sample half of the MI patients
could be detected. Level of education, vocational training,
regional and social mobility were equally distributed; occupations
differed to some extent with regard to public versus private
sector; white collars and skilled workers showed equal distributions, whereas un- or semiskilled workers were slightly overrepresented in the control group.

The rate of rejection was below 5% among patients, below 8% among controls. All data on MI patients were collected between 5 and 24 weeks after the onset of MI. The time interval between infarction and interview revealed no systematic trend. We also controlled for seasonal variations in the study group.

Because of unavoidable concentration on survivors, one bias factor exists which cannot be controlled, especially so, because the percentage of sudden cardiac death is still very high (23). This fact creates some difficulties for testing our hypotheses because patients who died of a sudden death without manifest prior illness may have been subjected, in their premorbid phase, to psychosocial stressors of a special strength (24). More details, as mentioned earlier, on the composition of the sample and statistical control for possible biases and intervening variables can be found in our final research report (29).

The following data have been collected:

(a) Clinical data included diagnosis of acute MI on the basis of EEG and enzymes, diagnosis of somatic risk factors by measuring blood pressure, body weight, cholesterol, triglycerides, diabetes, hyper-uricaemia, family history of CVD. Extensive information on smoking habits and on physical activity were obtained in the interview. Information on blood pressure and weight was only partially valid, as these measures were influenced by the course of the disease itself as well as by therapeutic intervention. The same holds true for measures of cholesterol and triglycerides. We tried to get inpatients, and we could show that measures taken from a subgroup during the first days after hospital admission did not differ significantly from measures taken after admission to the rehabilitation center. However we are aware of principal biases due to the retrospective study design.

In subgroup of N = 256, additional data on local-ization and extension of MI, on the degree of ischemia and the amount of ventricular premature beats (VPB) could be obtained and from 53 patients we could get data on coronary angiography. In the control group, data on blood pressure, body weight, smoking and physical activity were collected. Cases with previous manifest CVD (MI or angina pectoris) were excluded as well as persons who subjectively reported cardiac symptoms. Data on cholesterol, triglycerides and hyperuricaemia could not be collected in the control group.

(b) Sociological and psychological data first included a
structured interview with 71 questions on basic socio-
demographic data, on occupational career, on experiences of workload, on time budget, chronic difficulties
and social support, and on smoking and physical activity.
Shift work, rate fixing, workplace security, potential
stressors such as noise, heat, time pressure, inconsistent
demands, disruptions, limitations of one's activity,
responsibility and control were carefully explored.

A second instrument was developed in order to measure
frequency and subjective impact of life events during
the last 2 years. Using an inventory of 34 clearly
defined negative life events (ILE), we asked the subjects
to assess themselves their emotional reactions and coping
efforts according to the following dimensions:
controlability, predictability, position of the life event
in the subjective structure of relevance, interruption
of everyday routines, extent of situational vulnerability,
active coping, experienced social support, psychological
and social "costs" of adaptation, time period of impact.
This approach enabled us to calculate both the amount of
stressful events per selected subgroup or individual
and the respective subjective stress scores or their
mean value. Assuming a cumulative nature of the scores,
individuals could be assigned from 1 to 44 points
per event, with 44 points indicating extreme stress.
Accordingly, events could be classified following the
degree of subjectively perceived stress (for more details
see 19).

Psychological measures concentrated on the coronary-
prone behavior pattern which was assessed by a questionnaire of 21 items centering around overcommitment during
work, need for control and approval, impatience, speed
and time urgency. As pretest experiences with the German
version of the rating of statement list (RSL) developed
by van Dijl (25) were unsatisfactory, we developed an
own list of dichotomous statements along these lines.
Test statistical information about the first version of
this questionnaire is included in our final research
report (19). A second and more specific version, using
more rigorous statistical analysis, has been tested
in three different samples; results are not yet
published. In addition, denial as measured by MMPI-L-
scale and neuroticism as measured by a widely used
German personality inventory (FPI, 26) were included.

(c) The followup questionnaire contained questions on
the occupational and economic situation of cardiac

patients after rehabilitation, on social activities and
health behavior including self-help groups, on
information about the course of disease and subjective well-being. In addition, scales of coronary-
prone behavior were retested ($\underline{r}$ = .87).

## 3 RESULTS

### 3.1 Occupations and Coronary Risk

Studies which establish relationships between IHD and
occupational characteristics on the basis of mortality data
usually underestimate related health risks in blue-collar
occupations. This underestimation is due to a higher rate of
job-loss, of change of jobs or retirement in this group (18).
By concentrating on a large sample of subjects with first MI
and with occupational characteristics which were valid immediately
before disease onset, we are able to avoid at least partially
this bias. It is unknown, however, to what degree sudden death
following first MI is influenced by socio-economic characteristics.
Our data show occupations among white-collars and blue-collars
which are at highest coronary risk (see Figures 1 and 2).

These are, among others, technical assistants, air traffic
controllers and pilots, porters and guards, sales managers,
bank and insurance brokers and data processing specialists
in white-collar occupations, and metal workers, sawyers and
wood-working machinists, precision instrument makers, unskilled
workers, miners and furnace men in blue-collar occupations.

On the other hand, farmers, agricultural workers, foresters,
construction workers are among the most underrepresented groups
in the blue-collar sector, as are clergymen , soldiers, teachers,
and administrators in the white collar sector.

High noise and exposure to toxic substances have been
discussed as possible determinants of higher cardiovascular
risk in several blue-collar occupations, especially in metal
workers, miners, and sawyers (27-30). Mental workload produced
by time pressure, qualitative underload and other stressors
may be simultaneously present (see below). The latter
conditions are thought to be critical in the subgroup of
unskilled workers who experience poor working conditions, low
social status and a high degree of social instability (31).
In a few cases, the higher risk of technical assistants, sales
managers, bank and insurance brokers, air traffic controllers
and data processing specialists has been explored, and mental
workload was documented at least as one of several pathogenetic
factors (32-24).

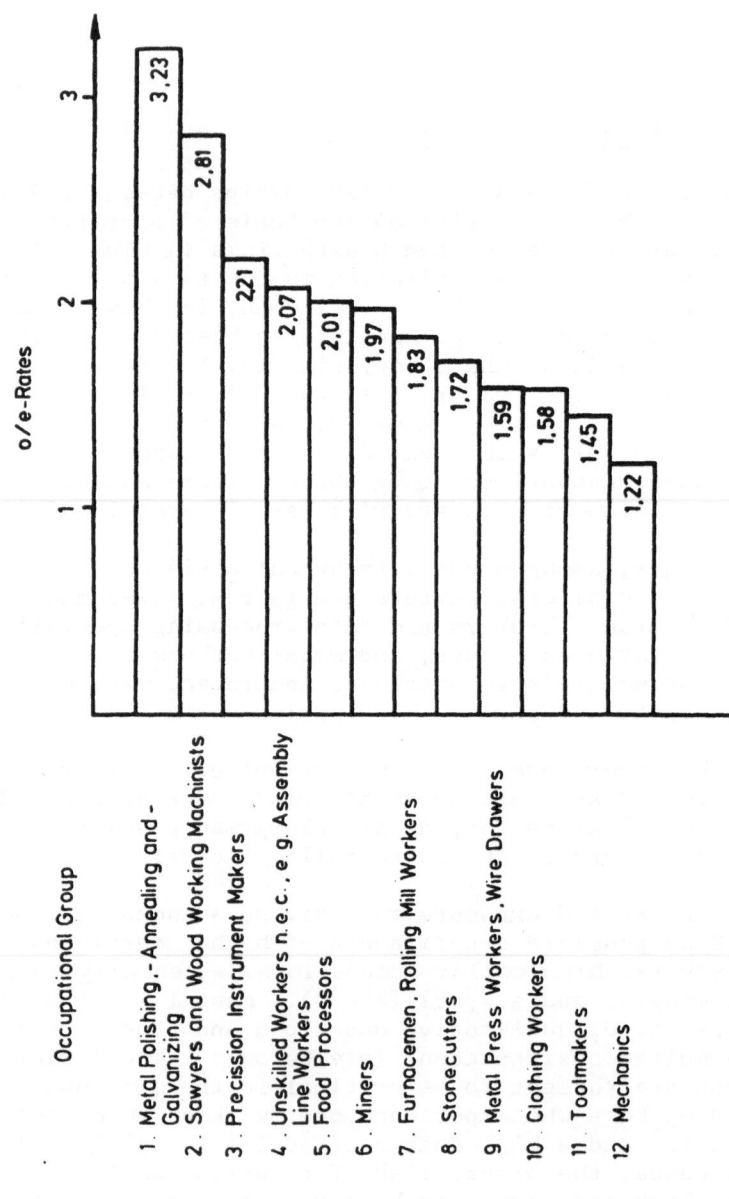

Figure 1: Blue Collar Jobs significant accumulated in Myocardial Infarction ( Men 35 - 64 j.. N = 10.482 )

o/e-Rates

Occupational Group

1. Metal Polishing.- Annealing and - Galvanizing   3.23
2. Sawyers and Wood Working Machinists   2,81
3. Precission Instrument Makers   2,21
4. Unskilled Workers n.e.c., e.g. Assembly Line Workers   2,07
5. Food Processors   2,01
6. Miners   1,97
7. Furnacemen, Rolling Mill Workers   1,83
8. Stonecutters   1,72
9. Metal Press Workers, Wire Drawers   1,59
10. Clothing Workers   1,58
11. Toolmakers   1,45
12. Mechanics   1,22

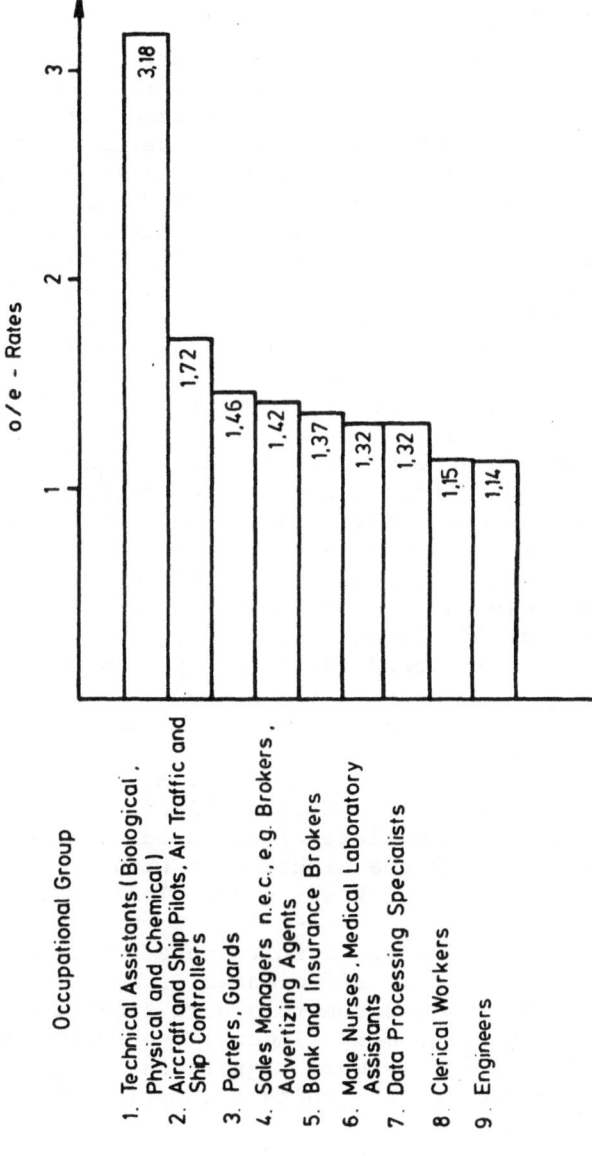

Figure 2: White Collar Jobs significant accumulated in Myocardial Infarction (Men 35-64 j., N = 12.207 )

Occupational Group

1. Technical Assistants (Biological, Physical and Chemical)
2. Aircraft and Ship Pilots, Air Traffic and Ship Controllers
3. Porters, Guards
4. Sales Managers n.e.c., e.g. Brokers, Advertizing Agents
5. Bank and Insurance Brokers
6. Male Nurses, Medical Laboratory Assistants
7. Data Processing Specialists
8. Clerical Workers
9. Engineers

Identification of stressful dimensions of work demands, however, could not be clarified to a sufficient degree on the basis of crude administrative data (35). We will concentrate on this issue in the next section.

## 3.2 White-Collar Work Setting and Coronary-Prone Behavior

In order to test subjective impact of more specific work settings, we present data from our retrospective study on middle-aged MI patients. It must be emphasized that our sample includes a wide range of occupations. Twenty percent of the MI subjects in the sample could be classified as unskilled or semiskilled workers, 23% as skilled blue-collar workers, 41% as white-collar workers, mainly employees, 10% as professionals and 6% as officials and higher ranks of civil service. Twenty-eight percent of the 380 subjects are in middle-echelon or in leading positions, and their work can be characterized by "coordination, organization, disposition, control and leadership". Blue-collar workers had their jobs mainly in private industrial plants. Every third worker experienced shift work, every fourth piece work.

In order to assess workload more adequately for the several groups, three different indices were constructed: Index I included all 34 characteristics of potential workload. The more characteristics were admitted by the interviewee as representative for his own regular work place, the higher the general workload was assumed to be. Index II concentrated on the subgroup of 27 characteristics of potential psychosocial workload, which included the majority of work-related items, whereas Index III measured the presence of more traditional physical work stressors (noise, heat, danger of accidents among others). It was postulated, first, that total amount of workload (Index I) was more pronounced in the MI group than in the control group, and second, that mental workload (Index II) was more pronounced in white collars as compared to blue collars in either population, but with the higher mean within MI white collars. In analogy, physical work stressors (Index III) were thought to be more prevalent among blue-collar workers than among white collars in either group. Results were consistent with the first and second assumption: differences of mean (Index I and Index II) between MI subjects and controls were significant at p = .001 level; differences of mean (Index II) between white-collar and blue-collar MI subjects were significant at p = .01 level. There was also evidence for the third assumption, but differences did not reach statistical significance.

In an analysis of very homogeneous small subgroups of the two samples of white and blue collars, similar results could be obtained, as demonstrated in Figure 3. Middle-echelon employees, supervisors and foremen in the MI and control group

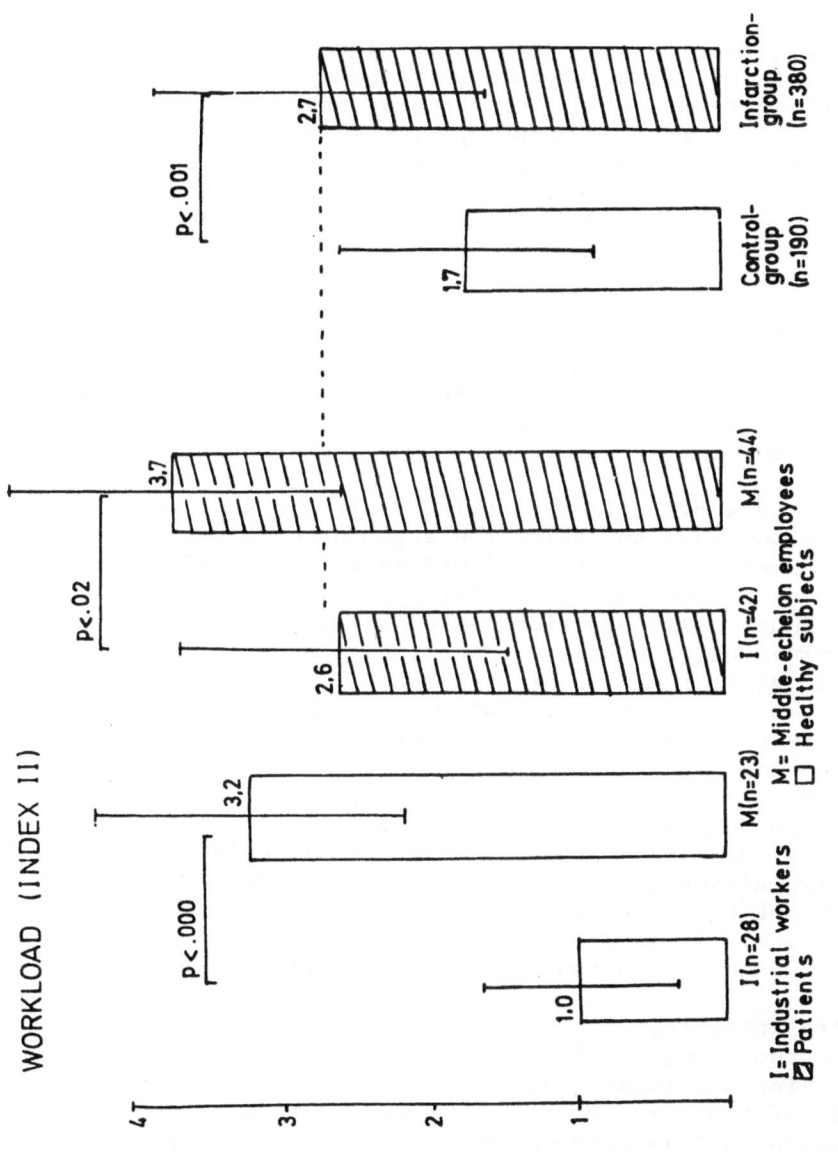

Figure 3: Workload (index II) in homogeneous occupational white-collar and blue-collar groups (MI-patients and healthy controls)

were compared to blue-collar workers with simple repetitive tasks.
As indicated, differences between the two subgroups in MI
patients and in healthy controls were significant. Among single
items of psychosocial workload, time pressure, interruptions
at work, high responsibility, concentration and inconsistent
demands were the ones with highest scores within MI patients.
Interestingly, these scores were again higher in a subgroup
of white-collar MI patients who experienced job insecurity
and cut-down in personnel during the last several years. Stressful
time pressure, for example, was experienced in 63% of this
group, as compared to 39% of white-collar MI patients without
experience of job insecurity; high concentrations labeled as
"stressful" was found in 80% of the group with job insecurity as
compared to 48%.

Interestingly, mean scores of CPB in these groups show a
very similar distribution; attitudes reflecting CPB are
significantly stronger in the group of middle-echelon employees
and foremen than in the group of workers with simple repetitive
tasks (Figure 4). Again, trends are more obvious in patients
than in healthy controls (p = .06 in the latter case).

Several interpretations of this result are suggested.
First, it is possible to follow the argument of Mettlin (37)
and to interpret higher scores of CPB in middle-echelon employees
as a result of professional competition, struggle and upward
mobility. Thus, self-selection caused by personality traits such
as job-involvement, competititiveness, hard-driving and
hostility might be the crucial variable. Yet, longitudinal
studies have not verified this interpretation to our knowledge.
A second interpretation points to interrelation between the two
measures; subjective workload, although assessed separately, may
be perceived in a specific way by subjects whose attributes
reflect a high degree of CPB. Pearson coefficients of correlations,
however, were .31 and .33 respectively for MI subjects and healthy
controls, explaining about 10% of total variance. Although the
argument cannot be ruled out, it is unlikely that amount of
subjective workload can be totally reduced to perceptions and
cognitions which are inherent in the CPB pattern.

A third interpretation is consistent with an interactional
approach to the study of CPB. The latter may be analyzed in
terms of coping strategies which are elicited by challenges
and demands of the work setting. Whereas much experimental
research supports this perspective (1,2,4), only a few studies
in real life settings are known to fit into this frame of
reference (38,39). A closer view to dimensions of Index II of
psychosocial workload reveals that threat to control and work
autonomy, inconsistent of demands, time pressure and interruptions
during responsible task-fulfillment are the most critical elements.

57

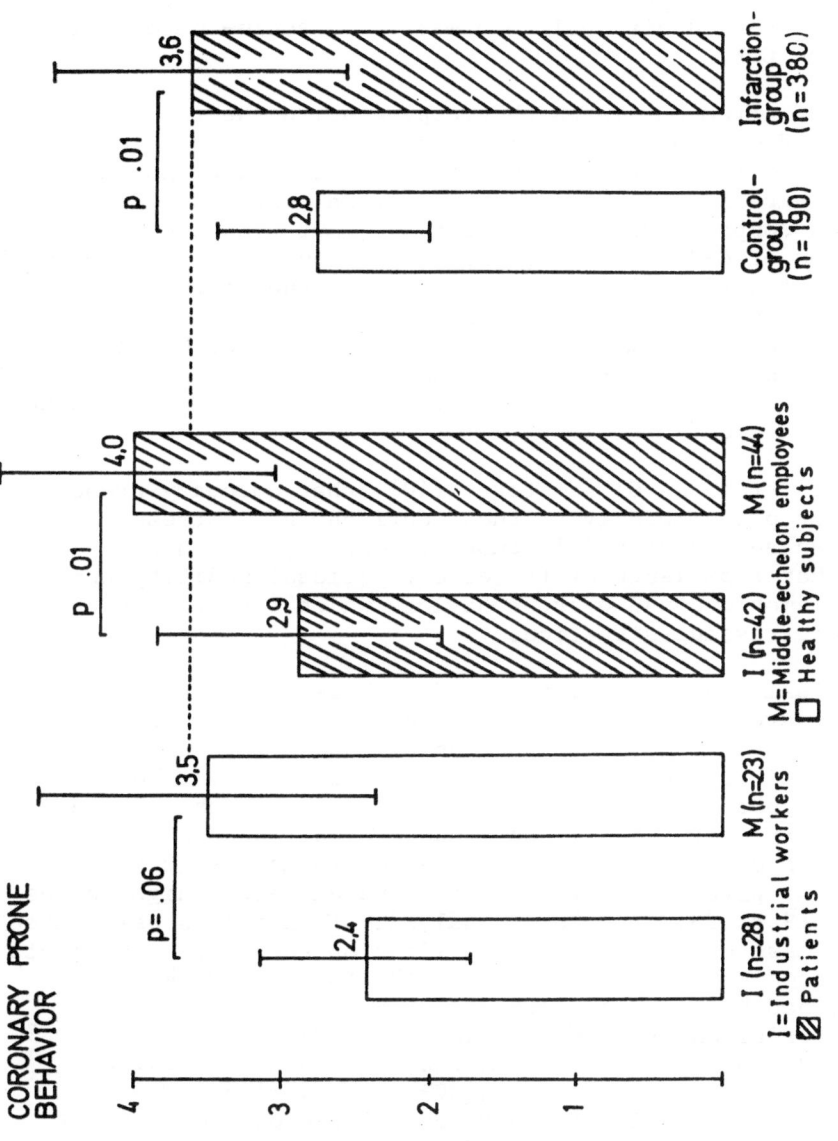

Figure 4: Coronary prone behavior in homogeneous occupational white-collar and blue-collar groups (MI-patients and healthy controls)

These features in the work setting can provoke the well-known cognitive, emotional, and overt beahvioral reactions that constitute the core of CPB. Before outlining a reconsideration of CPB in the framework of appraisal of demands and active coping, we present additional information on socio-contextual influences on CPB.

I. Weber, from our research group, studied the relation between forced occupational mobility and CPB in the sample described above (36). He not only found nearly twice as many MI subjects experiencing forced mobility, in most cases downward mobility, as compared to matched controls, but also significantly higher degree of CPB among this group, as compared to a group with stable occupational positions. For example, the percentage of MI subjects with high scores of CPB in the subgroup of forced mobility was 70%, as compared to 51% in the group with stable positions. A similar, but weaker trend was present in the control group (Figure 5). A statistical test based on LOGIT-model showed significant main effects.

If it is true, as Glass states (40), that coronary-prone persons react predominantly to those environmental stressors that threaten an individuals' sense of control, it can be concluded that experience of forced occupational mobility enhances cognitions, emotions and overt behaviors which try to seek control over this distressing situation.

As a final issue in the field of work setting and subjective coping, we address ourselves to the question of intrapersonal change of CPB over time as a function of exposure to challenges and threats. A followup of our initial MI sample over 18 months gave us the opportunity to analyze some aspects of this issue. First, and very unexpectedly, we found a significant increase in mean scores of CPB in MI subjects after 18 months ($t = 4.6$, $p = .01$). The percentage of subjects with extremely high scores raised from 19 to 33%. A closer analysis of variables associated with an increase of CPB after rehabilitation showed that subjects who experienced more actual strain in the field of work and health also had higher mean scores of CPB ($C = .45$, $p = .001$). A three-factorial analysis of variance with "age", "occupational status" and "actual strain" in the field of work and health" as related to "amount of change in CPB" was carried out in 110 MI subjects. Main effects were calculated on the basis of ANOVA procedure (41,42). Only 15.3% of total variance was explained by main effects ($F = 3.5$, $p - .01$), but out of these 13% could be attributed to the variable "actual strain" ($F = 7.4$, $p = .001$). A multiple classification analysis shows this effect for adjusted and unadjusted means of CPB (41) (Figure 6).

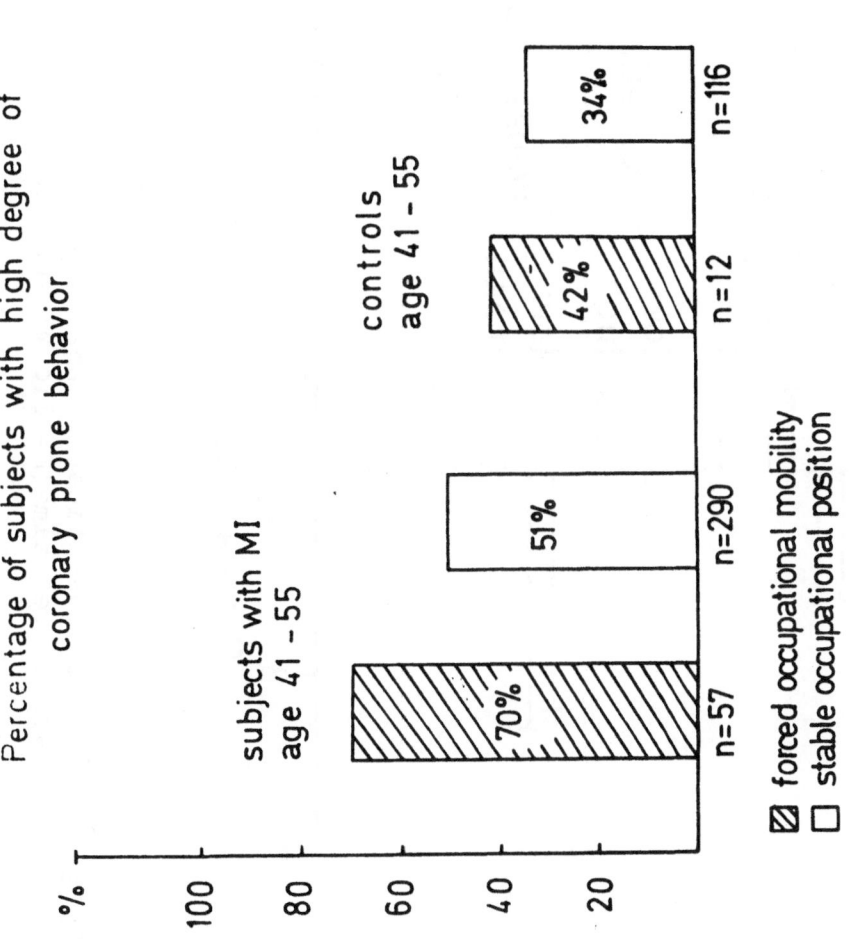

Figure 5 : Percentage of subjects with high degree of coronary prone behavior among MI and healthy controls, controlling for forced occupational mobility (LOGIT model)

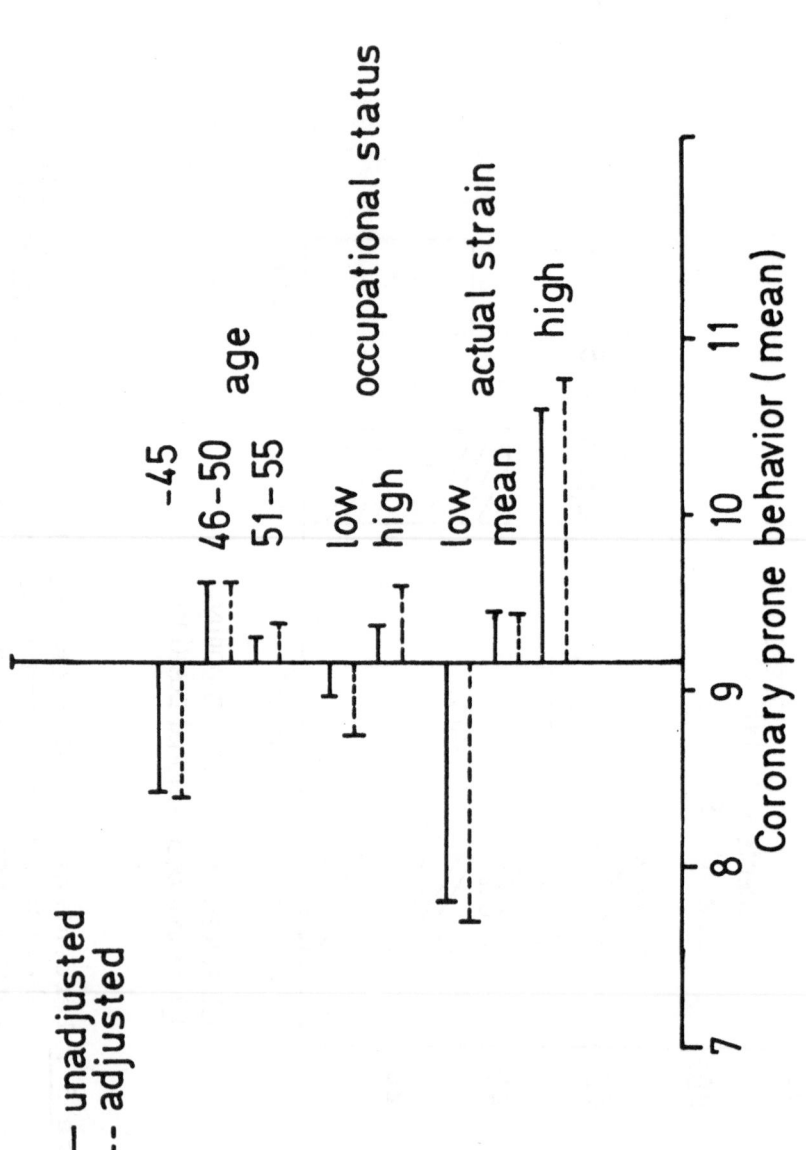

Figure 6: Multiple classification analysis:change in coronary prone behavior over time (N= 110 MI subjects)

The most important items of the index "actual strain" were
"being anxious about work and future" and "more vulnerable self-
esteem at work as compared to time before disease onset".
Thus, threat to one's occupational achievements may be answered
by improving the risky attitudes and behaviors of the CPB pattern.

Taken together, these results give some suggestive evidence
for an interactional approach to the study of CPB at least in the
white-collar work setting. We now want to ask whether psychosocial coronary risk constellations of a different nature can be
found among blue-collars.

## 3.3 Multiple Risks in the Blue-Collar Work Setting

First, physical stressors as well as mental stressors
associated with low occupational status are more prevalent among
unskilled and semi-skilled blue-collar workers than among higher
occupational levels, as illustrated in Figure 7. Marked
differences are found, as expected, in heat, noice, and heavy
physical work, but also in limitation of control and exposure to
interruption. On the other hand, mental work stressors that are
associated with tasks of coordination, organization, and
planning are more prevalent in white-collars (t=2.6, p= .01), where
CPB is higher as well, as demonstrated earlier (for the group
demonstrated in Figure 7 (t=3, p= .01).

The simultaneous presence of several work stressors seems
to be more typical for the blue-collar work setting. Sixty
percent of industrial workers with rate fixing experience
stressful levels of noise as an aggravating condition. A
similar result is obtained with shift-work. Simultaneous stressful
presence of noise and time pressure (C=.29, p = .001), of noise
and interruptions (C=.35, p = .001), of noise and heavy physical
work (C= .35, p = .001) have been documented. The same holds
true for physical stressors such as heat/cold (C=.51, p = .001),
and toxic substances ( C= .40, p = .001). It goes unsaid that
these coefficients would be much higher if only the subgroup
of blue-collar industrial workers (unskilled and semi-skilled)
had been analyzed. Again, blue-collar workers who were faced with
cut-down in personnel during the last years show higher means of
subjective workload than others, as was shown in white-collars.

Nearly half of the group of industrial blue-collars, not
including transportation and construction workers, could be
classified as belonging either to metal workers (turners, borers,
locksmiths and others) or to maintenance fitters, electricians,
and related occupations which are heavily exposed to physical
and mental work stressors. In addition, the vulnerability from
stressors outside the working life may be greater in blue-collars
both because of faulty coping mechanisms and because of exposure

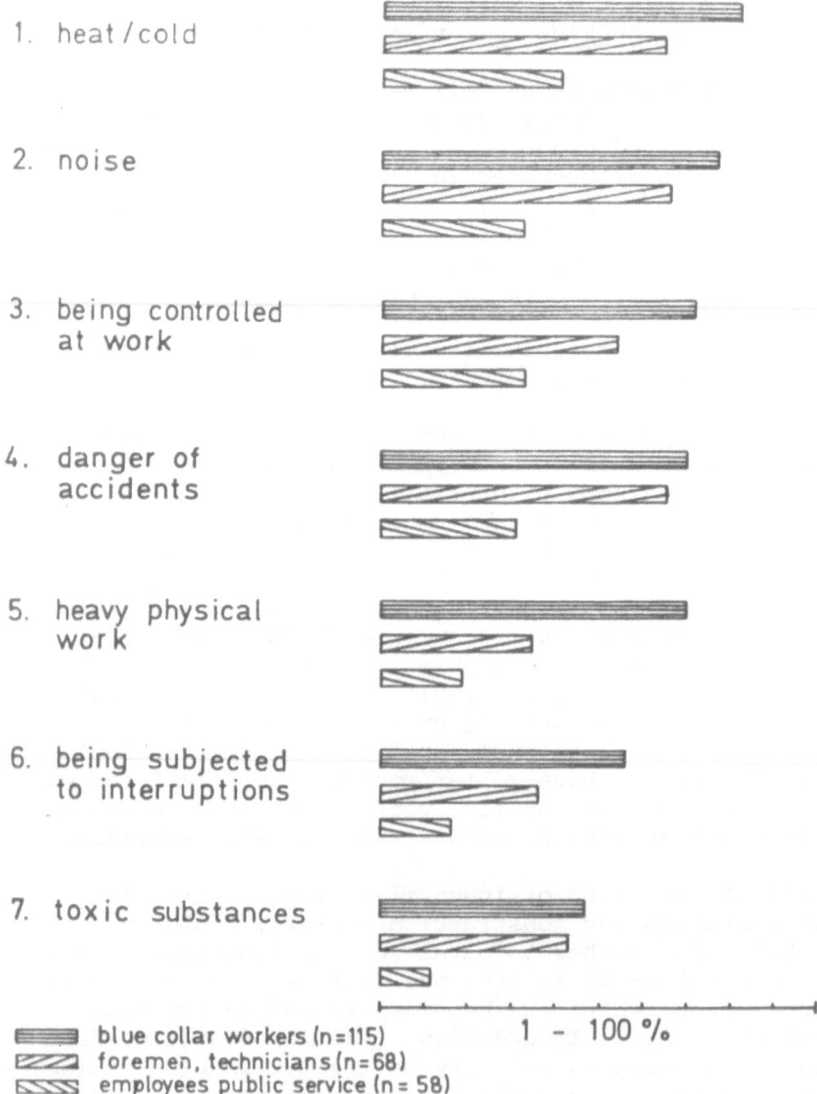

1. heat/cold

2. noise

3. being controlled
   at work

4. danger of
   accidents

5. heavy physical
   work

6. being subjected
   to interruptions

7. toxic substances

1 - 100 %

blue collar workers (n=115)
foremen, technicians (n=68)
employees public service (n=58)

Figure 7: Percentage of MI subjects experiencing stressful subjective workload (selective stressors) in different occupational subgroups

to more, and more serious, chronic difficulties and subacute
life changes. In our study, we could not demonstrate that blue-
collars experienced significantly more life events or more chronic
difficulties, but social support was somewhat weaker in this
group, and cumulative stressors were experienced as much as in
white-collars. In Table 1, for example, an analysis of variance
shows significant relationships between several working and living
conditions which are typical for blue-collars, and the amount
of subjective stress caused by life changes. For every one of
the eight variables, the same direction can be found; the higher
a chronic stressor is rated, the higher is the amount of subjective
impact caused by life events.

Explanations and possible biases of our scores of subjective
rating of the impact of life events have been discussed elsewhere
and cannot be analyzed in detail here (19, 21). On the basis of
our data it can be concluded that remarkable subgroups of
blue-collar workers with early manifestation of MI can be
characterized by psychosocial and physical risk constellations,
i.e., by the simultaneous presence of several risks whose
cumulative effects may overwhelm adaptive efforts of the individual
and, by this, precipitate cardiovascular breakdown.

After having presented empirical results from two studies
which support to some degree our basic assumption of a different
nature of psychosocial risk constellations in white-collar and
blue-collar occupations, we now search for a possible underlying
common denominator in terms of a psychoneuroendocrinological
analysis.


4   TOWARD A CONCEPT OF ACTIVE DISTRESS

4.1   A Psychoneuroendocrinological Hypothesis

The following considerations result from theorizing about
experience of distress as well as from review of recent literature.
Therefore, they should be considered with caution and as open as
substantial criticisms. The main reason to present them in this
context is the urge to draw additional and more specific links
between cognitive-emotional and physiologic processes in cardiovascular pathology.

The main argument can be summarized as follows:

4.1.1   It is possible to relate some of the most important
precursors of IHD (essential hypertension, atherosclerosis,
myocardial necrosis, spasms and ventricular premature beats),
at least partially, in a functional way to sustained neurohormonal
imbalance.

| Chronic Stressor | Life Event Score of subjective impact (ILE) | |
| --- | --- | --- |
| | F | p |
| NOISE | 7.8 | o.ool |
| TOXIC SUBSTANCES | 4.7 | o.ol |
| BEING CONTROLLED AT WORK | 11.4 | o.ool |
| HEAT/ COLD | 3.6 | o.o5 |
| BEING SUBJECTED TO INTERRUPTIONS | 7.2 | O.OO1 |
| HEAVY PHYSICAL WORK | 3.o | o.o5 |
| POOR ECONOMIC SAFETIES | 4.3 | o.ol |
| BAD HOUSING SITUATION | 7.4 | o.ool |

Table 1.   Analysis ov Variance Between Chronic and Subacute Stressors Typical for Blue-Collar Workers (N = 380 Myocardial Infarction Subjects).

4.1.2 Neurohormonal imbalance may be produced, among other processes, by synergistic activation of the sympathetic-adrenomedullary system (with enhanced release of catecholamines) and of the pituitary adrenal-cortical system (with enhanced release of ACTH and corticosteroids).

4.1.3 These synergistic effects are highly probable in situations which elicit two distinct behavioral patterns during a given time period or in short time intervals: the "fight-and-flight-reaction" and the "conservation-withdrawal reaction" (43, 44).

4.1.4 These evolutionary old patterns of coping with socio-environmental stressors are associated, in social mammals and also in humans, morphologically and functionally, with two neurohormonal systems and their somewhat separate morphological substrate: the "fight-and-flight reaction" being related to the amygdaloid complex in the limbic system of the brain and subsequently to the sympathetic-adrenal-medullary system, and the "conservation-withdrawal reaction" being related to the hippocampal complex of the limbic system and subsequently to the pituitary adrenal-cortical axis (45, 46).

4.1.5 The defense response, and the conservation-withdrawal response respectively, deal with experiences or anticipations of threat to socio-emotional bonds and affiliation and with experiences or anticipations of threat to maintenance of physical or social status. It is their relation to perceived loss of basic rewards and self-esteem which allows them to play an important role in the complex interactions between external world, higher nervous activity and somatic regulations. Frequency, duration, and intensity of these reactions may trigger pathological developments in the cardiovascular system via enhanced biosynthesis and release of related neurohormones (45, 46, 47).

4.1.6 Stressors which threaten socio-emotional bonds and/or maintenance of social status can be responded to by active or passive coping. During active coping, the individual has the feeling that it is necessary and possible to fight against threats predominance of the defense response), whereas passive coping can be characterized as giving-up reaction after experiences of powerlessness and/or helplessness (predominance of the conservation-withdrawal-reaction). Active coping without success, continuous struggle without reward, intense threat to one's efforts to control a relevant situation, and exorbitant or overwhelming demands upon one's adaptive capacities; these seem to be classes of critical experiences which create feelings of irritation, anger, frustration and dissatisfaction. It is probable that during these experiences both stress axes are activated, i.e., the sympathetic-adrenomedullary and the pituitary- adrenal-cortical system. We prepose to label these classes of critical experiences "active distress".

4.1.7 "Active Distress", or as labeled by M. Frankenhaeuser et al., "effort with distress" (48), has been shown to be elicited in experimental situations of task performance where degree of controlability was low (48, 49). This may hold for several characteristics of work settings as well as for critical life circumstances. Finally, subjects with coronary-prone behavior may react to experiences of active distress with special intensity, as they are obviously vulnerable to threats to personal control over demanding situations.

An empirical test of these thoughts includes, as far as cardiovascular pathology is concerned, the following steps:
1. Demonstration of sympathetic adrenal-medullary and pituitary adrenal-cortical activation in response to active distress in experimental as well as in real life situations;
2. Demonstration of clinical evidence and relevance of neurohormonal imbalance due to synergistic action of the two stress axes, i.e., demonstration of their impact on early and/or decisive stages in the development of precursors of ischemic heart disease;
3. Demonstration of epidemiologic links between situations and/or dispositions which mainly elicit active distress and the disease outcome postulated by theory.

As a first step into this direction, we present some preliminary evidence for the second postulate. The final part of this section deals, on a conceptual level, with one of several implications of the third postulate: the relationship between social and psychological characteristics which specifically elicit active distress. We propose to reconsider some features of CPB in this framework.

Figure 8 gives a selective overview over assumed relations between activation of the two stress axes, neuroendocrine responses and precursors of cardiovascular pathology, as computed by summarized recent information in related research. It goes without saying that this scheme is oversimplified and that evidence for the several mechanisms is very different at present. Its main purpose is to demonstrate that sympathetic adrenal-medullary and pituitary adrenal-cortical activation have been found in mechanisms leading to four well established precursors of IHD.

In the development of essential hypertension, a neurogenic type of blood pressure elevation has been documented at least in patients with high renin hypertension (high noradrenaline level and subsequent high plasma renin level (50), although available literature has paid inadequate attention to intervening variables such as thyroid function sodium balance, potassium and plasma

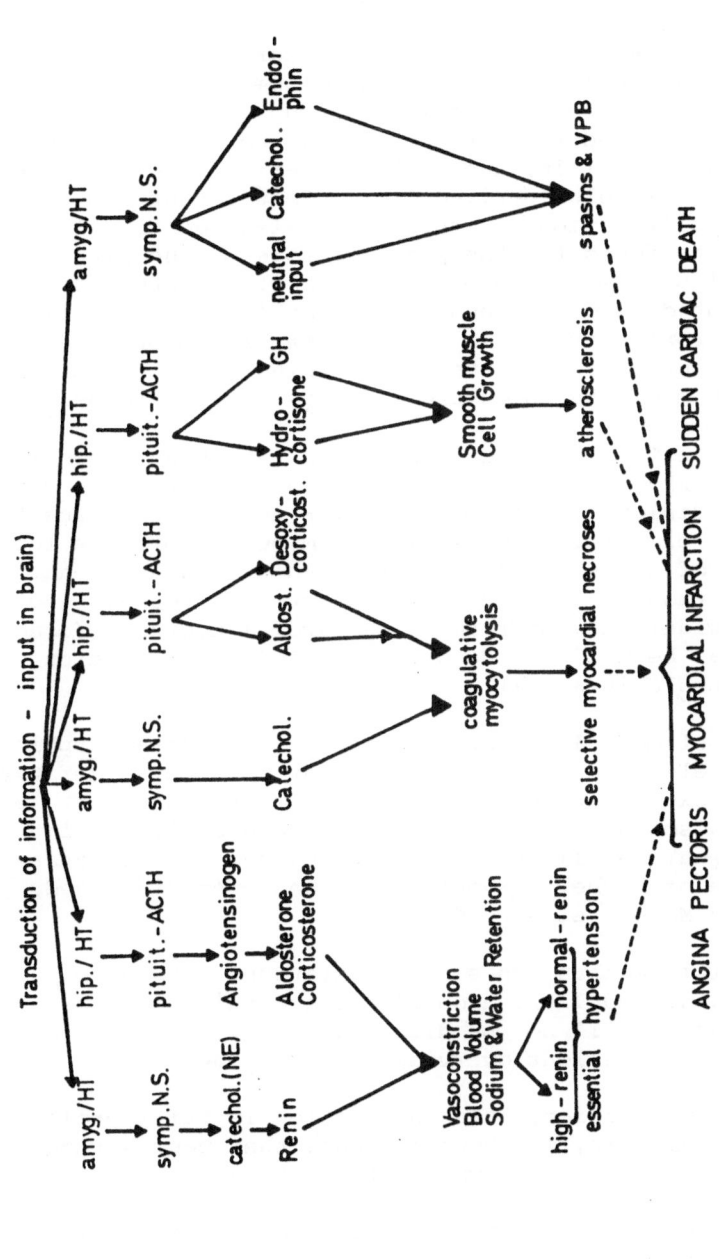

SELECTIVE RELATIONSHIPS BETWEEN NEUROENDOCRINE RESPONSES AND
CARDIOVASCULAR PATHOLOGY

Figure 8. Selective Relationships Between Neuroendocrine Responses and
Cardiovascular Pathology.

Abbreviations:  amyg.  = amygdala          symp.N.S. = sympathetic nervous
                hip.   = hippocampus                    system
                HT     = hypothalamus      pituit.   = pituitary
                GH     = growth hormone    VPB       = Ventricular premature
                                                       beats

volume (51). Influences of the pituitary-ACTH action on increase
in aldosterone and corticosterone (52) and a dissociation between
the renin-angiotensin system and aldosterone, induced by increased
adrenal sensitivity to angiotensin II have received increasing
attention during the last years (53, 54).

Hormonal requirements for growth of arterial smooth muscle
cells as a decisive early step in the development of atherosclerosis
has been demonstrated in vitro (55). Neurohormonal imbalance
in this process includes the action of ACTH and hydrocortisone,
of growth hormone, insullin, and platelet-derived growth factor,
among others. If platelet-derived growth factor controls the
smooth muscle proliferation of atherosclerosis, additional
evidence should be found for the possible role of the pituitary
adrenal cortical system. Immunological aspects of atherosclerosis
might be integrated into this analysis as well (56). Finally,
the finding of Troxler et al. is of considerable importance,
showing significantly raised levels of morning plasma cortisol
in subjects with moderate to severe coronary atherosclerosis (57).

Cardiotoxic effects of corticosteroids have been shown in
the pioneering work by Selye and Raab (58, 59). More recently,
selective myocardial necroses (myofibrillar degeneration due to
enhanced release of catecholamines in the myocardium) were found
in most victims of sudden cardiac death without a significant
narrowing (less than or equal to 50% of arterial vessels (60).
A specific and widely common form of myocardial necrosis (coagulative
myocytolysis) has been linked to overdrive and hyperfunction
induced by catecholamines (61).

Influences of medullary catecholamines and beta-endorphins
(62) on cardiac electrical properties appear to be considerably
less than those exerted by direct neural input to the heart (63),
but these mechanisms have in common an enhanced activity of the
sympathetic adrenal medullary system. With regard to coronary
spasms, the role of higher nervous system has been discussed,
among others, by Maserj et al. (64).

Other possible mechanisms such as relations between
sympathetic adrenal medullary arousal and hyperlipidemia or
platelet aggregation will not be discussed here. Further information
can be found in an excellent overview by Henry (56).

As pointed out earlier, this information is still preliminary.
In the present framework, it shows at least that neurohormonal
imbalance, possibly caused by synergistic activation of both
stress axes, can be linked to cardiovascular pathology if
sustained, prolonged or extremely intense mental stimulation
(due to experiences of active distress, as we assume) occurs.
Recent research in the field of brain peptides has provided some

information on powerful and far-reaching action of proteolytic
enzymes and prohormones which control biosynthesis and release
of a wider range of neurotransmitters (65). It may even be
that dissociation of the two stress axes is mediated by neuro-
modulatory impact and feedback (66). Obviously, many questions
calling for more interdisciplinary work evolve from these
observations.

## 4.2 Social Contexts of Active Distress and Coronary-Prone Behavior

After having suggested a psychoneuroendocrine and pathophysiologic framework for the study of individual experiences of
active distress, we want to recall the types of external situations
which reinforce these experiences. Thereafter, the role of CPB
which sustains or intensifies these reactions will be considered.

Social contexts which induce continuous activity (defense
response despite the individuals' limitations of adequate coping
can first be found in the working life. As mentioned earlier in
this paper, several work demands have been shown to be stressful
in this sense: quantitative overload (time pressure), high
responsibility in combination with limited resources or interruptions, structural limitations of one's autonomy (e.g., by
inconsistent demands, by narrowing job decision latitude
and control), forced inactivity by job-loss, to name the most
obvious ones. It should be noted that these characteristics are
related to the division of labor and to the formal structure of
roles and of power within the organization (e.g., industrial
plant), and that they are beyond the individuals' scope of
intervention. Quality and quantity of demands, and levels of
flexibility and change, however, differ considerably between
white- and blue-collar occupations, as we have demonstrated.
Important intervening variables, namely occupational sector,
ownership, size and location of companies, play a role, and the
process of economic change itself reinforces the action of the
stressors mentioned above, especially so during periods of rapid
economic growth. On the other hand, periods of "recession" of
the business cycle tend to create additional harmful effects,
mainly threats to social status by insecurity of work places and
job-loss, restriction upon social mobility, and overtime work due
to lower income (31). These economic and work conditions interfere
with social biographies of individuals in several ways, weakening
often socio-emotional support, increasing the potential for
marital discord and the vulnerability in the presence of critical
life events. Careers of chronic experiences of active distress
may precipitate, by recent life events, a breakdown in adaptive
efforts on a cognitive-emotional, behavioral and physiological
level (19).

It seems, at least among blue-collar workers with early MI, that CPB is not a prerequisite for links between workload, stress experiences and heart disease. But as an <u>aggravating condition</u>, it may play a critical role, especially among higher educational and occupational groups. This point has to be specified further.

The coronary-prone behavior pattern can be described as an "attempt to assert and maintain control over stressful aspects of one's environment. Type A's engage in a continuous struggle for control and, in consequence, appear hard driving and aggressive, easily annoyed and competitive" (40). These states of hyperresponsiveness can be followed by hyporesponsiveness in situations where individuals experience prolonged exposure to stressors which cannot be met by successful coping (40). This approach has been elaborated and tested in a series of interesting experiments by Glass and coworkers (1, 2, 40, 67). Yet some intriguing conceptual problems persist, as one of the authors himself points out: "We must define more precisely those behaviors in pattern A that are risk inducing...Efforts need to be directed toward a delineation of the classes of environmental stimuli that elicit the primary facets of the behavior pattern" (40). Another problem is: How can we explain recurrence and relative stability of this response pattern, even in the presence of unpleasant and annoying experiences?

In order to answer this question, we propose to concentrate on cognitive mechanisms. We hypothesize that Type A's tend toward an unrealistic appraisal of demanding situations and their related internal coping resources. Such an unrealistic appraisal can function in multiple ways. It seems that two forms can be easily depicted:

(a) Subjects overestimate given demands without being aware of their full coping resources. Inappropriately increased efforts are a probable behavioral consequence.

(b) Subjects underestimate given demands and, by doing so, expose themselves to possible overload. Perceptions of exhaustion and tiredness are suppressed, and internal coping resources are overestimated again and again.

In the long run, underestimation as well as overestimation of demands lowers the threshold of critical experiences of active distress. Subjects who tend to overestimate challenges and obligations experience an imbalance or misfit between invested efforts and pay-off with concomitant feelings of irritation, frustration, dissatisfaction, and hostility. It would be interesting, by the way, to interpret hostility, one of the crucial features of CPB, in terms of reactive coping with disappointment and lack of reward. Subjects who tend to underestimate demands and to overestimate their coping resources are likely to assume increased responsibility, to be work-addicted and to strive to fulfill all kinds of obligations and expectations. For quite a while, they are successful and experience rewarding feedback by significant others. But their burden increases, together with suppressed fatigue and exhaustion, and increased responsibility overwhelms their adaptive efforts. In this situation, intense active distress is very likely, and it may even be followed by depressive states of exhaustion with the possible outcome of psychological and physiological breakdown.

Our theoretical approach to CPB assumes that a specific link between cognition and performance may trigger psycho-neuroendocrine reactions which, in the long run, are harmful to the cardiovascular system. This link is analyzed as an intraindividual coping technique in the presence of demanding situations, a technique which starts by <u>unrealistic appraisal of challenges</u> and elicits overactivity at the behavioral and at the physiological level. Long-term payoff of this overactivity is assumed to be poor, and active distress is a probable emotional correlate.

Unrealistic appraisal of challenging situations is regarded as a relatively stable coping technique which is established over time. Three explanations which are not mutually exclusive are suggested:

(a) Unrealistic appraisal is the outcome of model learning during primary socialization. Children learn to appraise and behave in demanding situations the same way as their parents do (or one of them). Some experimental findings with coronary-prone children and their parents support this interpretation (69).

(b) Unrealistic appraisal can be understood as consequence of a specific motivation, i.e., a need for control and visible performance. This need may function as a compensation of experience or fears of low self-esteem or marginal socio-emotional status. It is thought to evolve during primary socialization, as related to, but not identical with achievement motivation.

(c) Unrealistic appraisal of demands is learned during secondary or tertiary socialization as an adaptive technique in dealing with increased work load. Under-estimation may be the more common reaction, given the routines of handling tasks and the perceptions of short-term reward associated with overcommitment and increased responsibility.

The approach outlined here has three general implications for an interactional analysis of CPB. First, given the existance of social stressors which induce active distress, CPB critically intensifies and aggravates these reactions. This situation calls for an integration of psychological and sociological analysis in the study of psychosocial risk constellations. Interactions as the ones demonstrated in the case of white-collar work settings and related high scores of individual CPB need to be studied more carefully by longitudinal study designs.

Second, it is probable to conclude that subjects with CPB bring themselves more often into challenging situations which stimulate their efforts. In this respect, CBP is not only a characteristic style of response to environmental demands, as Glass points out, but it also carries an element of active challenge-seeking, of intentional exposure to demands. General psychological coping theory has only recently recognized the importance of an individual's selective effort to create appropriate environmental settings (69). It might be interesting to explore similarities and differences between CPB and the "sensation-seeking person" (70).

Finally, if CPB is analyzed in terms of challenge and coping, it seems logical to assume that a change in intensity and duration of challenges results in a change of an individuals' level of CPB.

After having considered social contexts of active distress and possible cognitive and motivational mechanisms in coronary-prone subjects which sustain or intensify these experiences, we should mention that several topics of importance could not be touched by this analysis. Interactions between experiences of active distress and behavioral risks (e.g., smoking, drinking, faulty diet, lack of physical exercise) are an issue of high relevance, although available information indicates that these interactions are not simply linear ones. Another question points to the problem of disease specificity. Despite some evidence from neuroendocrinology and pathophysiology, it may well be that other parts than the cardiovascular system (e.g., the gastro-intestinal tract or the immune system, are affected by psychosocial risk constellations mentioned above. Some information on different disease outcome after exposure to active vs. passive distress is now available from a prospective study (71). Results show that risk of CVD is statistically associated with an interpersonal style of interaction which can be characterized as dominant, aggressive, or, as the authors call it, "emitting repression", whereas subjects who develop cancer are "receivers of repression", submissive and adjusting to non-rewarding interpersonal relationships.

As Table 2 shows, coefficients of correlations are low to
moderate, explaining only a small portion of total variance.
Yet it may be worth to design prospective studies which document
theoretically deduced disease outcome, based on psychosocial
predictors, and which control for intermediate neuroendocrine
and pathophysiologic processes. This type of study, although
crucial, has not yet been carried out to our knowledge.


## 5 CONCLUSION

Given the present state of knowledge in the field of work,
stress and heart disease, is it possible to design well-grounded
intervention strategies? We do not question the usefulness of
relaxation and related techniques of stress management, and it is
evident that socio-emotional support is a crucial resource in
dealing with distressing experiences. But it is unclear to
what degree they specifically protect against the disease under
study. And little is known about their efficacy in the presence
of powerful "at risk" contexts, especially in the work setting.
Interventions on a systems level are probably inevitable if
long-term success is the real goal. Take, for example, the multiple
risks of several blue-collar work settings. Protection against
noise, reduction of time-pressure and piecework, job enrichment
in lower positions, increase in occupational stability. These
are measures of primary importance in dealing with stress and work.
In white-collar positions, analogous propositions can be made:
reduction of amount of inconsistent demands in middle-echelon
positions, increase in work autonomy, changes in the reward
system (e.g., less rigid occupational careers, reward of qualities
such as trust, cooperation, and support instead of competitiveness,
mistrust, and individual struggle).

Perhaps, in the near future, we should concentrate our
scientific efforts on the realization and subsequent study of
such innovations efforts on the realization and subsequent study
of such innovations and their contributions to health and well-
being, as stated in the report of the Task Panel on support systems
submitted to the United States President's Commission on Mental
Health (72):.

 - Fund and establish within the Federal Government
 the continuing review, assessment, and interpretation
 of innovations in job and organizational design undertaken to improve the quality of work experience;

 - Develop criteria for the gradual enactment of
 Federal standards for the quality of employment;

 - Conduct experiments and demonstration projects to

74

| Subjects labeled at the beginning of the study | Subjects experiencing in their near - future | |
|---|---|---|
| | Cancer(n=2o4) | Circulatory and residual diseases(n=414) |
| Emittors of repression | -.13 | .28 |
| Emittors with long-lasting repression | § | .22 |
| Emittors with implicit repression | .o3 | .15 |
| Emittors without social support | -.11 | .25 |
| Emittors with high subjective impact | -.o2 | .16 |
| Receivers of repression | .35 | - .13 |
| Receivers with long-lasting repression | .36 | § |
| Receivers with implicit repression | .33 | - .o7 |
| Receivers without social support | .27 | .- .o9 |
| Receivers with high subjective impact | .21 | - .1o |

§ ) not ascertained

Table 2. Point-Biserial Coefficients of
Correlation Between Indicators
of Interpersonal Repression and
Incidence of Disease (Cancer vs.
Circulatory) in a Prospective
Study (N = 1,353).

test and to explain the contributions of work to mental health and well-being and to strengthen the natural supportive networks in places of work.

Perhaps we should move away from the "risk-paradigm" of scientific positivism towards a "benefit-paradigm" where scientists are actively involved in establishing better living (work) conditions.

REFERENCES

1. Krantz, D.S., D.C. Glass, M.A. Schaeffer, J.E. Davia. Behavior Patterns and Coronary Disease: A Critical Evaluation. Focus on Cardiovascular Psychophysiology (New York, Guildford Press, 1981).
2. Dembroski, T.M., S.M. Weiss, J.L. Shields, S.G. Haynes, and M. Feinleib (Eds.) Coronary Prone Behavior (New York, Springer, 1978) 129-136.
3. Rosenman, R.H. and M.A. Chesney. The Relationship of Type A Behavior Pattern to Coronary Heart Disease. Act. Nervosa Suppliment 22 (1980) 1-46.
4. Chesney, M.A. and R. H. Rosenman. Type A Behavior in the Work Setting. Current in Occupational Stress. (New York, J. Wiley, 1980) 187-212.
5. Rose, G. and M. Marmot. Social Class and Coronary Heart Disease. British Heart Journal 45 (1981) 13-19.
6. Koskenvuo, M., J. Kaprio, A. Kesaniemi, and S. Sarna. Differences in Mortality from Ischemic Heart Disease by Marital Status and Social Class. Journal of Chronic Disease 33 (1980) 95-116.
7. Holme, I. Paper unpublished. European Congress of Cardiology (1980) Paris.
8. Weinblatt, E., B. Ruberman, J.D. Goldberg, C.W. Frank, S. Shapiro, and B.S. Chandhary. Relation of Education to Sudden Death After Myocardial Infarction. New England Journal of Medicine 299 (1978) 60-65.
9. Zyzanski, S.J. Coronary Prone Behavior Pattern and Coronary Heart Disease: Epidemiologic Evidence. In Dembroski, T.M. et al. Coronary Prone Behavior. (New York, Springer-Verlag, 1978).
10. Rosenman, R.H., R.J. Brand, D. Jenkins, M. Friedman, R. Straus, and M. Wurm. Coronary Heart Disease in the Western Collaborative Group Study: Final Follow-Up Experience of $8\frac{1}{2}$ Years. Journal of the American Medical Association 233 (1975) 872-877.
11. Waldron, I., S.J. Zyzanski, R. Shkelle, C.D. Jenkins. Type A Behavior Pattern in Employed Men and Women. Journal of Human Stress 3 (1978) 2-18.

12. Kasl, S. Epidemiological Contributions to the Study of Work Stress. In Cooper, C.L. et al. Stress at Work. (New York, J. Wiley, Chichester, 1978) 3-48.

13. Haynes, S.G., M. Feinleib, and W.B. Kannel. Psychosocial Factors and CHD Incidence in Framingham-Results from an 8-Year Follow-Up Study. American Journal of Epidemiology 108 (1980) 229.

14. Rosenman, R.H., M. Friedman, R. Staus et al. A Prediction Study of Coronary Heart Disease. Journal of the American Medical Association 189 (1964) 103-110.

15. Theorell, T. Life Events, Job Stress and Coronary Heart Disease. In Siegrist, J. and M.J. Halhuber (Eds.) Myocardial Infarction and Psychosocial Risks. New York, Berlin, Heidelberg, Springer, 1981) 1-17.

16. Jenkins, C. Low Education: A Risk Factor for Death. New England Journal of Medicine 299 (1978) 95-97.

17. Bolm, U. Koronare Risikoberufe - Ergebnisse einer bundesweiten daten. (Med. Diss., Marburg, 1981).

18. Bolm, U., J. Siegrist. Occupational Morbidity Data in Myocardial Infarction - A Case Referent Study in West Germany. (Paper submitted for publication)

19. Siegrist, J., K. Dittmann, K. Rittner, and I. Weber. Soziale Belastungen und Herzinfarkt. (Enke, Stuttgart 1980).

20. Siegrist, J., K. Dittmann, K. Rittner, and I. Weber. Psycho-social Risk Constellations and First Myocardial Infarction. In J. Siegrist, M.J. Halhuber (Eds.) Myocardial Infarction and Psychosocial Risks. (Berlin, Heidelberg, New York, Springer 1981) 41-57.

21. Siegrist, J., K. Dittmann, K. Rittner, and I. Weber. The Social Context of Active Distress in Patients with Early Myocardial Infarction. Social Science and Medicine (in press).

22. Siegrist, J., K. Dittmann, and H. Weidenmann. The Role of Psychosocial Risks in Patients with Early Myocardial Infarction. Act. Nerv. Sup. (in press).

23. Smith, J.W. Mortality After Recovery from Myocardial Infarction. Journal of Chronic Disease 33 (1980) 1-4.

24. Rissanen, V. and M. Romo. Premonitory Symptoms and Stress Factors Proceeding Sudden Death from Ischemic Heart Disease. Acta. Med. Cand. 204 (1978) 389-396.

25. van Dijl, H. Myocardial Infarction and Work Attitudes. An Empirical Study. Journal of Psychosomatic Research 19 (1975) 197-202.

26. Fahrenberg, J., H. Hampel, and H. Selg. Das Freiburger Personlichkeitsinventar (FPI) (Hogrefe, Gottingen, 1973).

27. Rosenman, K.D. Cardiovascular Disease and Environmental Exposure. British Journal of Ind. Medicine 36 (1979) 85-97.

28. Khomulo, P.S., L.P. Rodionova, and A.P. Rusinowa. Changes in the Lipid Metabolism of Man in Protracted Effect of Industrial noise on the central nervous system. Kardiologie 7 (1967) 35-38.

29. Suvorow, G.A., E.I. Denisow, G.V. Ovakimow, Y.K. Tavtin.
    Correlations Between Hearing Losses and Neurovascular Impairments
    in Workers in Relation to the Level of Noise. Gig. Tr. Prof.
    Zabol. 7 (1979) 18-22.
30. Meinhardt, P. and U. Renker. Untersuchungen zur Morbiditat an
    Herz-Kreislauferkrankungen durch Dauerlarmexposition. Z. Ges.
    Hyg. 16 (1970) 853-857.
31. Brenner, M.H., A. Mooney, and T.J. Nagy (Eds.) Assessing the
    Contributions of the Social Sciences to Health. AAAS Symposium
    26 (Boulder, Colorado, Westview Press, 1980).
32. Kornitzer, M.D., M. Dramaix, and H. Gheyssen. Incidence of
    Ischemic Heart Disease in Two Belgian Cohorts Followed
    During 10 Years. European Journal of Cardiology 9 (1979) 455.
33. Cobb, S. and R.M. Rose. Hypertension, Peptic Ulcer and
    Diabetes in Air Traffic Controllers. Journal of the American
    Medical Association 224 (1973) 489.
34. Zorn, E., J.N. Harrington, and H. Goethe. Ischemic Heart
    Disease and Work Stress in West German Sea-Pilots. Journal
    of Occupational Medicine 19 (1977) 762.
35. Carruthers, M. Hazardous Occupations and the Heart. In
    C.L. Cooper, R. Payne (Eds.) Current Concerns in Occupational
    Stress. (New York, J. Wiley, 1980) 3-22.
36. Weber, I. Berufstatigkeit, Psychosoziale Belastung und
    Koronares Risiko. Doctoral dissertation (in preparation).
37. Mettlin, C. Occupational Careers and the Prevention of Coronary-
    Prone Behavior. Social Science and Medicine (1976) 367-372.
38. Howard, J.H., D.A. Cunningham, P.A. Rechnitzer. Work Pattern
    Associated with Type A Behavior: A Managerial Population.
    Human Relations 30 (1977) 825-836.
39. Burke, R.J. and T. Weir. The Type A Experience: Occupational
    and Life Demands, Satisfaction and Well-Being. Journal of
    Human Stress 4 (1980) 28-38.
40. Glass, D.C. Type A Behavior: Mechanisms Linking Behavioral
    and Pathophysiologic Processes. In J. Siegrist and M.J.
    Halhuber (Eds.) Myocardial Infarction and Psychosocial Risks.
    New York, Berlin, Heidelberg, Springer, 1981) 77-88.
41. Brockmeier, R. Katamnesen Psychosozialer Merkmale bei
    Herzinfarktpatienten. Diplomarbeit Soziologie: Unpublished.
    (Marburg, 1980).
42. Nie, N.H., C.H. Hull, J.G. Jenkins, K. Steinbrenner, and
    T.H. Bent. Statistical Package for the Social Sciences.
    (New York, McGraw Hill, 1975).
43. Ganong, W.F. Review of Medical Physiology. 8h Edition.
    (Los Altos, California, Lange Medical Publishers) 271-274.
44. Isaacson, R.L. Neural Systems of the Limbic Brain and Behavioral
    Inhibition. In R.A. Boakes, M.S. Halliday (Eds.) Inhibition
    and Learning. (London and New York, Academic Press, 1972)
    497-528.
45. Henry, J.P. and P. Stephens. Stress, Health and the Social
    Environment. (New York, Springer Verlag, 1977).

46. Henry, J.P., and J.P. Meehan. Psychosocial Stimuli, Physiological Specificity, and Cardiovascular Disease. In H. Weiner, M.A. Hoffer, A.J. Stundard, Brain,Behavior, and Bodily Disease. (New York, Raven Press, 1981) 305-333.

47. Henry, J.P. Present Concept of Stress Theory. In E. Usdin, R. Kvetnansky, I.J. Kopin (Eds.) Catecholamines and Stress Recent Advances. (New York, Amsterdam, Oxford, Elsevier, 1980) 557-571.

48. Frankenhaeuser, M. U. Lundberg. Psycho-Neuroendocrine Aspects of Efforts and Distress as Modified by Personal Control. In R. Sinz (Ed) Proceedings of Psychophysiology (Berlin (DDR) G. Fischer, in press).

49. Frankenhaeuser, M. Psycho-Neuroendocrine Approaches to the Study of Emotions as Related to Stress and Coping. In H.E. Howe, R.A. Dienstbier (Eds.) Nebraska Symposium on Motivation-1978. (Lincoln, University of Nebraska Press, 1979) 123-161.

50. Julius, S. L. Hansson, L. Andress et al. Borderline Hypertension. Acata Med. Scand. 208 (1980) 481-489.

51. Goldstein, D.S. Plasma Norepinephrine in Essential Hypertension. Circulation 3 (1981) 48-52.

52. Wallis, C.J., and M.P. Printz. Adrenal Regulation of Brain Angiotensinogen Content. Endocrinology 106 (1980) 337-342.

53. Sowers, J.M. Plasma Aldosterone and Corticosterone Responses to ACTH, Angiotensin, Potassium and Stress in Spontaneously Hypertensive Rats. Endocrinology 108 (1981) 1216-1221.

54. Ganten, D. The Brain Renin-Angiotensin System. In J.B. Martin, S. Reichlin, K.L. Bick (Eds.) Neurosecretion and Brain Peptides. (New York, Raven Press, 1981).

55. Weinstein, R., M.B. Steuerman, and T. Macaig. Hormonal Requirements for Growth of Arterial Smooth Muscle Cells In Vitro: An Endocrine Approach to Atherosclerosis. Science 212 (1981) 818.

56. Henry, J.P. Coronary Heart Disease and Arousal of the Adrenal Cortical Axis. Unpublished paper. (1981).

57. Troxler, R.G., et al. The Association of Elevated Plasma Cortisol and Early Atherosclerosis as Demonstrated by Coronary Angiography. Atherosclerosis 26 (1977) 151-162.

58. Selye, H. Stress in Health and Disease (London, Boston, 1970).

59. Raab, W. Preventive Myocardiology (Springfield: Thomas, 1970).

60. Reichenbach, D.M., N.W. Moss. Myocardial Cell Necrosis and Sudden Death in Humans. Circulation 51/52, Suppl. III. (1975) 60-62.

61. Eliot, R.S., F.C. Clayton, G.M. Pieper, and G.L. Todd. Influence of Environmental Stress on Pathogenesis of Sudden Cardiac Death. Federal Procedures 36 (1977) 1719-1724.

62. Wilson, S.P., K.J. Chang, and O.H. Viveros. Synthesis of Enkephalins by Adrenal Medullary Chromoffine Cells. Proc. Nat'l Acad. Sci., U.S.A. 77 (1980) 4364-4368.
63. Verrier, R.L. and B. Lown. Neural Influences and Sudden Cardiac Death. Adv. Cardiol. 25 (1978) 155-168.
64. Maseri, A., A. Pesola, M. Marzilli et al. Coronary Vasospasm in Angina Pectoris. Lancet I 8014 (1977) 713-719.
65. Krieger, D.T. and J.B. Martin. Brain Peptides. NEJM 302 (1981) 876-885.
66. Check, W.A. Old Hormones Reveal New Surprises. JAMA 243 (1980) 499-505.
67. Glass, D.C. Behavior Patterns, Stress, and Coronary Disease. (Hillsdale, 1977).
68. Matthews, K.A. Efforts to Control by Children and Adults with the Type A Coronary-Prone Behavior Pattern. Child Development 50 (1977) 842-847.
69. Roskies, E. and Lazarus, R.S. Coping Theory and the Teaching of Coping Skills. In P.O. Davidson, S.M. Davidson (Eds) Behavioral Medicine: Changing Health Life Styles. (New York, Brunner, Mazel, 1980).
70. Zuckerman, M. Sensation Seeking. (Hillsdale, 1977).
71. Grossarth-Maticek, R., J. Siegrist, and H. Vetter. Interpersonal Repression as a Predictor of Cancer. Soc. Sci. & Med. (in press).
72. Killilea, M. et al (Eds) Report of the Task Panel on Community Support Systems. Balimore, unpublished manuscript, 1978.

# RELATIONSHIPS BETWEEN CRITICAL LIFE EVENTS, JOB STRESS, AND CARDIOVASCULAR ILLNESS

Tores Theorell

National Institute for Psychosocial Factors
and Health
University of Stockholm
Stockholm, Sweden

## 1 EPIDEMIOLOGIC ASPECTS

Since Hinkle's (24,25) early studies on the impact of critical life events on illness and the publication of Holmes and Rahe's (26) schedule of recent experiences in 1968, a large volume of scientific evidence dealing with the interplay between life events and health have been published. In reviewing this voluminous literature, several questions can be asked: Has research on life events provided us with new knowledge in the area of specific illnesses such as cardiovascular disease; do we presently know more about the interplay between psychosocial environmental and individual factors in the pathogenesis of CHD? Has life event research been used in primary prevention? Has life event research been used in secondary prevention? This chapter is devoted to answering these questions.

### 1.1 New Knowledge

At the start of the 1970s, there was indirect evidence from a number of studies that important life events could be associated with increased mortality in coronary illness. Examples of such events, using a rather extensive definition of "events," include:

1.1.1 Migration: Persons moving from low incidence areas were shown to adopt the higher disease incidence (20,29).

1.1.2 Bereavement: Bereavement was shown to be associated with increased cardiovascular mortality particularly
within three months after the loss (38).

1.1.3 Disaster: Follow-up of populations who had
experienced natural disasters showed a marked elevation
of the prevalence of hypertension (22,33,44).

1.1.4 Night college: Hinkle and co-workers (24) showed
that periods of "night college" were associated with a
small, but significant excess of cardiac mortality.

Not all the reports were positive, however; Hinkle
et al. (25), for example, did not find any association
between objectively recorded job changes (promotions,
demotions, and transferrals) and risk for future CHD
death.

There have also been reports of possible association
between marital divorce and cardiovascular illness, but
it is not clear whether being divorced or becoming divorced was important.

In general, theories about social and physiological
mechanisms linking events to CHD were missing. Hinkle,
on the basis of empirical observations, was impressed
that serious life events (crises) did not result in
harmful health changes in the majority of people (25)
and he formulated the general theory that favorable life
attitudes are illness protective in a life crisis situation. Later, several groups have constructed general
frameworks (6,28,30,32,42,47) in which the following
factors have been taken into account: (a) genetic predisposition, (b) previous experiences which may have
relevance to either somatic risk factors or psychological
coping, (c) social factors surrounding the event itself
such as social support, (d) perception(s) of the event,
and (e) physiological reactions.

Methodological problems must also be considered.
Holmes and Rahe's (26) original idea was to provide an
instrument indicative of total "objective" amount of
social change taking place during a period of an indiv-
ual's life. However, a number of problems arose as
research progressed. First, there is the problem of
memory artifacts and other problems associated with the
time factor. Low test-retest scores have been found
(9,51), deteriorating with the time that has elapsed
since the event occurred. As expected, trivial events

show more memory artifacts than important ones. Furthermore, the pathophysiological effects of events may
decrease (27) or perhaps even increase with time passage.

Second, events which are clearly out of a person's
control are more truly environmental than those which
could be controlled or avoided by the person. The latter
group of events is more confounded by the individual's
own personality (16).

Third, as with control, the possibility of antici-
pating a change that is about to occur may drastically
alter the impact of that change (16).

Fourth, the desirability of a change may also have
great significance. Several studies have shown that
undesirable events are more important than desirable
events in the pathogenesis of psychological and psychophysiological symptoms (28,36,39).

Fifth, Paykel's studies (39) have shown that loss
events, such as death of a family member, are more closely
associated than gains, such as addition of a new family
member, with development of depression.

Sixth, there is the issue of threat vs. non-threat
inherent in the event. Brown (5) has pointed out that
the social circumstances surrounding the life event may
make a marked difference. That is, certain supportive
factors such as someone to talk to may make a loss of a
loved one much less depressing. Retrospective studies
of life events preceding myocardial infarction point in
this same direction (8,46).

The methodological issues combine to cast some
serious doubt(s) on the meaning of adding standard
weights (derived from normal populations) of reported
items on the schedule of recent events during a given
time period across individuals. Suggestions for
improvement of this instrument include: (a) providing
total scores obtained from self-rated rather than
standard weights (8,28,34,41,46) of reported events;
(b) correcting the life event score for the time that
has elapsed since the event occurred (27); (c) using
negative weights for undesirable and positive weights
for desirable events, as well as a self-rated combined
measure of desirability and impact (28,36); and, (d)
using upset caused rather than adjustment required by
the event as a basis for weighting.

Self-rated weights have generally produced stronger correlations with health change outcome(s); however, the results are more difficult to interpret since the scores are more confounded by personality factors. This, while mathematical precision is perhaps gained, theoretical precision is lost!

Paykel (39) found amount of emotional upset more important than amount of adjustment in retrospectively discriminating depressed patients from controls. We had similar results in discriminating patients with MI from healthy controls (34).

Brown (7) and Totman (60) have more recently proposed a different approach to measuring the impact of life event stress on illness, albeit an approach that is time-consuming and less applicable to large scale, epidemiologic studies.

The physiologic consequences of various, specific events have been noted in several instances. For example, job loss was studied among workers during a shut-down of two factories in Michigan, USA. The urinary excretion of noradrenaline was observed to increase particularly when several months had passed after the event. Blood pressure levels also increased, but stayed elevated only as long as the workers were unemployed (11). Similarly, blood pressure elevations were noted in newly divorced men over a period of several months (23). Migration from low (CHD) risk areas to high risk areas results in elevation in blood pressure, which seems to occur rather rapidly, in both children and adults, a consequence that appears unrelated to changes in salt intake (3,10). A subsequent increase in prevalence and incidence of MI is also seen years after the migration. As pointed out by Marmot and Syme (35), acculturation is an important mediating factor. Subjects who retain their old psycho-social lifestyle seem to derive protection against CHD regardless of conventional risk factors. A study of reverse migration (from a high risk area to a low risk area), in this case from Finland to Sweden, was recently carried out by our research group (1). All cases of male MI were identified during a three-year period in one region of Stockholm. Two control subjects (three in the lowest age strata) matched for age, sex and area of residence were ramdomly selected for each case. Age-adjusted relative risks of developing MI were calculated for Finnish immigrants versus native Swedes with partic-ular emphasis on duration of stay in Sweden. Finnish

immigrants who had stayed in Sweden for less than 10
years did not have any significant excess of CHD risk.
This may be due to the fact that those who decide to
migrate are more healthy than other subjects (48).
For those who stayed in Sweden for between 10 and 20
years, a sizeable and significant excess risk was
observed.  After 20 years, no excess risk was observed.
These trends could not be explained on the basis of
differences in ethnic origin (Swedish or Finnish speaking
Finns), place of birth, social class or marital state.
We do not know whether a psychosocial crisis situation
10-20 years after migration caused the elevation(s) of
MI risk during that period.

At least two studied have been published which are
relevant to the impact of life events on MI risk in
women.  The retrospective study of women who had suffered
MI in Goteborg (4) indicated that more objective life
events were reported for the years preceding MI than
during the same period in the control group.  A retrospective study of life events preceding cardiac death
in Baltimore, USA, (15) showed that loss by death of a
"significant other" was clearly more frequently reported
for those who had died in this fashion than for the
control group.  So far, it may seem that the association
between "objective" events and myocardial infarction is
more clear-cut for women than men.

One cannot also ignore the age factor.  As pointed
out by Coddington (13), the impact of a given life event
may change drastically with age.  Even from the age of
40 to 60 years, the yearly incidence of reported changes
in one's life varies considerably (see Figure 1).  This
figure shows the yearly incidence of selected self-
reported life events in a five-year age strata in the
"non-absence group" of the building construction workers.
As clearly demonstrated, the age differences are quite
large despite the relatively narrow age range that was
studied.  There appear to be two distinct groups of
events:  (a) those which diminish with increasing age,
such as "start of extra job" or "increased responsibility
at work" and (b) those which decrease with advancing age,
such as "death of a close relative" or "unemployment."
Events which occur "out of place" with regard to age
would be more likely to result in undesirable health
changes, e.g., MI.

In the follow-up of health change in these same
workers, only those who did not clearly suffer from the

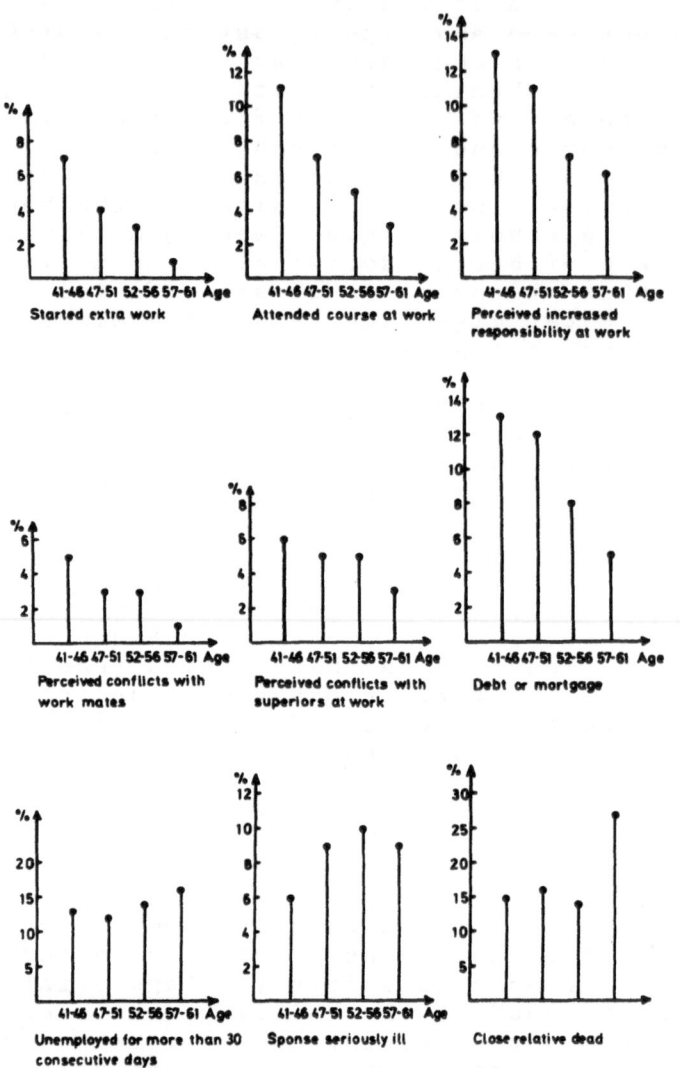

Fig. 4. Retrospectively reported one-year incidence of recent life events in 5155 fulltime working building-construction workers.

Figure 1. Retrospectively reported one-year incidence of recent life events in 5,155 full-time working building-construction workers

illness already at the start were included. In the follow-up of MI, those who had been absent from work during the preceding year because of symptomatic CHD (MI, angina pectoris, hypertension, or diabetes) were excluded. For the identification of MIs, we used the death registry and the hospital registries were used. Thirty-two cases of MI occurred during the first year and 29 during the second year of follow-up of this group (total n = 6,723).

The total life change score based upon "standard upset weights" was not predictive of MI. The only life event that was significantly predictive for the first year of follow-up was "increased responsibility at work last year". However, when the workers were divided into age groups, it became evident that "increased responsibility" was important only after age 50. This could perhaps be seen against the "normal aging" hypothesis: When increased responsibility takes place at an age when most building-construction workers do not expect it, it may be of more significance than at a younger age. It should be pointed out that reported "increased responsibility" may have no "objective" background. For instance, we did not find that newly appointed foremen had elevated risk of developing MI (54).

The only life event that approached significance in predicting MI during the second year of follow-up was death of a close relative. This finding may illustrate that we do not know what the "brought forward time" (7) or the "incubation period" may be for different events.

By means of factor analysis, clusters of variables were sought without reference to the outcome MI. Three clusters of psychosocial factors were found: (a) "work load" during the previous 12 months including conflicts and responsibilities at work, extra work, and threat of unemployment; (b) recent change in family structure; and, (c) chronic family difficulties. These clusters were tested in relation to MI. For example, a subject who had reported at least one item belonging to the work load cluster was considered to have "work load". A multiple regression was performed using a number of dichotomized variables as predictors including: age, smoking, density of living arrangements, the three clusters noted above, and MI during the first two years of follow-up (n = 61) as the dependent variable. All prediciting variables were constructed in such a way that at least 25% of the subjects were in the category with the smallest number (55).

The results indicated that it was easier to predict

MI when the deaths were excluded, i.e., easier to predict the surviving cases by means of psychosocial predictors. The most important variables were psychosocial work load, age, and "concrete work" (which is the most physically demanding building-construction work).

A complex web of causation may explain this, such as: Group piece wage puts a strain on each individual worker. When he gets older, he must make extra physical effort in order not to diminish the earnings for himself and for his friends. When he cannot keep up any more, the work mates start ostracizing him. This may create deteriorating psychosocial climate and thus accelerate onset of MI.

Illnesses other than MI were also considered in our follow-up study. The Swedish compulsary insurance system was used for identification of all cases of sickness leave for at least 30 consecutive days in the part of the population that lived in the city of Stockholm. As can be seen in Table 1, "low back pain" and "neurosis" are the only categories of prospective illness that really show a striking association with changes in general. "Work load", on the other hand, was important only in the prediction of myocardial infarction. Thus, there may be some specific mechanisms involved which link psychosocial work processes to risk of MI.

Elsewhere, in a study of air traffic controllers (43), subjects observed to be hypertensive in a population subjected to a screening procedure tend to report relatively low rates of life change, as judged by means of a self-rating modified version of the SRE. It should be pointed out that high blood pressure is normally not perceived as an illness (12) by the subject himself. The observation of a low average life change score in this group may either reflect a tendency not to report changes or to have fewer events. Our group has recently analyzed the systolic blood pressure levels which had been examined in 74,000 18-year-old men living in greater Stockholm and going through the compulsory recruitment for military service. These subjects were living in 63 different residential areas at the time of examination. A significant variation was observed across these areas with regard to average systolic pressure. Areas with low average SBP were those with socially stable conditions (e.g., inner city areas with a high median income and low rates of subjects on social welfare). Areas with high average SBP were those in which marked social changes

Table 1.  Life changes associated with excess risk of
          chronic (greater than 30 consecutive days)
          illness during first year of follow-up.

---

Illness:       Myocardial Infarction (n = 32)

Life Change: Increased responsibility in work[*]

---

Illness:       Ulcer or chronic gastritis  (n = 54)

Life Change: None

---

Illness:       Degenerative joint disease  (n = 188)

Life Change: Spouse seriously ill[**]
             Change in sex habits[*]
             Decreased physical activity[*]

---

Illness:       Neurosis  (n = 32)

Life Change: Unemployment for 30 consecutive days[***]
             "Other change at work[*]
             Close friend seriously ill[*]
             Change in sex habits[*]
             Chronic somatic illness[**]

---

[*]p less than 0.05;  [**]p less than 0.01;  [***]p less 0.001

Neurosis here is defined as follows: anxiety syndromes,
asthenia without obvious organic illness and neurotic-
depressive reactions causing work absenteeism for at
least 30 consecutive days.

were going on, either with high rates of immigration or
newly erected suburbs.  In the latter groups of areas,
low median income and a high proportion of subjects on
social welfare were common.  Relative overweight was an
important mediating factor (59).

Three samples of subjects evidencing high (greater
than 146 mmHg), normal (between 124 and 131 mmHg), and

low (between 100 and 106 mmHg) were subjected to a life
event interview, using Brown's (7) methodology. The
interview covered the subject's whole life. The mean
number of self-reported life events increased with age
for all three groups, ranging from an average of 1 - 2
events per year at age 3 to an average of 8 - 10 events
per year at age 18. The "high pressure" group reported
low rates of life events and the "low pressure" group
high rates of events, although the differences were not
statistically significant. When the subjects were asked
to classify the events into "positive" or "negative"
categories, the "high pressure" group tended to report
less positive and more negative or non-classifiable
events than other groups, although again the differences
were not significant (49). The number of positive events
reported in the "low pressure" group increased more with
increasing age than in the other groups (p less than
0.05).

Thus, the development of high blood pressure in a
longitudinal perspective may have more to do with too
few life events than with too many. This is also consistent with the observation that the young "high
pressure" group was on average significantly more anxious
and aggression-inhibited than the other groups (50).
One interpretation of this may be that an environment
that provides few opportunities for learning diversified
coping strategies may contribute to non-healthy coping
later in life and therefore accelerate hypertensive
development.

To summarize: The most easily interpretable information so far has been obtained from studies which have
focussed on specific events. This information may also
be the most useful for purposes of primary prevention.
In the studies of change in general, the theoretical
and practical problems are still prominent.

## 1.2  Primary Prevention

Life changes in the work sphere seem to be of
particular importance in the precipitation of MI although
the associations are neither specific nor strong. It
seems that the elevation of near-future MI risk after
critical life events in the job could be prevented by
a number of factors which need further exploration.
Karasek and Theorell (31) and Alfredsson et al. (1)
have pointed out that influence over one's own work
situation and possibilities for growth and development
may reduce the impact of psychosocial work demands on

MI risk. Elsewhere in this volume, House discusses the protective role of social support in mediating stress in the work environment.

To my knowledge, no effort has been made to utilize life event information in order to postpone or prevent CHD illness episodes. Two methods seem to be theoretically possible: (a) to identify persons in specific crisis situations such as newly bereaved and then increase social support to them. The psychiatric benefits of such a procedure have already been demonstrated in a controlled trial in London (37). Such specific crisis situations have been subjected to intervention trials in relation to CHD. This, however, would possibly be a fruitful area of future research. (b) to teach subjects in a population to identify their own undesirable and threatening crisis situations and tell them to seek social support in them. Both of these approaches could be used in controlled epidemiologic trials.

## 1.3 Secondary Prevention

A clinical impression is that subjects who are given the opportunity to discuss the life events that have occurred during the period before an MI benefit from doing so. This has not been subjected to any controlled investigation although a number of studies have indicated that extensive group discussions after MI may favorably affect psychiatric and in some studies even medical prognosis. The great strength in the life event strategy lies in its face value, i.e., the concept is easily understood by most people.

## 1.4 Summary Conclusions

Epidemiological life event research focussing on CHD seems to indicate:

1.4.1 that methods of recording events in general are either theoretically obscure or practically unfeasible on a large scale.

1.4.2 that life events per se are less significant in the pathogenesis of CHD than in the pathogenesis of psychiatric illness and that different kinds of events are important to different kinds of groups of subjects and illnesses. For Swedish middle-aged men, for instance, changes at work seem to have particular relevance to the development of myocardial infarction.

1.4.3 that personality factors and social circumstances interact with life events in such a way that interpretations of demonstrated associations are difficult.

1.4.4 that the purpose of future life event research in this area must be clearly formulated.

1.4.5 that teaching and discussing the impact of certain kinds of life events may be fruitful strategy in future primary and secondary prevention research.

2   PSYCHOPHYSIOLOGICAL AND CLINICAL ASPECTS

Once CHD has become overt, e.g., after a first MI, the question arises as to what the significance of life events may have for the risk of re-infarction.

The most frustrating experience I ever had as a clinician was with a 45-year-old clerk, an immigrant from a country in southern Europe, who had suffered an MI and was subsequently controlled medically by me. He returned to work two months after the infarction but suffered from frequent attacks of angina pectoris. In addition, he reported arguments with his teen-aged son and conflicts with his boss. These arguments tended to aggravate his cardiac condition. More than a year after his first MI, he was driving his own car and had a minor collision with another motorist. He became so upset with the situation that he started a physical fight with the other driver. The police were called, and my patient was arrested. He turned out to have too much alcohol in his blood. A law suit followed. He was sentenced to a short jail term which was a disaster for him. He would loose his job if the jail term came to his employer's attention. I tried to make the judge pardon him while he waited for one year to serve his jail sentence. The negotiations lasted for many painful months. I made two firm statements, the last one indicating that my patient would die if jailed. He was informed that he would not be pardoned. The same day he was taken to the hospital with re-infarction. Recurring ventricular fibrillations occurred in the hospital, and he died that day. Autopsy showed a recent septal MI of only a few hours' duration.

This clinical example illustrates: (a) that acute arousal may not be a sufficient cause of MI, not even in the presence of obvious predisposition, i.e., the patient did not suffer re-infarction at the time of the traffic accident. Rather, he suffered the infarction after serious humilation, which took place over a period of several months (chronic stress), and immediately after the final flow had been inflicted, what might be regarded as the extreme "vital exhaustion" situation (2). A combination of several weeks of psychological strain followed by acute arousal for a very short period has been hypothesized to precede a significant proportion of sudden coronary death (17). The physiological basis for this is not known. Animal experiments have indicated that a long period of elevated corticosteroid levels in the blood may deplete Magnesium and Potassium from the myocardium and increase its vulnerability to necrosis formation when exposed to catecholamines (40,45). The case also suggests (b) that even when the physician explicitly predicts serious consequences of an event that is to occur, he may not have sufficient power to prevent it!

Statistically significant associations on a group level between events and near-future recurrence risk were made on a group of coronary patients whose clinical information was gathered during an 8-year period in Oklahoma City, USA. Eighteen of the patients died of CHD during the course of the study. These patients were matched retrospectively with 18 patients of corresponding age and sex. The clinical interviews of the patients were re-analyzed blindly by an independent investigator who had no access to the clinical observations. Statistically significant build-up of life changes (total scores according to Holmes and Rahe SRE), particularly at work, were observed in the death group 7-12 months prior to death. No similar build-up was observed in the group of survivors. Regardless of the mechanisms involved, it was obvious that reports about accumulated frustration, conflicts, and other changes, again primarily at work, were more common among those CHD patients who were destined to die a near-future death. In this particular case, the "incubation period" was sufficiently long (in most cases more than 6 months); secondary prevention would have been possible, at least from a theoretical standpoint.

What action would be adviseable in such a case? When one is dealing with an individual patient, a careful analysis of the individual situation is necessary. Possibilities for secondary preventive intervention might include: (a) actions directed toward the environment (e.g., the patient is encouraged to discuss with superiors

94

and colleagues at work how he might beneficially alter his work situation) and/or (b) actions directed towards the psychophysiological reactions of the afflicted patient (e.g., using biofeedback, autogenic training, or psychopharmacological remedies to directly alter blood pressure, heart rate, and other relevant physiological parameters for CHD death).

From both a diagnostic and therapeutic standpoint, it is valuable to show the patient how his/her cardiovascular system reacts during discussions about specific (stressful) life events.

We know that patients with lower degrees of "socialization" (those who are less willing to talk than other patients) react with more pronounced cardiovascular reactions to discussions about events (58). What psychophysiological reactions take place seems to be governed to some extent by genetic factors. In a study of middle-aged and older male twins with varying degrees of coronary heart disease (17 monozygotic and 13 dizygotic pairs) we observed that the blood pressure levels and finger plethysmographic amplitudes as well as the plasma growth hormone levels showed increasing similarity within monozygotic pairs during the course of a discussion about events (53).

A longitudinal study of 21 CHD patients followed at weekly intervals demonstrated in most cases a statistical association between the amount of events that had taken place during the past week and the urinary excretion of adrenaline during the last day of this week. About one third of the patients did not show such an association, which again illustrates the necessity of individual analysis of the psychophysiological reactions (56).

Events that take place after the onset of overt CHD seem to have great clinical significance. If they are monitored at regular intervals, the clinician may be able to take more efficient secondary preventive action. This is a field which needs further exploration.


REFERENCES

1.   Alfredsson, L., Karasek, R.A., and T. Theorell.
     Myocardial Infarction Risk and Psychosocial Work

Environment - An Analysis of the Male Swedish
Working Force. Social Science and Medicine (1981)
in press.
2.  Appels, A. The Syndrome of Vital Exhaustion and
Depression and Its Relationship to Coronary Heart
Disease. In J. Siegrist and M.J. Halhuber (Eds.)
Myocardial Infarction and Psychosocial Risks.
(Berlin, Springer, 1981).
3.  Beaglehole, R., E. Eyles, and I. Prior. Blood Pres-
sure and Migration in Children. International
Journal of Epidemiology 8 (1979) 5-10.
4.  Bengtsson, C. Ischaemic Heart Disease in Women. Acta
Med. Scand. suppl. 549 (1973) chapter 10.
5.  Brown, G. Methodological Research on Stressful Life
Events. In B.S. Dohrenwend and B.P. Dohrenwend
(Eds.) Stressful Life Events, Their Nature and
Effects. (New York, Wiley, 1974).
6.  Brown, G.W. and T. Harris. Social Origins of Depression - A Study of Psychiatric Disorder in Women.
(London, Tavistock, 1978).
7.  Brown, G.W., F. Sklair, T.O. Harris, and J.L.T. Bir-
ley. Life Events and Psychiatric Disorders.
Psychological Medicine 3 (1973) 74 and 159.
8.  Byrne, D.G., and H.M. Whyte. Life Events and Myocardial Infarction Revisited: The Role of Measures
of Individual Impact. Psychosomatic Medicine 42
(1980) 1-10.
9.  Casey, R.L., M. Masuda, and T.H. Holmes. The Validity
of Life Change Measurement. Journal of Psychosomatic Research 11 (1967) 239.
10. Cassel, J. Studies of Hypertension in Migrants. In
O. Paul (Ed.) Epidemiology and Control of Hypertension. (New York, Stratton, 1975).
11. Cobb, S. Physiologic Changes in Men Whose Jobs Were
Abolished. Journal of Psychosomatic Research 18
(1974) 245-258.
12. Cochrane, R. Neuroticism and the Discovery of High
Blood Pressure. Journal of Psychosomatic Research
13 (1969) 21-25.
13. Coddington, R.D. The Significance of Life Events as
Etiological Factors in the Diseases of Children
- II. A Study of a Normal Population. Journal of
Psychosomatic Research 16 (1972) 205.
14. Connolly, J. Life Events Before Myocardial Infarction.
Journal of Human Stress 2 (1976) 3-17.
15. Cottington, E.M., K.A. Matthews, E. Talbott, and
L.H. Kuller. Environmental Events Preceding Sudden
Death in Women. Psychosomatic Medicine 6 (1980)
567-573.

16. Dohrenwend, B.S. and B.P. Dohrenwend. (Eds.) Stress-ful Life Events, Their Nature and Effects. (New York, Wiley, 1974).

17. Engel, G.L. Sudden and Rapid Death During Psychological Stress. Folklore or Folk Wisdom? Annals of Internal Medicine 74 (1971) 771.

18. Fairbank, D.T. and R.L. Hough. Life Event Classifications and the Event - Illness Relationship. Journal of Human Stress 5 (1979) 41-47.

19. Friedman, M. and R.H. Rosenman. Association of a Specific Overt Behavior Pattern with Blood and Cardiovascular Findings. JAMA 169 (1959) 1286.

20. Garcia-Palmieri, M.R., R. Costas, M. Cruz-Vidal, M. Cortez-Alicea, D. Patterne, L. Rojas-Franco, P.D. Sorlie, and W.B. Kannel. Urban-Rural Differences in Coronary Heart Disease in a Low Incidence Area. The Puerto Rico Heart Study. American Journal of Epidemiology 107 (1978) 206-216.

21. Glass, D.C. Behavior Patterns, Stress, and Coronary Disease. (New York, Wiley, 1977).

22. Graham, J.D.P. High Blood Pressure After Battle. Lancet 1 (1945) 239-240.

23. Harburg, E., et al. A Longitudinal Study of Blood Pressure in Men Who Go Through Marital Separation. CVD Newsletter, January (1980).

24. Hinkle, L.E. The Effect of Culture Change, Social Change and Changes in Interpersonal Relationships on Health. In B.S. Dohrenwend and B.P. Dohrenwend (Eds.) Stressful Life Events, Their Nature and Effects. (New York, Wiley, 1974).

25. Hinkle, L.E., W.N. Christenson, F.D. Kane, A. Ostfeld, W.N. Thetford, and H.G. Wolff. An Investigation of the Relation Between Life Experience, Personality Characteristics and General Susceptibility to Illness. Psychosomatic Medicine 20 (1958) 278-295.

26. Holmes, T.H. and R.H. Rahe. The Social Readjustment Rating Scale. Journal of Psychosomatic Research 11 (1967) 213-218.

27. Horowitz, M., C. Schaefer, D. Hiroto, N. Wilner, and B. Levin. Life Event Questionnaires for Measuring Presumptive Stress. Psychosomatic Medicine 39 (1977) 413.

28. Johnson, J.H. and I.G. Sarason. Recent Developments in Research on Life Stress. In V. Hamilton and D.M. Warburton (Eds.) Human Stress and Cognition: An Information Processing Approach. (Chichester, England, Wiley, 1979).

29.  Kagan, A., T. Gordon, and G.G. Rhoads. Some Factors
     Related to Coronary Heart Disease Incidence in
     Honolulu Japanese Men: The Honolulu Heart Study.
     International Journal of Epidemiology 4 (1975)
     271-279.
30.  Kagan, A.R. and L. Levi. Adaptation of the Psycho-
     social Environment to Man's Abilities and Needs.
     In L. Levi (Ed.) Society, Stress and Disease.
     The Psychosocial Environment and Psychosomatic
     Diseases. (London, Oxford University Press, 1972).
31.  Karasek, R.A. and T. Theorell. Psychosocial Factors
     and Coronary Heart Disease - Swedish Prospective
     Findings and US Prevalence Findings Using a New
     Occupational Inference Method. Advances in Card-
     iology (1981) in press.
32.  Lazarus, R.S. Stress and Coping in Adaptation Ill-
     ness. In Z.J. Lipowski, D.R. Lipsitt, and P.C.
     Whybrow (Eds.) Psychosomatic Medicine: Current
     Trends and Clinical Applications. (New York,
     Oxford University Press, 1977).
33.  Logue, J.N. and H.A. Hansen. Case-Control Study of
     Hypertensive Women in a Post-Disaster Community:
     Wyoming Valley, Pennsylvania. Journal of Human
     Stress 6 (1980) 28-34.
34.  Lundberg, U. and T. Theorell. Scaling of Life
     Changes: Differences Between Three Diagnostic
     Groups and Between Recently Experienced and Non-
     Experienced Events. Journal of Human Stress 2
     (1976) 7-17.
35.  Marmot, M.G. and Syme, L.G. Acculturation and Cor-
     onary Heart Disease in Japanese-American Men.
     American Journal of Epidemiology 104 (1976) 225-
     247.
36.  Myers, J.K., J.J. Lindenthal, and M.P. Pepper.
     Social Class, Life Events and Psychiatric Symptoms,
     a Longitudinal Study. In B.S. Dohrenwend and B.S.
     Dohrenwend (Eds.) Stressful Life Events, Their
     Nature and Effects. (New York, Wiley, 1974).
37.  Parkes, C.M. Bereavement Counselling - Does It
     Work? British Medical Journal 281 (1980) 3-6.
38.  Parkes, C.M., B. Benjamin, R.G. Fitzgerald. Broken
     Heart, a Statistical Study of Increased Mortality
     Among Widowers. British Medical Journal 1 (1969)
     740.
39.  Paykel, E.S. Life Stress, Depression and Attempted
     Suicide. Journal of Human Stress 2 (1976) 3-12.
40.  Raab, W. Prevention of Ischemic Heart Disease.
     (Springfield, Charles C. Thomas, 1966).

41. Rahe, R.H. Epidemiological Studies of Life-Change and Illness. International Journal of Psychiatry in Medicine 6 (1975) 133-146.
42. Rahe, R.H. The Pathway Between Subjects' Recent Life Changes and Their Near-Future Illness Reports: Representative Results and Methodological Issues. In B.P. Dohrenwend and B.S. Dohrenwend (Eds.) Stressful Life Events, Their Nature and Effects. (New York, Wiley, 1974).
43. Rose, R.M., L. Hurst, and C.D. Jenkins. Air Traffic Controller Health Change Study. Boston University School of Medicine, rep. FFA Contract No DOT-FA 73WA-3211 (1978).
44. Ruskin, A., O.W. Beard, and R.L. Shaffer. Blast Hypertension. Elevated Arterial Pressure in the Victims of the Texas City Disaster. American Journal of Medicine 4 (1948) 228-236.
45. Selye, H. and F. Bajusz. Conditioning by Corticoids for the Production of Cardiac Lesions with Nor-adrenaline. Acta Endocrin. 30 (1959) 183.
46. Siegrist, J. Cardiovascular Disease and the Sympa-thetic Nervous System. Lancet 2 (1980) 1195-1196.
47. Siegrist, J., K. Dittmann, K. Rittner, and I. Weber. Soziale Betastungen und Herzinfarkt - Eine Medizin-Soziologische Fall-Kontroll-Studie, Fer-dinand Enke Verlag, Stuttgart (1980).
48. Smedley, B. and A. Ericson. Perinatal Mortality Among Children of Immigrant Mothers in Sweden. Acta Paediatr. Scand. suppl. 275 (1979) 41-46.
49. Svensson, J. Cardiovascular Effects of Anxiety Induced by Interviewing Yound Hypertensive Male Subjects. Psychosomatic Medicine (1981) in press.
50. Svensson, J. and D. Schalling. Personality and Blood Pressure in Young Men. Unpublished manu-script (1981).
51. Theorell, T. A Study of the Validity of Life Change Measurement in Hospital Patients. In T. Theorell (Ed.) Psychosocial Factors in Relation to the Onset of Myocardial Infarctia and to Some Metabolic Variables - a Pilot Study. Academic Thesis, Karolinska Institute, Stockholm (1970).
52. Theorell, T. Selected Illnesses and Somatic Factors in Relation to Two Psychosocial Stress Indices - A Prospective Study of Middle-Aged Construction Building Workers. Journal of Psychosomatic Research 20 (1976) 7-20.
53. Theorell, T., U. de Faire, D. Schalling, U. Adamson, and F. Askevold. Personality Traits and Psycho-physiological Reactions to a Stressful Interview

in Twins with Varying Degrees of Coronary Heart
Disease. Journal of Psychosomatic Research
23 (1979) 89-99.

54. Theorell, T. B. Floderus, and E. Lind. The relationship of Disturbing Life-Changes and Emotions
to the Early Development of Myocardial Infarction
and Other Serious Illnesses. International
Journal of Epidemiology 4 (1975) 281.

55. Theorell, T. and B. Floderus-Myrhed. Workload and
Risk of Myocardial Infarction. A Prospective
Psychosocial Analysis. International Journal of
Epidemiology 6 (1977) 17-21.

56. Theorell, T., E. Lind, J. Froberg, C.G. Karlsson,
and L. Levi. A Longitudinal Study of 21 Coronary
Subjects - Life Changes, Catecholamines and
Related Biochemical Variables. Psychosomatic
Medicine 34 (1972) 505.

57. Theorell, T. and R.H. Rahe. Life Change Events,
Ballistocardiography and Coronary Death - A
Longitudinal Clinical Study. Journal of Human
Stress 1 (1975) 18.

58. Theorell, T., D. Schalling, and T. Akerstedt. Cir-
culatory Reactions in Coronary Patients During
Interview - A Noninvasive Study. Biological
Psychology 5 (1977) 233.

59. Theorell, T., J. Svensson, and B. Aulborg. Blood
Pressure Variations Across Areas in the Greater
Stockholm Region - Analysis of 74,000 18-year-old
Men. Social Science and Medicine (1981) in press.

60. Totman, R. What Makes Life Events Stressful? A
Retrospective Study of Patients Who Have Suffered
a First Myocardial Infarction. Journal of Psychosomatic Research 23 (1979) 193-201.

# TYPE A BEHAVIOR PATTERN

Marcel Kornitzer

Laboratory of Epidemiology and Social Medicine
Free University
Brussels, Belgium

## 1  INTRODUCTION

Type A behavior pattern is an overt style of reactions, characterized by some of the following:  intense striving for achievement, competition, easily provoked impatience, time urgency, abruptness of gesture and speech (explosive voice), hyper-alert posture, overcommitment to vocation or profession, excesses of drive and hostility.  This behavior pattern was first described by Friedman and Rosenman (11), at the end of the 1950s in the United States.  Friedman describes the type A pattern as an "action-emotion complex" that is exhibited by those individuals who are engaged in a chronic incessant struggle in order to achieve more and more in less and less time, thus giving rise to a sense of time-urgency, and who usually, but not always, exhibit a free floating but well rationalized hostility.  For a long time, this behavior pattern has been extensively studied in the United States (7) whereas lately methods for measuring type A behavior have been validated in Europe, and prevalence data on European populations have been published (1, 16, 19, 30).  As we were interested in type A behavior, as well as in other variables in their relation to coronary heart disease, we introduced them in most of our major epidemiological prospective studies (20, 27).  Some of the results presented here were published or are in press and reflect a collaborative undertaking with colleagues G. De Backer, F. Kittel, and M. Dramaix.

## 2  TECHNIQUES FOR EVALUATING TYPE A BEHAVIOR

In the original study, type A behavior was assessed by means of a structured taped interview: those type A subjects who appeared to exhibit the pattern in its most extreme form were designated as type A-1 in contrast to type A-2, the less afflicted subjects; conversely those type B subjects who exhibit almost complete tranquility (the "easy-going type") were disignated as type B-4 in contrast to type B-3, the less extreme type B subjects. Finally, an intermediate class AB or X was used for those subjects in whom classification in A or B was not possible.

In the Belgian Heart Disease Prevention Project (20), the structured interview (SI) was administered to 726 middle-aged males at work: 4.1% were found to exhibit type A-1 behavior, whereas 4.4% exhibit the extreme type B-4 behavior. More than one-fifth of all interviews yielded uncertain behavior patterns. Slightly more French speaking subjects exhibited the type A pattern (Table 1).

In the original study of type A behavior in the United States, the Western Collaborative Group Study (WCGS), type A pattern was also assessed by means of two other techniques:

## 2.1 The Jenkins Activity Survey for Health Prediction (JAS)

In the 1969 version, the JAS is a self-administered question-naire composed of 64 questions. Four weighted scores are derived: an overall type A score or JAS-AB, a score for "speed and impatience" or JAS-S, a score for "job-involvement" or JAS-J and, finally, a score for "hard-driving" or JAS-H.

In the WCGS, an agreement of 73% between the SI and JAS has been achieved. In the Belgian Heart Disease Prevention Project, we did utilize both techniques and reached an overall agreement of 69.8% (19). In the WCGS, the JAS has been found to be predictive of CHD (18).

## 2.2 The Bortner Scale

Here, we have 14 bipolar scales of the type "always too late - never too late" or "always in a hurry (for eating, walking) - does things always relaxed". This questionnaire is administered in the presence of a technician who explains the technique and gives one example. The 14 scores are summed up and the higher the score the more the subject is in the type A direction. Like in the WCGS, we reached an overall agreement with the SI of over 70% (Table 2) (24).

Other techniques for assessing type A pattern have been utilized in different groups. Haynes et al. (15) devised a specific structured interview for the Framingham Study; Matthews and Angulo

Table 1. Distribution of behavior types as determined by standardized interview among French- and Dutch-speaking persons in Belgium

| | BEHAVIOR TYPE | | | | | | TOTAL |
|---|---|---|---|---|---|---|---|
| | $A_1$ | $A_2$ | Uncertain | $B_3$ | $B_4$ | | |
| FRENCH | 5.4% (11) | 39.6% (80) | 22.3% (45) | 30.2% (61) | 2.5% (5) | | 202 |
| DUTCH | 3.6% (19) | 32.1% (168) | 22.5% (118) | 36.6% (192) | 5.2% (27) | | 524 |
| TOTAL | 4.1% (30) | 34.1% (248) | 22.4% (163) | 34.8% (253) | 4.4% (32) | | 726 |

(23) assessed three important components of type A behavior in
children:  competitiveness and impatience, anger, and aggression,
helped in part by the childrens' teachers.  Waldron and her colleagues (5) have developed a short interview that has been used
primarily with adolescents.  Glass (14) developed a self-
administered questionnaire derived from the JAS for assessment of
type A behavior in college students.  Last but not least, Jenkins
developed a questionnaire for housewives and non-working men.
Finally, let it be said that in the case of the structured interview,
final type assessment relies on self-perception of type A behavior
and observed type A behavior exhibited during the interview. However,
the JAS and the Bortner Scale must rely on self-perceptions only.

Table 2.  Bortner Scale and Structured Interview

| SI | A-1 | A-2 | B-3 | B-4 | A | B |
|---|---|---|---|---|---|---|
| Bortner Scale | 198 | 185 | 151 | 140 | 186 | 149 |

Overall correct classification = 70.8%

## 3  TYPE A PATTERN IN RELATION TO OTHER VARIABLES

### 3.1  Socio-cultural Variables

Type A behavior seems to be part of the American way-of-life,
rooted in American middle to upper class white males.  Regional
differences are observed in Belgium:  French speaking subjects are
more type A than Dutch speaking subjects.  The same holds true for
the JAS-S, -J and -H (Table 3).

Like Shekelle and colleagues (26) in the United States, we
observed a very significant positive correlation of type A behavior
with social (socioprofessional) class (Table 4).

A strong positive correlation is also observed between educational (study) level and scores on both the Bortner Scale and the
JAS (Table 5).

Both social class and educational level yield an independent
and significant correlation with type A behavior as can be seen
in Table 6.

Married subjects score higher on the JAS-AB, -S and -J as
compared to subjects classified as "alone" (single, divorced, and

Table 3.  Type A behavior and language.

| Psychological variable | Language | $\bar{X}$ | $\pm$ S.D. | F |
|---|---|---|---|---|
| Bortner Scale | French | 185.00 | 41.17 | 194.00[***] |
| | Dutch | 161.40 | 41.25 | |
| J.A.S.-AB | French | - 1.83 | 9.61 | 69.34[***] |
| | Dutch | - 5.07 | 9.56 | |
| J.A.S.-S | French | - 3.99 | 10.27 | 89.49[***] |
| | Dutch | - 7.99 | 10.41 | |
| J.A.S.-J | French | - 9.20 | 7.53 | 99.50[***] |
| | Dutch | -12.07 | 7.01 | |
| J.A.S.-H | French | - 0.46 | 6.91 | 11.70[***] |
| | Dutch | - 1.31 | 5.97 | |

[***] P < 0.001

Table 4. Type A behavior and socio-professional class.

| Psychological variables | Socio-professional class | $\bar{X}$ | $\pm$ | SD | F |
|---|---|---|---|---|---|
| Bortner Scale | Executives | 194.60 | | 37.56 | 288.00[***] |
| | White-collars | 172.20 | | 40.41 | |
| | Blue-collars | 157.30 | | 40.59 | |
| JAS -AB | Executives | 2.35 | | 9.15 | 269.27[***] |
| | White-collars | -3.31 | | 9.39 | |
| | Blue-collars | -6.07 | | 9.24 | |
| JAS -S | Executives | -0.58 | | 10.76 | 232.04[***] |
| | White-collars | -5.86 | | 10.80 | |
| | Blue-collars | -8.98 | | 9.84 | |
| JAS -J | Executives | -2.16 | | 7.97 | 1103.43[***] |
| | White-collars | -9.95 | | 6.55 | |
| | Blue-collars | -13.61 | | 5.79 | |
| JAS -H | Executives | -0.54 | | 6.61 | 28.78[***] |
| | White-collars | -1.16 | | 5.97 | |
| | Blue-collars | -1.37 | | 6.08 | |

[***] $p < 0.001$

Table 5. Type A behavior and study level.

| Psychological variables | Study level | $\bar{X}$ $\pm$ SD | | F |
|---|---|---|---|---|
| Bortner Scale | Elementary Secundary Universitary | 155.80 175.60 199.40 | 40.18 41.04 38.02 | 261.00*** |
| JAS -AB | Elementary Secundary Universitary | - 6.60 - 2.15 4.17 | 9.11 9.62 8.51 | 280.96*** |
| JAS -S | Elementary Secundary Universitary | - 9.44 - 4.99 1.66 | 9.78 10.67 10.40 | 245.03*** |
| JAS -J | Elementary Secundary Universitary | -13.82 - 8.89 - 0.38 | 5.48 7.61 7.85 | 839.12*** |
| JAS -H | Elementary Secundary Universitary | - 1.45 - 0.83 0.19 | 6.04 6.21 6.86 | 13.29*** |

*** $P < 0.001$

Table 6.  Independent correlation of study level and socio-professional class with type A behavior.

| Behavioral variables | Socio-professional class | STUDY LEVEL | | | F |
|---|---|---|---|---|---|
| | | Universitary | Secundary | Elementary | |
| Bortner Scale | Executives | 202.40* | 192.70*** | 178.40*** | *** |
| | White-collars | 190.20 | 179.30 | 163.60**** | *** |
| | Blue-collars | 173.00 | 166.70 | 154.20 | *** |
| JAS-AB | Executives | 4.80* | 1.54*** | 0.83**** | *** |
| | White-collars | 1.83* | - 1.61 | - 5.53**** | *** |
| | Blue-collars | - 0.80 | - 3.88 | - 6.81 | *** |

* $P < 0.05$ ; *** $P < 0.001$

widowers) (Table 7).

Table 7.  Type A pattern and marital status.

| Psychological variables | Marital status | X | + | SD | F |
|---|---|---|---|---|---|
| Bortner Scale | Married Alone † | 164.70 156.50 | | 41.95 41.51 | 20.00*** |
| JAS -AB | Married Alone | - 4.54 - 6.45 | | 9.59 9.69 | 21.18*** |
| JAS -S | Married Alone | - 7.42 - 8.92 | | 10.47 10.32 | 11.17*** |
| JAS -J | Married Alone | -11.58 -13.04 | | 7.20 6.27 | 22.30*** |
| JAS -H | Married Alone | - 1.15 - 1.17 | | 6.11 6.34 | NS |

*** $P < 0.001$ ; NS = Not significant

No correlation with physical fitness (work-load for a heart rate of 150 bpm or more) has been observed whereas a significant positive correlation with a score of total leisure time activity has been found (Table 8).

## 3.2  Coronary Risk Factors

Small, mostly non-significant correlation coefficients are observed for heart rate, systolic blood pressure, diastolic blood pressure, serum cholesterol, HDL-cholesterol and body mass index (Table 9).

Smoking habits are related to the JAS-S, -J and -H whereas they are not to the overall JAS-AB (Table 10).

## 3.3  Other Psychosocial Variables

Type A behavior pattern is significantly related to a self-perceived job-stress or work-load score (Table 11) and to scores of anality (A), obsessionality (B), neuroticism (N) and social

110

Table 8. Type A behavior, physical leisure time activity and physical fitness.

| | | JAS-AB | P | JAS-S | P | JAS-J | P | JAS-H | P |
|---|---|---|---|---|---|---|---|---|---|
| Work-load quartiles | 1. | - 1.27 | | - 4.43 | | - 8.39 | | - .43 | |
| | 2. | - 1.29 | | - 4.50 | | - 8.14 | | - 1.20 | |
| | 3. | - 1.36 | | - 4.02 | | - 8.22 | | - 1.33 | |
| | 4. | - 1.86 | NS | - 4.16 | NS | - 8.16 | NS | - 1.38 | NS |
| Leisure time activity quartiles (of an activity metabolic index) | 1. | - 2.36 | | - 4.64 | | - 9.65 | | - .98 | |
| | 2. | - 1.36 | | - 3.97 | | - 8.57 | | - 1.01 | |
| | 3. | - .86 | | - 4.27 | | - 8.06 | | - .96 | |
| | 4. | - .56 | ** | - 2.85 | * | - 8.17 | ** | - .31 | NS |

* $P < 0.05$ ; ** $P < 0.01$.

Table 9.  Type A behavior and bioclinical variables.
Pearson correlation coefficients (N=2298).

| J A S | BIOCLINICAL VARIABLES | | | | | | |
|---|---|---|---|---|---|---|---|
| | Heart rate | Systolic blood pressure | Diastolic blood pressure | Cholesterol | HDL-cholesterol | Triglycerides | BMI |
| JAS-AB | -.006 NS | .014$^{NS}$ | .005$^{NS}$ | .095$^{***}$ | .046$^{*}$ | -.014$^{NS}$ | -.039$^{*}$ |
| JAS-S | -.013 NS | -.015$^{NS}$ | .006$^{NS}$ | .051$^{**}$ | .022$^{NS}$ | .005$^{NS}$ | .052$^{***}$ |
| JAS-J | -.008 NS | -.024$^{NS}$ | .024$^{NS}$ | .102$^{***}$ | .065$^{***}$ | .012$^{NS}$ | -.006$^{NS}$ |
| JAS-H | .007 NS | .008$^{NS}$ | -.008$^{NS}$ | .085$^{***}$ | .051$^{**}$ | -.020$^{NS}$ | -.045$^{*}$ |

* P < 0.05 ;  ** P < 0.01 ;  *** P < 0.001

112

Table 10.  Type A and smoking behavior (N = 2302)

| VARIABLE | CATEGORY (%) | JAS–AB | JAS–S | JAS–J | JAS–H |
|---|---|---|---|---|---|
| Smoking Habits | Smokers (49) | −1.32 | − 4.20 | −9.36 | − .45 |
| | Non-smokers(21) | −1.73$^{NS}$ | − 4.84** | −7.38*** | −1.01* |
| | Ex-smokers (30) | − .89 | −2.86 | −8.23 | −1.25 |

* P < 0.05 ; ** P < 0.01 ; *** P < 0.001.  NS = Not significant.

Table 11.  Job-stress and type A pattern.
          Pearson correlation coefficients

| ↓ Job-stress score | JAS–AB | JAS–S | JAS–J | JAS–H |
|---|---|---|---|---|
| Total (N=2066) | .28*** | .26*** | .22*** | .17*** |
| Blue-collars (N= 983) | .24*** | .24*** | .10*** | .16*** |
| White-collars(N= 757) | .32*** | .24*** | .27*** | .16*** |
| Executives (N= 326) | .16*** | .25*** | .21*** | .14*** |

*** P < 0.001.

conformism (L) (9, 25) (Table 12).

Table 12.    JAS and S.H.-E.P.I. Pearson Correlation
            Coefficients

| | R | −AB | −S | −J | H |
|---|---|---|---|---|---|
| **S. H. / E. P. I.** A | A | .143*** | .059*** | .075*** | .158≡*** |
| B | B | .294*** | .317*** | .108*** | .169*** |
| N | N | .453*** | .454*** | .104*** | .259*** |
| E | E | .012NS | .006NS | −.040* | .038* |
| L | L | −.219*** | −.260*** | −.184*** | −.028NS |

(N=7398)  * P ⩽ .05 ;    ** P ⩽ .01 ;    *** P ⩽ .001


     In multiple regression analysis entering 16 variables, we
observed the following:

3.3.1  JAS-AB:  correlates independently with job-stress, professional
status, educational level, serum cholesterol, triglycerides (negative
correlation) and marital status (negative correlation).  No correlation was observed with smoking behavior, body mass index, age, heart
rate, systolic blood pressure, diastolic blood pressure, HDL-
cholesterol, work-load, total leisure time AMI and heavy leisure time
AMI.  The total explained variance is less than 12% (Table 13).

3.3.2  JAS-S:  correlates independently with job-stress, professional
status, marital status (negative correlation), smoking habits and
educational level (Table 14).  Less than 10% of the total variance
of the JAS-S is explained by means of these variables.

3.3.3  JAS-J:  correlates with educational level, professional status,
job-stress, quartiles of heavy leisure time activity and marital
status (negative correlation) (Table 15).  More than 25% of the total

114

Table 13.  Multiple regression analysis
          Dependent variable : JAS-AB (N=1282)

| V A R I A B L E S | β COEFFICIENTS | $R^2$ | F TEST |
|---|---|---|---|
| Job-stress score | .2364 | .076 | 76.8**** |
| Professional status (blue-collars,white-collars, executives) | .1013 | .099 | 11.1**** |
| Study level (primary,secondary, universitary) | .0882 | .105 | 8.4* |
| Cholesterol | .0810 | .108 | 8.4* |
| Triglycerides | -.0683 | .112 | 6.1* |
| Marital status (married, alone) | -.0561 | .116 | 4.5* |

NS : Smoking,BMI,Age,heart-rate,systolic blood pressure,diastolic blood
     pressure,HDL-cholesterol,workload,heavy AMI,total AMI.

Table 14. Multiple regression analysis
. Dependent variable : JAS-S (N=1282)

| V A R I A B L E S | β COEFFICIENTS | $R^2$ | F TEST |
|---|---|---|---|
| Job-stress score | .2358 | .069 | 74.6[***] |
| Professional status | .0717 | .080 | 5.5[+] |
| Marital status | -.0671 | .084 | 6.3[+] |
| Smoking habits (smokers, non-smokers) | .0642 | .088 | 5.8[+] |
| Study level | .0698 | .092 | 5.1[+] |

NS : BMI,age,heart-rate,systolic blood pressure,diastolic blood pressure, cholesterol, HDL-cholesterol,triglycerides,workload,AMI,heavy AMI.

116

Table 15. Multiple regression analysis
Dependent variable : JAS-J.

| V A R I A B L E S | β COEFFICIENTS | $R^2$ | F TEST |
|---|---|---|---|
| Study level | .2748 | .179 | 96.5[****] |
| Professional status | .2320 | .226 | 69.5[****] |
| Job-stress score | .1282 | .242 | 26.9[****] |
| Quartiles heavy AMI | .0905 | .250 | 13.7[****] |
| Marital status | -.0628 | .254 | 6.7[***] |

NS : BMI,heart-rate,systolic blood pressure, diastolic blood pressure,
cholesterol,HDL-cholesterol,triglycerides,workload,AMI,age,smoking.

variance of the JAS-J is explained by means of those variables,
where educational (study) level is the strongest correlate.

3.3.4 JAS-H: correlates only with job-stress and smoking habits;
the total explained variance is less than 4% (Table 16).

Table 16. Multiple regression analysis.
Dependent variable : JAS-H.

| VARIABLES | COEFFICIENT | $R^2$ | F TEST |
|---|---|---|---|
| Job-stress score | .1733 | .028 | 38.4*** |
| Smoking habits | .0706 | .032 | 6.4** |

NS : BMI, Heart Rate, Systolic blood pressure, cholesterol,
HDL-cholesterol, triglycerides, workload, AMI, heavy AMI,
professional status, study level, age, marital status.
*** $P < 0.001$ ; ** $P < 0.01$

3.3.5 Comments: The type A behavior pattern has strong sociocultural as well as psychological correlates. The most important
are social class, educational level, neuroticism and job-stress.
The significant correlation of type A behavior with social class
sets a, as yet not solved, fundamental question: Are subjects
with this behavior pattern preferably promoted in the work setting
of industrialized countries or, alternatively, is this work-setting
favorable to the emergence of type A behavior in the middle to
upper social classes?

Again, for the correlation of type A pattern with educational
(study) level, one can ask: Are type A subjects favored in their
studies reaching, hence, the highest educational levels or, alternatively, is the educational institution promoting the emergence
of the type A pattern? Lengthy follow-up studies of children should
eventually be able to answer the latter.

When performing case-control studies, one should be cautious
about these socio-cultural correlates; multivariate adjustment
should be the rule.

## 4   TYPE A PATTERN AND CORONARY HEART DISEASE (CHD)

### 4.1   Prevalence Studies

Whereas prevalence studies are not suited for causality infer-
ence, they are the first "hint-givers" or indicators.  In the
Belgian Heart Disease Prevention Project, we studied the JAS-AB
and JAS-S in relation to different groupings of CHD (21) (Table 17).

In an overall univariate classification, subjects free of CHD
had the lowest scores both on the JAS-AB and JAS-S whereas the
highest JAS-AB scores were observed  in those subjects with ECG
modifications, without angina but aware of their status, and highest
JAS-S scores were found in those subjects with both angina and ECG
modifications (Table 18).

Mean score of CHD cases was significantly higher on the JAS-AB
and -S as compared to subjects free of CHD (Table 19).

Table 19.   Univariate analysis.

|  | Free of CHD (N=5434) | All CHD cases (N=678) | t Test |
|---|---|---|---|
|  | $\overline{M}$ | $\overline{M}$ |  |
| JAS-AB | - 4.87 | - 3.06 | +++ |
| JAS-S | - 7.71 | - 6.01 | +++ |

+++ P < 0.001.

The same was true for all angina cases (Table 20), whereas no
significant differences were observed between subjects free of CHD
and those with positive ECG findings without angina (Table 21).

In a multiple stepwise discriminant analysis including the JAS-
AB that variable discriminated significantly all CHD-cases, all angina
cases and ECG findings without angina from subjects free of CHD
(Table 22).

When the JAS-S was included that variable discriminated all CHD
cases, all angina cases, all ECG findings without angina and ECG
findings without angina in subjects unaware of their condition, from
subjects free of CHD (Tables 23 and 24).

Table 17.   Flow chart representing the grouping of cases and controls.

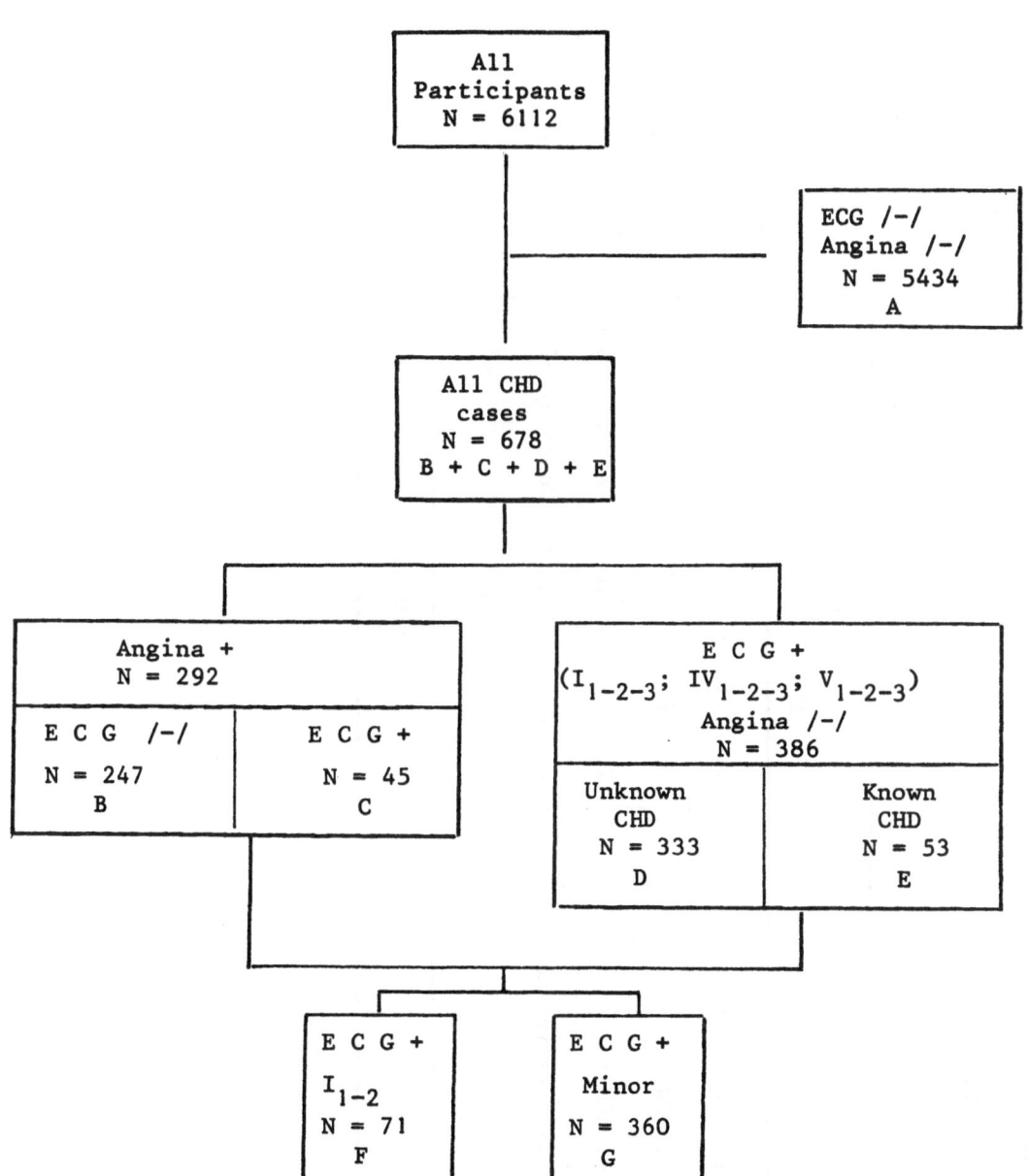

120

Table 18. Univariate analysis

| J A S -AB GROUPS | M̄ | J A S -S GROUPS | M̄ |
|---|---|---|---|
| E. ECG +, Angina /−/(Known) | − .99 | C. Angina +, ECG + | −4.54 |
| B. Angina +, ECG /−/ | −1.14 | B. Angina +, ECG /−/ | −4.60 |
| C. Angina +, ECG + | −2.74 | E. ECG +, Angina /−/(Known) | −4.65 |
| D. ECG +,Angina /−/(Unknown) | −4.87 | D. ECG +,Angina /−/(Unknown) | −7.47 |
| A. Free of CHD | −4.87 | A. Free of CHD | −7.71 |
| P < 0.001 | | P < 0.001 | |

Table 20.  Univariate analysis.

|  | Free of CHD (N=5434) | All angina cases (N=292) | t Test |
|---|---|---|---|
|  | $\overline{M}$ | $\overline{M}$ |  |
| JAS-AB | − 4.87 | − 1.38 | ✦✦✦ |
| JAS-S | − 7.71 | − 4.59 | ✦✦✦ |

✦✦✦  $P < 0.001$.

Table 21.  Univariate analysis.

|  | Free of CHD (N=5434) | ECG + Angina /−/ (unknown − known) (N=386) | t Test |
|---|---|---|---|
|  | $\overline{M}$ | $\overline{M}$ |  |
| JAS-AB | − 4.87 | − 4.33 | NS |
| JAS-S | − 7.71 | − 7.08 | NS |

NS = Not significant.

Table 22. Multiple stepwise discriminant analysis

| G R O U P S | V A R I A B L E S | F |
|---|---|---|
| Free of CHD versus All CHD cases | Age<br>Systolic blood pressure<br>JAS-AB<br>Cholesterol | +++<br>+++<br>+++<br>++ |
| Free of CHD versus All angina | Age<br>JAS-AB | +++<br>++ |
| Free of CHD versus ECG + Angina /-/ (heart condition known) | Age<br>Socio-professional class<br>Systolic blood pressure<br>Smoking /-/<br>JAS-AB | +++<br>+<br>+<br>+<br>+ |

+ P < 0.05 ; ++ P < 0.01 ; +++ P < 0.001.

Table 23.  Multiple stepwise discriminant analysis

| G R O U P S | V A R I A B L E S | F |
|---|---|---|
| Free of CHD<br>    versus<br>        all CHD cases | Age<br>Systolic blood pressure<br>JAS-S<br>Cholesterol | +++<br>+++<br>+++<br>++ |
| Free of CHD<br>    versus<br>all angina cases | Age<br>JAS-S<br>JAS-H | +++<br>+++<br>+ |

+ P < 0.05 ; ++ P < 0.01 ; +++ P < 0.001.

Table 24.  Multiple stepwise discriminant analysis

| G R O U P S | V A R I A B L E S | F |
|---|---|---|
| Free of CHD<br>    versus<br>ECG + Angina /-/<br>(heart condition known<br>or unknown | Systolic blood pressure<br>Age<br>Cholesterol<br>JAS-S | +++<br>+++<br>++<br>+ |
| Free of CHD<br>    versus<br>ECG + Angina /-/<br>(heart condition<br>unknown) | Systolic blood pressure<br>Age<br>Cholesterol<br>JAS-J /-/<br>JAS-S | +++<br>+++<br>++<br>+<br>+ |

+ P < 0.05 ; ++ P < 0.01 ; +++ P < 0.001.

4.1.1 <u>Comments</u>: Case-control and prevalence studies are primarily used to generate hypotheses, while prospective studies should test them. Prevalence studies of the type A behavior pattern could be misleading and produce methodological errors due to the following reasons:

4.1.1 The behavior pattern may change after the occurrence of coronary disease; this change could be in either direction regardless of whether differences in behavior between cases and controls are or are not observed.

4.1.2 The relationship of the behavior pattern to CHD may be different in fatal and nonfatal cases; the differences obtained between cases and controls might not exist when fatal or nonfatal cases are compared, or vice versa. Yet in the WCGS, the type A pattern predicted both fatal and nonfatal incidents, angina pectoris or myocardial infarction. Prospective studies can only resolve the issue of antecedence and consequence.

## 4.2 Incidence Studies

Those are the important ones used to assess causal relationship. The first, and most important, is the WCGS (4) where it has been shown both for the type "A", SI and JAS that they are predictors of CHD. We have shown a relation between type A behavior and incidence of CHD in three different studies.

4.2.1 <u>The three cohort study</u> (Brussels-Ghent, Marseilles, Paris). In that study (22), the Bortner Scale was used in 2,811 middle-aged male subjects free of CHD at entry. Classical coronary risk factors predicted new hard events (Table 25) and, less so, new soft events (Table 26).

The Bortner type A scale was related to hard ($\underline{p}$ = 0.10) and total events ($\underline{p}$ = 0.05) (Table 27).

In a multivariate analysis, the Bortner type A scale was an independent predictor of hard and total CHD events (Table 28).

4.2.2 <u>The physical fitness study</u>. In this Belgian prospective study (27), searching for clues relating physical activity and physical fitness with CHD incidence, the JAS was utilized at the baseline screening. Preliminary results indicate a relation of CHD incidence in subjects free of CHD at entry, with both the JAS-AB and JAS-S scores (Figure 1).

4.2.3 <u>The Belgian heart disease prevention project</u>. In this study (20), 10% of the control group received the JAS, the Bortner Scale and passed the SI at their baseline examination. Whereas incidence

Table 25.  Bioclinical risk factors and incidence of CHD (Hard events).

| | BRUSSELS-GHENT | | MARSEILLES | | PARIS | | TOTAL | |
|---|---|---|---|---|---|---|---|---|
| | Free of CHD | Hard Events | Free of CHD | Hard Events | Free of CHD | Hard Events | Free of CHD | Hard Events |
| Number | 622 | 26 | 684 | 14 | 1393 | 19 | 2699 | 59 |
| Age (yrs) | 48.0*** | 51.9 | 48.1° | 50.4 | 45.9 | 46.2 | *** | |
| SBP (mmHg) | 141* | 148 | 136° | 144 | 137*** | 149 | *** | |
| Cholesterol (cg/l) | 231* | 246 | 223 | 232 | 224* | 242 | ** | |
| Smoking (%) | 63 | 58 | 65 | 85 | 66*** | 100 | ** | |

°P = .10 ; * P = .05 ; ** P = .01 ; *** P = .001.
From : Lellouch, Kornitzer et al., (22).

e 26. Bioclinical risk factors and incidence of CHD (Soft events).

| | BRUSSELS-GHENT | | MARSEILLES | | P A R I S | | TOTAL | |
|---|---|---|---|---|---|---|---|---|
| | Free of CHD | Soft Events | Free of CDH | Soft Events | Free of CHD | Soft Events | Free of CHD | Soft Events |
| Number | 622 | 37 | 684 | 11 | 1393 | 5 | 2699 | 53 |
| Age (yrs) | 48.0 | 48.8 | 48.2* | 50.9 | 45.9* | 48.2 | | ++ |
| SBP (mmHg) | 141 | 139 | 136 | 137 | 137 | 150 | | |
| Cholesterol (cg/l) | 231+ | 245 | 223 | 216 | 224 | 246 | | + |
| Smoking (%) | 63 | 67N | 65° | 91 | 66 | 60 | | |

° P = .10 ; + P = .05 ; ++ P = .01.
From Lellouch, Kornitzer et al., (22).

Table 27.  Bortner scale and incidence of CHD.

| | Brussels-Ghent N / $\bar{M}$ | | Marseilles N / $\bar{M}$ | | Paris N / $\bar{M}$ | | Total |
|---|---|---|---|---|---|---|---|
| Free of CHD | 622 | 168 | 684 | 186 | 1393 | 181 | |
| Soft events | 37 | 176 | 11 | 190 | 5 | 198 | P = .13 |
| Hard events | 26 | 177 | 14 | 193 | 19 | 190 | ° |
| Total CHD | 63 | 176 | 25 | 192 | 24 | 192 | ✦ |

° P = .10 ;  ✦ P = .05

Table 28.  Multivariate analysis of bioclinical risk factors and
Bortner Scale  (All three cohorts).

| SOFT   EVENTS | HARD   EVENTS | TOTAL   CHD |
|---|---|---|
| Age          ✦✦ | Age          ✦✦✦ | Age          ✦✦✦ |
| Bortner | SBP          ✦✦ | Smoking      ✦ |
| Smoking | Smoking      ✦✦ | Bortner      ✦ |
| Cholesterol | Cholesterol  ✦ | Cholesterol  ✦ |
| SBP | Bortner      ✦ | SBP |

✦ P = .05 ;  ✦✦ P = .01 ;  ✦✦✦ P = .001

Table 29. Type A behavior and incidence of CHD.

| | JAS–AB | P | JAS–S | P | JAS–J | P | JAS–H | P |
|---|---|---|---|---|---|---|---|---|
| Free of CHD | -3.62 | | -6.79 | | -10.60 | | -0.92 | |
| New soft events (N = 82) | -1.41 | <0.04 | -3.51 | <0.006 | -10.81 | NS | -0.24 | NS |
| New hard events (N = 27) | -0.29 | <0.07 | -3.49 | <0.10 | -11.07 | NS | 0.50 | NS |
| Total events (N=109) | -1.13 | <0.009 | -3.50 | <0.002 | -10.88 | NS | -0.07 | NS |

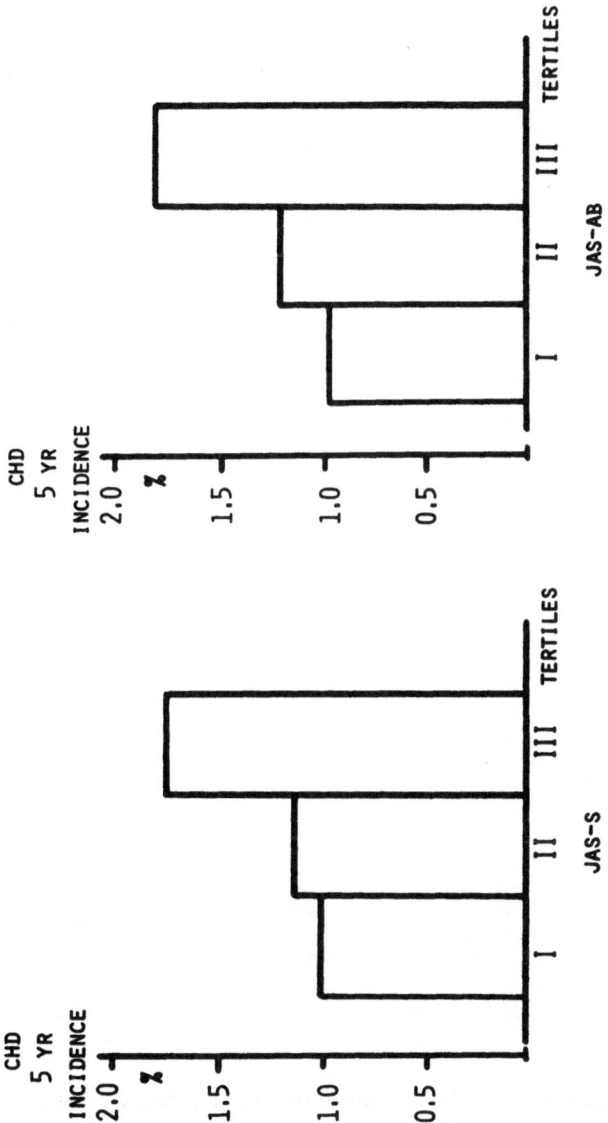

Figure 1. Relationship of prospective CHD incidence to JAS-AB and JAS-S scores at entry.

of soft events was only marginally higher in type A subjects, assessed by means of the SI, as compared to type Bs, incidence of hard events (fatal or nonfatal myocardial infarction or sudden deaths), was almost twice as high in type A subjects as compared to type Bs (figure 2).

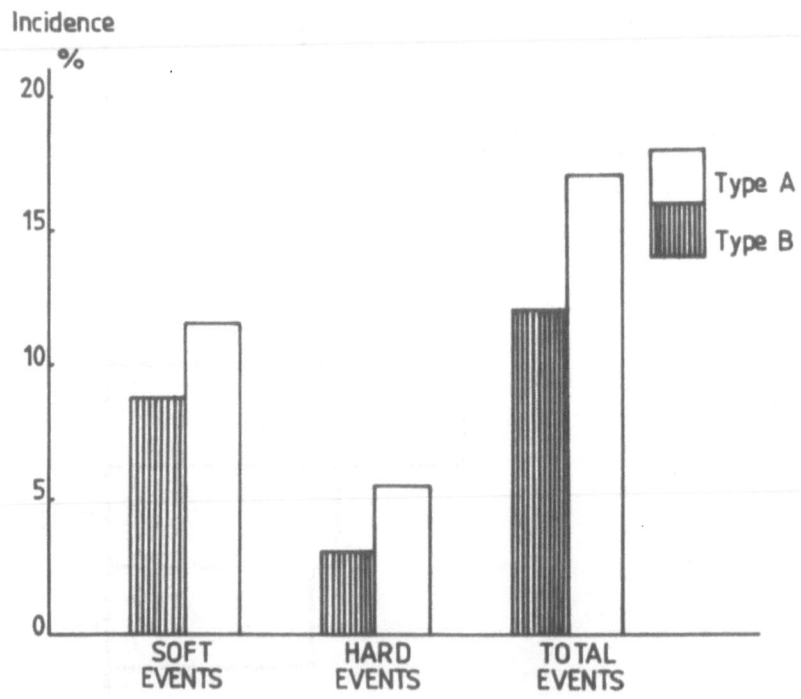

BELGIAN HEART DISEASE
PREVENTION PROJECT

TYPE A – BEHAVIOR and INCIDENCE
OF
CORONARY HEART DISEASE

Figure 2.   Incidence of soft, hard, and total events
for type A vs. B subjects.

When subjects are classified according to intensity of type A or B behavior, a gradient is observed with a 9 times higher incidence of all new coronary events in type A-1 as compared to type B-4 subjects (Figure 3).

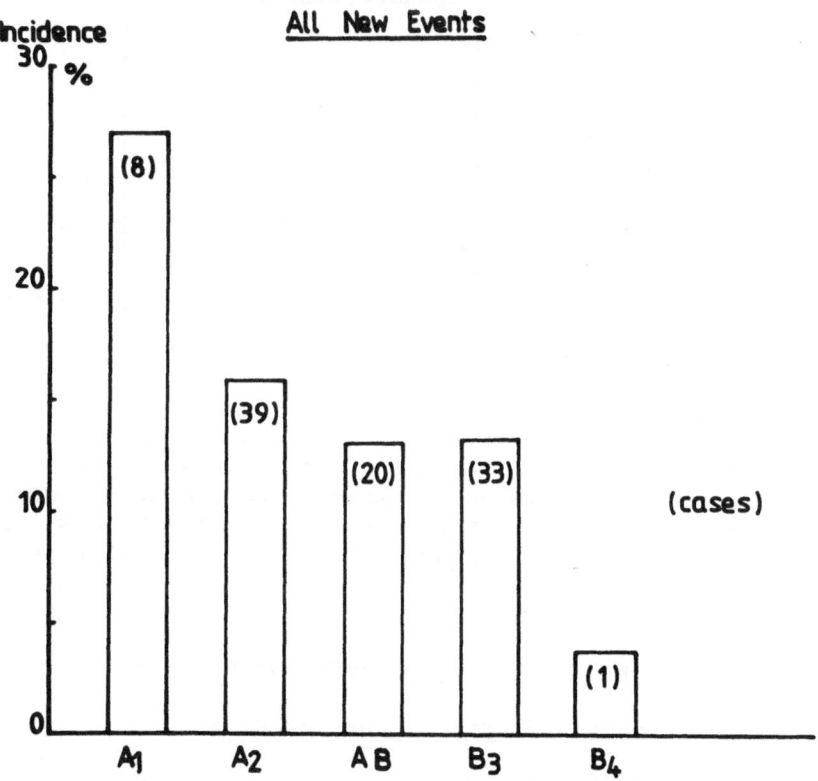

Figure 3.  Prospective incidence of new coronary events as a function of type AB pattern.

Using the JAS, we observed a significantly higher mean baseline JAS-AB for subjects with new soft and total events as compared to those remaining free of CHD; highest mean JAS-AB was observed in those subjects with a hard coronary event. Mean JAS-S score (speed and impatience) was significantly higher in subjects with new soft events as well as in those with any new event, whereas no significant relation was found for the JAS-J (job-involvement) or the JAS-H (hard-driving) (Table 29).

As for the Bortner Scale, subjects with a new coronary event had significantly higher baseline scores as compared to those remaining free of CHD (Table 30).

Table 30.  Type A behavior and Bortner Scale

|  | Base-line value | P |
|---|---|---|
| Free of CHD | 167 |  |
| New soft events | 174 | NS |
| New hard events | 180 | = 0.10 |
| Total events | 176 | < 0.05 |

4.2.4  Comments:  Those are, as far as we know, the first European incidence results showing a relation of type A behavior pattern with the incidence of CHD.  In the three cohort study (French-Belgian study) type A behavior is an independent predictor of CHD.  Those results strengthen the American observations in the WCGS and Framingham studies and seem to show that the relation of type A pattern with CHD is cross-cultural.


5  PATHOGENESIS OF CHD AND TYPE A BEHAVIOR PATTERN

5.1  Atherosclerosis and Type A Behavior Pattern

During the 1970s, several groups have published data concerning a positive correlation of type A behavior and major coronary vessel narrowings on the angiograms.  Most of those data referred to the SI (2, 10, 29).  We did not observe a significant relation using the

Bortner Scale (Tables 31 and 32).

Table 31.  Angiographic coronary score.

| | < Median N = 58 | ≥ Median N = 58 | P |
|---|---|---|---|
| Age | 47.7 | 49.6 | NS |
| Serum cholesterol (mgr/dl) | 245.0 | 285.0 | < .01 |
| Multiple logistic function | .0174 | .0271 | < .02 |
| Bortner Scale (Type A pattern) | 202 | 201 | NS |

5.1.1  Comment:  Methodological problems like case-referring according to place and time could play a role.  Nevertheless, the important
discrepancy between the SI and JAS or Bortner Scale in relation to
coronary lesions could be a point in favor of a more valid assessment
of the coronary-prone behavior pattern by means of the former.

## 5.2  Type A Pattern and Catecholamine Excretion

Whereas Friedman et al. (12) observed a significant difference
in catecholamine between type A vs. B subjects during their working
hours, we did not in the Belgian Heart Disease Prevention Project
(6).

5.2.1  Comment:  Most of our subjects were not A or B extreme types
whereas this was the case in the American study.

## 5.3  Reactivity During Challenge in Type A vs. B Subjects

Dembroski and co-workers (8), as well as Gastorf (13), observed
that whereas blood pressure levels did not differ during baseline
conditions, type A subjects showed a significantly greater increase
compared to type Bs under challenging conditions in the laboratory.
We defined groups of "high-stress and low-stress" medics and para-

134

Table 32. Coronary artery stenosis [+]

| | None N=22 | One N=33 | Two or Three N=62 | P |
|---|---|---|---|---|
| Age | 45.4 | 47.8 | 49.9 | <.05 |
| Serum cholesterol (mgr/dl) | 262 | 236 | 282 | <.02 |
| Cigarette smoking (%) | 27.4 | 48.5 | 51.7 | NS |
| Systolic blood pressure (mmHg) | 129 | 140 | 139 | NS |
| Multiple logistic function | 0.147 | 0.240 | 0.277 | NS |
| Bortner score | 211 | 197 | 201 | NS |

[+] Coronaro-stenosis = narrowing of 50% or more.

Table 33. Type A pattern and modification of SBP, DBP and HR in HS[*] and LS[**] Groups

| BORTNER SCALE | H S GROUP | | | L S GROUP | | | P | | |
|---|---|---|---|---|---|---|---|---|---|
| | $\Delta$ SBP A | $\Delta$ DBP B | $\Delta$ HR C | $\Delta$ SBP A | $\Delta$ DBP B | $\Delta$ HR C | A | B | C |
| < Median (Type B) | .30 | 2.33 | -5.30 | .06 | -1.11 | -3.33 | NS | <.05 | NS |
| ⩾ Median (Type A) | .83 | 1.17 | -2.21 | -1.40 | .63 | -1.29 | NS | NS | NS |
| P | NS | NS | <.05 | NS | NS | NS | | | |

[*] High-stress ; [**] Low-stress ; $\Delta$ = Mid-day value – Morning value.

Table 34. Type A pattern and modification of SBP, DBP and HR in HS and LS Groups. (Extreme quartiles).

| BORTNER SCALE | HS GROUP | | | LS GROUP | | | P | | |
|---|---|---|---|---|---|---|---|---|---|
| | Δ SBP A | Δ DBP B | Δ HR C | Δ SBP A | Δ DBP B | Δ HR C | A | B | C |
| First quartile (Type B) | - .68 | .45 | -4.0 | .55 | .90 | - .41 | NS | NS | NS |
| Fourth quartile (Type A) | 1.09 | 2.24 | -3.5 | -1.0 | -.66 | -2.99 | NS | <.05 | NS |
| P | NS | NS | NS | NS | NS | < .10 | | | |

medics according to Russeks' classification.

High-stress: anesthesiologists, surgeons, nurses working in coronary or intensive care units.

Low-stress: pathologists, dermatologists, ward-nurses.

Blood pressure and heart rate were measured early in the morning and at noon whereas type A behavior was assessed by means of the Bortner Scale. We observed significant differences in modification of diastolic blood pressure between HS and LS groups. Differences in blood pressure and HR in high-stress type A and B individuals were not significant although in the expected direction (Table 33), at least when first and fourth quartiles of distribution were compared (Table 34).


6  GENERAL CONCLUSIONS

Lately a respected panel convened by the American Heart Association (28) concluded that a probable causal relationship exists between type A behavior pattern and CHD although panel members raised several, as yet unsolved, questions about the cross-cultural validity of both the behavior pattern (definition) per se and its presumed pathogenetic mechanism. It is our impression that our group has tried to contribute, in a modest way, to answer some of their questions.

REFERENCES

1. Appels, A., W. de Haas, and J. Schuurman. Een Test Ter Meting van het 'Coronary-Prone Behaviour Pattern' Type A. Ned. T. Psychol. 34 (1979) 181.
2. Blumenthal, J.A., et al. Type A Behavior Pattern and Coronary Atherosclerosis. Circulation 58 (1978) 439.
3. Bortner, R.W. A Short Rating Scale as a Potential Measure of Pattern A Behavior. Journal of Chronic Disease 22 (1969) 87.
4. Brand, R.J. et al. Multivariate Prediction of Coronary Heart Disease in the Western Collaborative Group Study. Circulation 53 (1976) 348.
5. Butensky, A. et al. Elements of the Coronary-Prone Behavior Pattern in Children and Teenagers. Journal of Psychosomatic Research 20 (1976) 439.
6. De Backer, G. et al. Relation Between Coronary-Prone Behavior Pattern, Excretion of Urinary Catecholamines, Heart Rate, and Heart Rhythm. Preventive Medicine 8 (1979) 14.

138

7. Dembroski, T.M. et al. Coronary-Prone Behavior (New York, Springer-Verlag, 1978).
8. Dembroski, T.M. et al. Effect of Level of Challenge on Pressor and Heart Rate Responses in Type A and B Subjects. Journal of Applied Social Psychology 9 (1979) 209.
9. Eysenck, H.J. Manual for the Eysenck Personality Inventory (San Diego, Education and Industrial Testing Service, 1968).
10. Frank, K.A., S.S. Heller and D.S. Kornfeld. Type A Behavior Pattern and Coronary Angiographic Findings. Journal of the American Medical Association 240 (1978) 761.
11. Friedman, M. and R.H. Rosenman. Association of Specific Overt Behavior Pattern with Blood and Cardiovascular Findings. Journal of the American Medical Association 169 (1959) 1286.
12. Friedman, M. et al. Excretion of Catecholamines 17-Ketosteroids, 17-Hydroxycorticoids and 5-Hydroxyindole in Men Exhibiting a Particular Behavior Pattern (A) Associated with High Incidence of Clinical Coronary Artery Disease. Journal of Clinical Investigation 39 (1960) 758.
13. Gastorf, J.W. Physiologic Reaction of Type A's to Objective and Subjective Challenge. Journal of Human Stress (1981) 16.
14. Glass, D.C. Behavior Patterns, Stress, and Coronary Disease (Hillsdale, N.J., Erlbaum, 1977).
15. Haynes, S.G. et al. The Relationship of Psychosocial Factors to Coronary Heart Disease in the Framingham Study. II. Prevalence of Coronary Heart Disease. American Journal of Epidemiology 107 (1978) 384.
16. Heller, R.F. Type A Behavior and Coronary Heart Disease. British Medical Journal 2 (1979) 368.
17. Jenkins, C.D., R.H. Rosenman and M. Friedman. Development of an Objective Psychological Test for the Determination of the Coronary Prone Behavior Pattern in Employed Men. Journal of Chronic Disease 20 (1967) 371.
18. Jenkins, C.D., R.H. Rosenman and S.J. Zyzanski. Prediction of Clinical Coronary Heart Disease by a Test for the Coronary-Prone Behavior Pattern. New England Journal of Medicine 290 (1974) 1271.
19. Kittel, F. et al. Two Methods of Assessing the Type A Coronary-Prone Behavior Pattern in Belgium. Journal of Chronic Disease 31 (1978) 147.
20. Kornitzer, M. et al. Regional Differences in Risk Factor Distributions, Food Habits and Coronary Heart Disease Mortality and Morbidity in Belgium. International Journal of Epidemiology 8 (1979) 23.
21. Kornitzer, M. et al. The Belgian Heart Disease Prevention Project: Type A Behavior Pattern and the Prevalence of Coronary Heart Disease. Psychosomatic Medicine 43 (1981) 133.
22. Lellouch, J. et al. Ischemic Heart Disease and Psychological Patterns: Prevalence and Incidence Studies in Belgium and France. Advances in Cardiology 29 (1981) in press.

23. Matthews, K.A. and J. Angulo. Measurement of the Type A Behavior Pattern in Children: Assessment of Children's Competitiveness, Impatience-Anger, and Aggression. Child Development 51 (1980) 466.
24. Rustin, R.M. et al. Validation de Techniques d'Evaluation du Profil Comportemental "A" Utilisees dans le Projet Belge de Prevention des Affections Cardiovasculaires. Rev. Epidem. Sante Publ. 24 (1976) 497.
25. Sandler, J. and Hazari, A. The Obsessional on the Psychological Classification of Obsessional Character Traits and Symptoms. Journal of Medical Psychology 33 (1960) 113.
26. Shekelle, R.B., J.A. Schoenberger and J. Stamler. Correlates of the JAS Type A Behavior Pattern Score. Journal of Chronic Disease 29 (1976) 381.
27. Sobolski, J. et al. Physical Activity, Physical Fitness and Cardiovascular Diseases: Design of a Prospective Epidemiological Study. Cardiology 67 (1981) 38.
28. The Review Panel on Coronary-Prone Behavior and Coronary Heart Disease: A Critical Review. Circulation 63 (1981) 1199.
29. Zyzanski, S.J. et al. Psychological Correlates of Coronary Angiographic Findings. Archives of Internal Medicine 136 (1976) 1234.
30. Zyzanski, S.J., K. Wrzesniewski and C.D. Jenkins. Cross-Cultural Validation of the Coronary-Prone Behavior Pattern. Social Sciences and Medicine 13A (1979) 405.

# TYPE A BEHAVIOR PATTERN AND THE ANAL-OBSESSIVE TIME ATTITUDE

Jacques A. M. Winnubst

Workgroup in Psychology and Organization
University of Nijmegen
The Netherlands

## 1 INTRODUCTION

It would seem that in highly industrialized countries, a
certain personality mechanism is of the greatest importance to an
individual in maintaining himself. Above all he must possess
the capacity of accurately timing behavior. One might almost
assert that our economic preoccupations imply that time becomes
a purely economic factor, a commodity that is scarce in the sense
that many people experience that they suffer increasingly from
lack of time. One could say: they are anxious about the flow
of time. This attitude toward time has other implications too;
the higher the position on the social scale, the more this
commodity is economized upon, for example by employing such
aids as calendar, memorandum book, planmaster and clock. It
is noticeable that unpunctuality with regard to appointments often
gives rise to considerable irritation; on the other hand, some
highly qualified persons, amongst whom we might consider certain
professors, seem to consider it their prerogative to let others
wait.

After this short sketch of one aspect of everyday life, I
have come to the theme of this paper, which is time attitude,
time anxiety and the relationship of these aspects to coronary-
prone behavior and A/B typology. Above all, I hope to convince
you that A/B typology is rooted in psycho-analytic theory.
Attitude toward time is the attitude of individuals toward the
physical reality of time and the various aids that are employed
in its accurate measurement and description. My assumption is
that persons can and do differ in their attitude about time.
Some indeed will look upon time as a scarce commodity which must

be used economically; others will look upon time as a less
relevant factor which should not be taken into consideration.


## 2 THE ANAL CHARACTER

Especially the former attitude, the economic, rigid and
systematic handling of time, has led me to some theme's in
psychoanalytical personality theory, in particular that of the
anal personality and of obsessive-compulsive neurosis.  Freud
(9) described an interesting series of characteristics which,
as he noticed in his practice, always occurred together, namely,
parsimony, obstinacy and orderliness.  Theoretical work and
research conducted by Jones (19), as theorist, and Pettit (27)
and Kline (23) as researchers, are notable.  They have gradually
made it clear that the adoption of an anal syndrome is justifiable
and that the findings have interesting consequences for the
concept of time attitude.

It seems possible to relate the concept of time attitude
to the theory of anality and in fact this possibility has been
explored by a number of investigators.  Primarily important are
the following questions:  What does the anal syndrome look like,
i.e., what are its constituent elements?  How can we explain
its origin?  What relationship exists between anality and a
certain attitude to time?  Of essential importance in my approach
will be the question whether the theorizing has been properly
done and what status may be ascribed in this respect to the
psychoanalytic theory of personality.  Because I consider an
empirical attitude towards psychoanalytic theory of great
importance, the answer to the questions stated above will
strongly depend upon research on the anal personality and upon
the relationship between anality and time attitude.

In this psychoanalytic practice, Freud had noticed that
the above mentioned combination of personality traits chiefly
appeared in persons who were late in toilet training and who,
moreover, always postponed their bowel motion.  The explanation
Freud gave was that such persons derived a high degree of lust
from this behavior.  This explanation fit in with his 1905 treatise
(8) on the various psychosexual stages.  The derivement of lust
through bowel motion indicates an anal erotic preoccupation in
the child.  Because in later life this interest often completely
disappears, it must be assumed that in the course of libido
development, anal  sexuality becomes the impulsive drive for
the anal personality.

This may be understood, says Freud, if one considers that
in western cultures anal eroticism is fenced in with a strict
taboo and in its original form it has very little scope in later

life. This is why the anal preoccupation is displaced from
its original objective in the period of sexual latency (between
5 and 11 years of age) and deflected into sublimations or into
reaction formations. These processes of deflection of drive energy
in accordance with obtaining morals, in origin anal erotic,
ultimately result in the typical trio of personality traits, i.e.,
orderliness, parsimony and obstinacy.

The inevitableness of the interrelationship was not very
clear to Freud at this stage. He arrived at the following
description: orderliness, cleanliness and dependability may
be seen as a reaction formation to the original interest in the
unclean, the dirty, the childish and the alien to the body (in
this context Freud quotes an English proverb: "Dirt is matter
in the wrong place."). Obstinacy he found more difficult. For
the time being, Freud held the opinion that the small child
for the first time in his life has a chance to show something of
his own will in toilet training; at the same time his bottom is
the place where for the first time in his life he may experience
some sort of punishment. The concept parsimony is clearer;
according to Freud, the relationship between motions and interest
in money is well documented. Firstly, he says, there is the
constant constipation suffered by some neurotics, constipation
which not even hypnosis can cure. Furthermore, in primitive
thought, e.g., in myth, fairy tale, superstition, dreams and
neurosis and in unconscious thought, there is always a strong
tie between money (also gold) and exrements.

A further point of interest is that Freud in his paper
Die Disposition zur Zwagsneurose (10) refers to the anal sexual
stage to explain not only the origin of anal personality but also
that of compulsive neurosis. In compulsive neurosis there is
a regression to the pregenital, auto-erotic stage; it could be
said that there is a reversion to an early fixation on this
developmental period. Freud considers this explanation plausible
since expressions of hate and anal sexuality so freqently occur
in the compulsive neurosis. Furthermore, the neurosis often
manifests itself in an embarrassing, meticulous wash and
cleanliness compulsion, which can only be accounted for as a
reaction formation against anal erotic stimuli. The cleansing
ritual is characterized by repetition and a fixed rhythmic pattern.

The above short summary of the compulsive neurosis is
intended to make clear that the compulsive neurosis and the anal
character theoretically have the same origin, though Freud himself
hardly associated the two concepts.

It will have become clear from the above that, after
describing and interpreting the fundamental three traits of the
anal personality, Freud in fact came no further than his first

intuition.  A whole series of authors have since contributed
to working out Freud's basic idea.  Older contributions are
those by Abraham (1), Ferenzi (6), Jones (19), Menninger (25),
Sadger (30).  More recent studies include those by Gottheil (12),
Heimann (16), and Kline (23).


3 RESEARCH ON THE ANAL PERSONALITY

The kernel question of research into anality is whether
there is in fact a constellation, or something like it, of
personality traits in which parsimony, orderliness, and obstinacy
are predominant; in other words, does an anal syndrome exist?

The first research on the triad of anal traits took place
after the second world war.  Barnes (2) conducted a factor
analytic investigation over a number of items which were
supposed to represent different psychosexual stages, including
the anal.  His supposition that these different stages would
yield separate factors was not confirmed.  However, his Factor I
does remind one of anality; it is indicated by the concept
meticulousness, of which the characteristic traits were given as
orderliness, neatness, trustworthiness and a sense of duty.
Data on the reliability and validity of this investigation are
quite absent.

Beloff (3) studied both the structure of the anal personality
and the origins of it.  In this section we shall concentrate
on the structure.  His hypothesis on this point reads, "That a
psychological, functional entity exists, corresponding to the
anal character, as described by psychoanalysis" (p. 150).  After
close examination of the psychoanalytic literature, Beloff arrived
at the following  rather broad series of anal traits:  obstinacy,
thrift, craze for collecting, orderliness, cleanliness, punctuality, tendency to postpone, sadism in personal relationships,
scrupulousness, pedantry, feeling of superiority, irritability,
wish to dominate, desire for autonomy.

On the basis of this series of personality traits, a
questionnaire was compiled in which it was assumed that the
questions would indeed measure overt behavior and attitudes to
anality.  In constructing the scale, 35 men and 40 women
were involved.  The items analysis yielded 28 items of which
the mean $\underline{rt}$ = $-.71$ and of which the range was .93 to .53.

In order to obtain an insight into the validity, 28 items
were presented anew to 120 subjects and furthermore the same list
was presented to 4 friends of each subject who were requested to
fill in how they thought the subject in question would score.
Centroid factor analysis on self-ratings as well as on peer-

ratings as well as on peer-ratings both resulted in one general factor on which 22 and 21 items respectively had a significantly high load. Beloff correctly regarded this result as a positive argument for the validity, which is ever strengthened by the significant correlation of .48 between peer-ratings and self-ratings. Of importance was also the fact that the items with the highest load were: feeling of superiority, wish to dominate, sadism, irritability, scrupulousness and obstinacy. Traits such as thrift, cleanliness, and craze for collecting contributed a great deal less to the total variance. This scale thus pictured especially an authoritarian attitude, i.e., an inclination towards the manipulation of people; to a lesser degree the manipulation (possession or collection) of things was involved.

Also the factor analysis performed by Lazare et al. (24) yielded this picture. These authors obtained a factor that was composed of orderliness (load: .74), strong superego (load: .62), obstinacy and perseverance (load: .54). Likewise, in the latter study it appeared that thrift and cleanliness are apparently less basic to the anal syndrome than was originally assumed.

In all the studies mentioned, validity remains a problem of continuous concern. The merit of Kline's (20, 21, 22) work is that it has always focused on this problem. His starting point was a 30 item scale (Ai 3) which was subjected to a careful item analysis and which was checked for acquiescence and social desirability.

Subsequently, Kline performed three studies to investigate construct validity. I shall briefly summarize these: Validation 1. This study was carried out using the 16 PF test by Cattell and the EPI by Eysenck (varimax rotation). The Ai 3 loaded (.52) on only one factor, termed the superego factor by Kline. The dimensions were: Cattell's G (superego), load: 165, C (ego-strength), load: .47, Q 3 (self-control), load: .54, Q 4 (id pressure), load: -.28, Eysenck's EPI, load: .69. Kline considered this first result as a substantial confirmation of the anal personality because the latter is regarded as a defense mechanism against anal sexuality mediated by the super-ego and executed by the ego. The Ai 3 according to Kline is clearly dependent on the important personality variables extra-version and neuroticism. Validation 2. The Ai 3 was subjected to factor analysis (varimax rotation) with the anality scales by Beloff (3) and Hazari (15). The Ai 3 loaded only on the second factor named obsessive traits and not on the first factor named general emotionality and instability. Validation 3. Factor analysis (varimax rotation) was applied to Ai 3 and Grygier's (14) DPI. Anality loaded .62 on the superego dimension of the scale exclusively,

On the basis of these results, i.e., independence of important personality dimensions and correspondence with other anality scales, Kline arrived at the conclusion that his Ai 3 is a valid test. Apart from the construct validity Kline also obtained information on the concurrent validity through judgments made by others on experimental subjects. Testing for reliability resulted in an internal consistency of .67.

The most important contributions to the subject of the anal syndrome have now been discussed. Indeed, various other authors have been engaged in demonstration the anal structure, namely Finney (7), Hazari (15), Pichot and Perse (28), Sandler and Hazari (31), but I shall refrain from further discussion of this research. For the time being it seems sufficient to quote Kline's statement, "There is firm evidence for the anal character" (23), p. 29), this in contrast, it may be noted in passing, to the status of oral and other psychosexual syndromes (34).

## 4 ANALITY AND TIME ATTITUDE

The next question regards the relationship between anality and time attitude. It was Jones (19) who first drew attention to the symbolic content of time. His comments on the subject are short but significant. Time, says the psychoanalyst Jones, can represent a value for a person, just as money can. A certain personality type is typified by a remarkable sensitivity to the way in which others handle time. These people wish to remain in charge of their own time, demand however a large part of the time of other people and do not tolerate interference with their own behavioral time-tables. Noteworthy is Jones' opinion that the above attitude to time is closely connected to obsessive compulsive neurosis; the individual, frustrated in his temporal scheme, displays reactions that range from irritability to fierce aggressiveness.

The interest in money, according to Abraham (1), can be deflected into an interest in time. Many neurotics are constantly worried about the problem of time. Only the time spent alone or working is considered by them as well spent. Delay or interruption of work makes them very irritated and they greatly dislike inactivity and relaxation. Just as was the case with money, these patients save time on a small scale, at other moments they waste it on a large scale. The propensity for saving time is mainly exhibited in the attempt to do two things at once.

Summing up, we may state that according to psychoanalytical theory, the relationship between time, time anxiety and anality is expressed in the following traits:

(a) An attitude of possessiveness with respect to one's own time,
(b) The idea that only the time spent alone and at work it worthwhile,
(c) An inability to relax,
(d) A tendency to save time on a small scale while wasting it on a large scale,
(e) The feeling of constantly lacking time,
(f) The propensity for time and work budgeting,
(g) Irritation and aggression resulting from delay or interruption of work, and
(h) An attitude of submissiveness to social norms about time, accompanied by internal rebellion against the same norms.

In psychoanalytic theory, one can find many remarks too about the time-aspects of compulsive neurosis (or obsessive-compulsive behavior). Jones (19) pointed out the anal-erotic background of compulsive neurosis, and Von Harnik (33) derived interesting case material from compulsive neurosis histories. It is probably time to say, however, that compulsive neurosis has a more pathological accent than the theme of anality and is connected more easily with anxiety.

As the cause of compulsive neuroses Bonaparte (4) regards a premature introduction of time awareness in the child, and, as I interpret it, an unduly strict toilet training. Her description of compulsive neurotics shows the similarity with the anal personality so well that it is worth quoting literally.

"They have a horor of clocks, but at the same time they labour under a compulsion to take note of the most minute details concerning the hours, minutes and seconds. The flight of time is especially horrifying to them; they would gladly forget or deny its reality if they could but do so."

The more "classical" psychoanalysts made clear the common basis of anality, compulsive neurosis and time anxiety.

In view of the above, Kline's (23) remark that he could hardly discover any difference in his factor analytic research between anal and obsessive-compulsive traits will not cause any surprise too. Gorman and Katz (11) state, in accordance with Kline, that this is possibly also true for the temporal aspects of anality and obsessive-compulsion.

Summing up, we may state that the relationship between time, time anxiety and the obsessive style is expressed in the following traits:

(a) The constant feeling that time flows away,
(b) A chronic feeling of lack of time,
(c) The experience that time passes too quickly and is wasted
(d) A compulsive preoccupation with minutes and seconds,
(e) Anxiety about clocks,
(f) Feelings of depression and disturbance of concentration, and
(g) Great fear of death.

## 5 RESEARCH ON ANALITY AND TIME ATTITUDE

The most important investigation in the context of the present paper is doubtless that by Pettit (27). This author explicitly aimed at a test of the supposed relationship between the anal personality and (a specific) time attitude. His theorizing is based on Freud's anality theory and the way this has been worked out in the direction of the time attitude concept as proposed by Abraham (1), Ferenczi (6), and Jones (19).

Pettit also assumes there is a negative relationship between anal personality traits and spontaneous behavior; people with an anal personality structure will always want an orderly arrangement of their experiences such that these are always organized and clearly defined. They will have a dislike for diffuse, inarticulated impressions. Thus, time can become "more figure than ground". Because he will continuously attempt to impose structure and to exert control, it may be assumed that the anal personality will reject spontaneous events and surprises.

The purpose of the investigation was to test: (a) whether a positive relationship exists between anal personality structures and a worried, meticulous and obstinate attitude towards time; and (b) whether a negative relationship exists between anal personality structures and spontaneity.

To this end, four scales were used: the Time Scale, the Composite Anality Scale (32), the Grygier Anality Scale and finally the Grygier Spontaneity Scale (the latter two scales are described in Grygier (13). The Time Scale appeared to correlate very significantly with both the Composite Anality

Scale ($r$ = .64) and the Grygier Anality Scale ($r$ = .51).  Moreover, the Time Scale showed a negative correlation with the Grygier Spontaneity Scale ($r$ = -.32).  The two anality scales were, as might be expected, highly correlated ($r$ = .57).  It was not really clear why the Grygier Spontaneity Scale correlated negatively with the Grygier Anality Scale, while hardly showing any relationship with the other anality scales, viz. the Composity Scale.

Pettit was still of the opinion that his results supported his hypotheses, but he did recognize certain objections which might be brought forward against his investigation.  A primary objection might be that the scales used could have a pronounced social desirability character.  Though Pettit presents several arguments which imply that a disturbing effect of this kind is unlikely, he does admit that a closer check be desirable.

Another possible objection is that the relationship between anality and time attitude may be regarded as being mediated by cultural factors; in this case anality is no longer seen as a reaction formation to early anal impulses.  Pettit's opinion is that both factors play a role and that longitudinal as well as experimental investigations will be needed to settle the question.  According to Pettit, the psychoanalytic view gives an insight into the way in which cultural values are passed on to the child at the very early age during which toilet training is given, and also how this is achieved through a process of symbol formation.  Pettit thus appears to have inclination towards the latter psychoanalytic view.  At any rate his research implied an important advance in various respects.

The significance of the research done by Gorman and Katz (11) lies on the one hand in the fact that it effectuated a replication of Pettit's investigation and, on the other hand, that in it Calabresi and Cohen's (5) important specification of the time attitude concept played a major role.  Gorman and Katz set out from the criticism they had on the research by Pettit.  (a) Anal character traits and the corresponding time attitudes are parts of the dominant western value pattern. For this reason, social desirability might well be a crucial intermediary variable in the relationship anality and time attitude. (b) Calabresi and Cohen (5) showed that at least four orthogonal factors of time attitude can be distinguished:  time anxiety, time submissiveness, time possessiveness, and time flexibility. The important question then is which factor, or combination of factors are related to the anality concept.  (c) Finally, they posed the question whether the relationship between time and anality could not be brought under the more general theoretical constructs of rigidity, ego-strength or obsessive-compulsive mode.  In this context they referred to research by Kline (22) in which there appeared to be agreement between the anal and the compulsive neurotic traits.

The replication was set up as follows. There were 110 students (54 male, 56 female) who were given the following questionnaires: (a) The Time Attitude Scale by Calabresi and Cohen; (b) Pettit's Time Scale; (c) The Composite Anality Scale (also used by Pettit); (d) The Marlowe-Crowne Social Desirability Scale; (e) The Gough-Sanford Rigidity Scale. The product-moment correlation between the scales was calculated, and subsequently a factor analysis (principal components) was performed. The result was a single factor. Except for the social-desirability scale, all the scales loaded significantly on this factor. Gorman and Katz named the factor Obsessive-Compulsive mode and concluded moreover from their result that there was good reason to regard anality as belonging to the construct regidity. Social desirability appeared furthermore to have no effect on the investigated relationship. It appeared possible, however, to expose a close relationship, in agreement with Pettit's results, between anality and several forms of time attitude.

Especially the time submissiveness subscale yielded some very significant results, viz. ($\underline{r}$ = .48) with Pettit's time scale ($\underline{r}$ = .41) with the Composite Anality Scale, and ($\underline{r}$ = .52) with the rigidity scale. This led Gorman and Katz to believe that the relation between anality and time attitude was primarily concerned with reaction formation against the expulsive stage. This is a stage in which the desire to freely expel and manipulate feces is transformed into the opposite type of behavior in which conformity to what is socially desirable precominates. This conclusion is enhanced by a total lack of connection between the retentive wish to save time (time possessiveness subscale) and anal retentive personality traits (Composite Anality Scale).

## 6 TIME ANXIETY AND A/B TYPOLOGY

Till now I developed the theoretical line and research concerning the anal and compulsive theme. Now I intend to work out the connection between this line and my own empirical research about time anxiety and the relationship with A/B typology and other behavioral variables.

In 1975 I completed a five-year project about time variables in psychology, and wrote a book entitled, "The Western Time Syndrome". In that work I described the most important molar time variables: time perspective, delay of gratification, time anality, and time competence. I developed an instrument, "The Western Time Attitude Scale" (WTAS), consisting of eleven scales. In this way it was possible for me to study the relationship between these eleven dimensions and other variables.

In the same period, Dr. Ad Appels drew my attention to the
fact that the theme of time anality, at a theoretical level,
is connected in a special way to the A/B typology of Rosenman
and Friedman (29). These cardiologists described a hurried,
competitive and impatient style of behavior, and they considered
this style to be an important cardiac risk factor. My "own"
time anxious persons experience time as flowing too fast, time
is very threatening for them, they see time as a tyrant and they
are accelerating themselves constantly, they feel very guilty
for spilling time.

Rosenman and Friedman described in 1959 for the first time
this coronary prone behavior pattern (29). Type A behavior
is an overt style of reaction with the following aspects: intense
achievement striving, impatience, competitiveness, time-urgency,
hyper-alertness, overcommitment to work, excessive hostility.
Type A behavior seems to be associated with higher prevalence
of the symptoms of coronary disease for both men and women. A
recent review by Jenkins (17) mentions eight prospective studies
and 16 cross-sectional and retrospective studies about the
relationship between coronary-prone behavior pattern and CHD.
Nearly all of them confirmed the hypothesis.

When we look at another recent article about coronary-
prone behavior (18), we see some striking resemblances between
our own work about the anal-obsessive time attitude and the
studies about A/B typology.

Some aspects of A-types out of the 1978 article of
Jenkins et al.:

(a) they held two or more jobs simultaneously for
a period of more than four years,
(b) they were never late for appointments,
(c) they were particularly conserving of time in that
they often carried work materials with them and worked
while waiting for people,
(d) they like to hurry up slow speakers, and
(e) they were very impatient with persons who do
things slowly.

The accepted label for this behavior is "time urgency".
It seems to me that the time urgent person is a strongly goal-
directed person; other persons are seen by this person as a
threat for their available time. I think these people are
suffering increasingly from lack of time. Time is a scarce
commodity for them. It is clear that they are anxious about
the flow of time too.

Jenkins' items do not contain this anxiety tendency.  Should
it not be interesting to study the relationship between the "time
urgency" of A/B typology and the "time anxiety" of the Western
Time Syndrome?  We thought so.

The Western Time Anxiety Scale (WTAS) is constructed out
of several existing scales.  The WTAS consists now of eleven
independent sub-scales which are anchored in four theorectical
concepts:  time perspective, delay of gratification, time
anality, and time competence (34).

In a factor analysis (Kaiser-Cafrey Alpha) about the above
mentioned eleven scales, two time anality scales emerged:

1.  Time anxiety (time obsession):  time is experienced
by persons as going too fast.  They have the feeling that
they don't have enough time, they are panicky about this,
time shortage is a continuing threat, they are pressed and
hurried people.  Some items:

    p - 110   I get almost panicky when I don't have
              enough time.
    p - 114   I seem to be more pressed for time than
              most people.
    p - 169   It bothers me to think how fast time
              goes.

2.  Time submissiveness (punctuality):  persons are
characterized by a scrupulous attitude about time,
they are very punctual.  They are worried about clocks
and agendas.  They are always on time.  Time is a
normative affair for them; they are ruled by time.
Some items:

    p - 131   I would be lost without a watch.
    p - 138   I would rather have a definite schedule
              and stick to it.
    p - 145   I like to have a definite schedule and
              stick to it.

When we consider the place of the two anality dimensions
in the network of other time-variables, we see the following
pattern (Figure I):

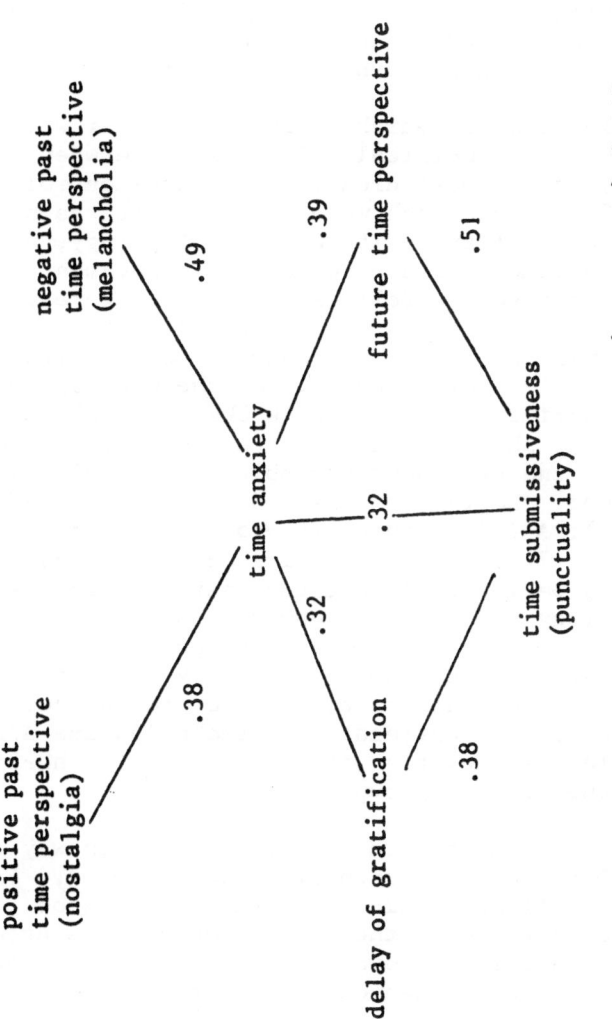

Figure 1.  Western Time Syndrome.

I call this pattern: the Western Time Syndrome. You can
see the central place of time anxiety in this network. Time
anxiety, the worrying attitude toward time is commuted with the
tendency to plan ahead and to schedule things, to postpone
gratification, save money for rainy days, with punctuality and
with the tendency to be more occupied with both positive  and
negative aspects of the past.  These persons are dwelling more
in the future and in the past.  In the here-and-now they are
deeply worried about a lack of time to fulfill all their plans
and dreams.  I think we are looking here at highly motivated
people with a certain, nearly neurotic, attitude toward time.
I think it will be interesting now to look at relationships
between A/B typology and Western Time Syndrome.

By developing some research in 1978, together with Nass
and Verhagen (26), the empirical relationship between A/B typology
and time anxiety became more clear.  In a case-control study
two groups of 58 subjects each were compared with each other
on a number of personality variables:  A/B typology, depression,
rigidity, Western Time Attitude Scale and achievement motivation.
The groups were composed as follows:  The cases were male
myocardial infarction patients, who have had their infarctions not
longer than one year before.  The controls were healthy persons.
All persons were male, white, Dutch, and the mean age was 46 years.
By means of a discriminant-analysis (Wilks) we could see which of
the independent variables (scales) traced best the difference in
the categories of the dependent variables.  The following pattern
of results emerged:  Depression (F=15.04, p = .01); JAS (A/B scale)
(F=11.09, p= .01); A/B (interview)(F=8.54, p= .01); (Positive)
Fear of failure (F=7.51, p = .01); Time anxiety (F=6.40, p= .05);
Rigidity (F=4.73, p= .05).  I conclude that the Depression Scale
and the A/B typology are the best describers of the differences
between coronaries and controls.  For our purpose it is important
to have proven the value of the time anxiety scale as a discriminating scale with a certain cardiovascular relevance.  Another
interesting point is the correlation between Jenkins A/B scale and
my own time anxiety scale: $r$ = .54 in the group of heart patients
and $r$ - .53 in the control group.

A specific attitude toward time and a certain way of handling
time are central aspects of coronary-prone behavior.  Friedman
and Rosenman, as well as Jenkins, are the pioneers of the A/B
typology and they have shown the importance of time urgency as
an element with special cardiovascular relevance.  My own
contribution lies in the "diagnosis" that this urgency is highly
correlated with time anxiety, and that this last mentioned
theme is rooted in psychoanalytic theory and especially in anal
and compulsive theory.  So there is to my opinion a strong, but
overlooked connection between the psychoanalytic theory about
anal-compulsive behavior and the work of Friedman and Rosenman.

REFERENCES

1. Abraham, K.  Contributions to the Theory of the Anal
   Character.  In K. Abraham, Selected Papers (London,
   Hogarth Press, 1921.
2. Barnes, C.A.  A Statistical Study of the Freudian Theory
   of Levels of Psychosexual Development.  Genetic Psychology
   Monographs.  45 (1952) 109-174.
3. Beloff, H.  The Structure and Origin of the Anal Character.
   Genetic Psychology Monographs 55 (1957) 141-172.
4. Bonaparte, M.  Time and the Unconscious.  International
   Journla of Psychoanalysis 21 (1940) 427-468.
5. Calabresi, R. and J. Cohen.  Personality and Time Attitudes.
   Journal of Abnormal Psychology 78 (1968) 431-440.
6. Ferencai, S.  Zur Ontogenie des Geldinteresses.  In Ferenczi,
   S., Schriften zur Psychoanalyse.  I. (Frankfurt am Main,
   S. Fischer Verslag, 1914).
7. Finney, J.C.  Maternal Influences on Anal or Compulsive
   Character in Children.  Journal of Genetic Psychology 103
   (1963) 351-367.
8. Freud, S.  Drei Abhandlungen zur Sexualtheorie.  Gesammelte
   Werke, Band V.(London, Imago Publishing Company, 1905).
9. Freud, S.  Charakter und Analerotik.  Gesammelte Werke,
   Band VII.  (London, Imago Publishing Company, 1908).
10. Freud, S.  Die Disposition zur Zwagsneurose.  Gesammelte
    Werke, Band VIII.  (London, Imago Publishing Company,
    1913).
11. Gorman, B. and B. Katz.  Temporal Orientation and Anality.
    Proceedings of the 79th Annual Convention, APA (1971)
    367-368.
12. Gottheil, E.  An Empirical Analysis of Orality and Anality.
    Journal of Nervous and Mental Disease 141 (1965) 308-
    317.
13. Grygier, P.  The Personality of student nurses:  A Pilot
    Study Using the DPI.  International Journal of Social
    Psychiatry 2 (1956) 105-112.
14. Grygier, T.G.  The Dynamic Personality Inventory. (London,
    N.F.E.R., 1961).
15. Hazari, A.  An Investigation of Obsessive-Compulsive
    Character Traits and Symptoms in Adult Neurotics.
    (London, University of London, 1957).
16. Heimann, P.  Notes on the Anal Stage.  International Journal
    of Psychoanalysis 43 (1962), 406-414.
17. Jenkins, C.D.  Behavioral Risk Factors in Coronary Artery
    Disease.  Annual Review of Medicine 29 (1978), 543-562.
18. Jenkins, C.D., S.J. Zyzanski, and R. H. Rosenman.  Coronary-
    Prone Behavior:  One Pattern or Several?  Psychosomatic
    Medicine 40 (1978) 25-43.
19. Jones, E. Anal-Erotic Character Traits.  In Jones, E. Papers on
    psychoanalysis. (London, Bailliere, Tindall & Cox, 1918).

156

20. Kline, P.   An Investigation Into the Freudian Concept of the
    Anal Character.   (Manchester, University of Manchester,
    1967).
21. Kline, P.   Obsessional Traits, Obsessional Symptoms and Anal
    Erotism.   British Journal of Medical Psychology 41 (1968)
    299-305.
22. Kline, P.   The Anal Character:   A Cross-Cultural Study in Ghana.
    British Journal of Social and Clinical Psychology 8 (1969)
    201-210.
23. Kline, P.   Fact and Fantasy in Freudian Theory.   (London,
    Methuen, 1972).
24. Lazare, A., G.L. Klerman, and D. J. Armor.   Oral, Obsessive
    and Hysterical Personality Patterns:   An Investigation of
    Psychoanalytic Concepts by Means of Factor Analysis.
    Archives of General Psychiatry 14 (1966) 624-630.
25. Menninger, W.D.   Characterologic and Symptomatic Expressions
    Related to the Anal Phase of Psychosexual Development.
    Psychoanalytic Quarterly 12 (1943) 161-193.
26. Nass, C., F. Verhagen, and J.A.M. Winnubst.   A/B Typologie,
    de Protestantse Ethiek en het Westers Tijdssyndroom.   Een
    Empirische Studie.   Gedrag, Tijdschrift voor Psychologie
    7 (1979) 41-57.
27. Pettit, T.F.   Anality and Time.   Journal of Consulting and
    Clinical Psychology 33 (1969) 170-174.
28. Pichot, P. and J. Perse.   Analyse Factorielle et Structure
    de la Personalite. (Lund, University of Lund, 1967).
29. Rosenman, R.H. and M. Friedman.   Type A Behavior and Your
    Heart.   (Greenwick, Connecticut, Fawcett, 1974).
30. Sadger, R.   Analerotik und Analcharakter.   Die Heilkunde
    1910.
31. Sadler, J. and A. Hazari.   The Obsessional:   On the
    Psychological Classification of Obsessional Character
    Traits and Symptoms.   British Journal of Medical Psychology
    33 (1960) 113-121.
32. Schlesinger, V.J.   Anal Personality Traits and Occupational
    Choice - A Study of Accounts, Chemical Engineers and
    Educational Psychologists.   Unpublished Ph.D. thesis.
    (Michigan, University of Michigan, 1963).
33. Von Harnik, J.   Die Triebhaft-affektiven Momente im Zeitgefuhl.
    Internationale Zeitschrift fur Psychoanalyse 10 (1924),
    33-35.

BARRIERS TO WORK STRESS: I. SOCIAL SUPPORT

James S. House

Department of Sociology and Epidemiology
University of Michigan
Ann Arbor, Michigan

1  INTRODUCTION

In the last decade, the concept of "social support" has become
increasingly prominent in both scientific and applied or policy-
related discussions of stress and health.  By the mid-1970s in the
United States, social support was the topic of invited addresses
to the American Public Health Association and Psychosomatic Society
by two of our most distinguished social epidemiologists, the late
John Cassel (5) and Sidney Cobb (6) respectively.  The very first
recommendation of the 1978 report of our President's Commission
on Mental Health (28, p. 15) was that:  "A major effort be developed
in the area of personal and community supports which will:  (a)
recognize and strengthen the natural network to which people belong
and on which they depend; ...".

The current fascination with social support stems from its
being, as I have argued elsewhere (13), a potential "triple threat"
in the battle to alleviate the impact of stress on health (Figure
1).  That is, social support is believed both to reduce the
experience of stress and to enhance levels of health and well-being.
Most importantly, social support has been hypothesized to have the
capacity to mitigate or "buffer" the impact of stress on health.
That is, social support can reduce or eliminate the deleterious
health effects of life stresses, even when we either can not or will
not reduce levels of stress to which people are exposed.  Since
stress is a ubiquitous feature of life and work, and may even have
beneficial effects in some situations (1, 29), strategies for
minimizing the deleterious health effects of irreducible stresses
at work and elsewhere have special appeal.

This potential ability of social support to buffer the impact of stress on health has repeatedly been identified as its key feature. Thus Kaplan, Cassel and Gore (19) went so far as to assert that "social supports are likely to be protective only in the presence of stressful circumstances," and Cobb (6) also noted that "one should not expect dramatic main effects (on health) from social support." Both Cobb (6) and Cassel (5) felt their reviews documented the ability of social support to buffer the impact of stress on health.

The enthusiasm for social support of the early and mid-1970s has given way in the last few years to increasing skepticism. Critics have correctly diagnosed a number of problems in the extant literature on social support (7, 12, 31). First, no clearly agreed upon definition of social support exists, and not infrequently the term is used without any definition, or only a tautological one. Cassel's (5) APHA address is one of the most cited in the literature on social support, yet Cassel used the concept repeatedly without ever defining it. A more recent paper (21) defines social support as "support accessible to an individual through social ties," or, in essence, social support is support which is social. Secondly, the critics note, that even if an author or study provides a clear and meaningful definition of support, there is often little correspondence between this definition and commonly used operational measures. In his Presidential address to the Psychosomatic Society, Cobb (6) defined support as "information leading the subject to believe that he is cared for and loved ... that he is esteemed and valued (or) ... that he belongs to a network of communication and mutual obligation." The definition clearly suggests that support must be measured on terms of what people "believe." Yet none of the more than a dozen studies reviewed by Cobb measured support in this way. Other studies include everything but the kitchen sink in their measure of "social support," for example, job satisfaction (21) or social status and ego strength (23).

Finally, critics have increasingly noted that the evidence is not always strong and consistent for the most vaunted property of social support, namely its ability to buffer the impact of stress on health, and that the purported effects of support on stress and health may even be spurious products of other variables (e.g., personality) which predispose people to experience more stress, poorer health, and less social support. In this regard, it is telling that despite the emphasis of both Cassel (5) and Cobb (6) on the buffering properties of social support, at best only three or four of the dozen or so studies each reviews document true buffering and many are amenable to alternative causal interpretations.

We are witnessing a natural and understandable reaction to
the somewhat excessive scientific and policy claims which may have
been made in the initial enthusiasm for the concept of social
support.  This is, after all, not such a new idea (6).   Others
have emphasized the positive benefits of similar concepts for some
time:  sociologists speaking of social integration; psychologists,
of affection and attachment; philosophers and theologians, of
love.  Still there is something novel in the idea that certain
types of social interactions and relationships can reduce stress
and buffer its impact on health and well-being.  Proponents of
social support may have seemed to tout it as a new panacea for
problems of stress and health, but the current critiques of the
literature on social support run the risk, I fear, of throwing
out the baby with the bath water.  What I would like to do in this
paper is to provide an overview of the current status of work on
social support, focusing on problems of work stress and health
(13).  Specifically, I seek:

(a)   to briefly define what I think social support is and
      how it is related to stress and health, with special
      focus on the idea of buffering;

(b)   to suggest how I think we should measure support and
      test its effects;

(c)   to indicate why I think there is a substantial body
      of evidence showing not only main or additive effects
      of support on both stress and health but also sub-
      stantial buffering effects on relationships between
      stress and health;

(d)   to review in some detail work I have been involved
      in on occupational stress, social support, and
      health, which has a number of desirable features
      absent in other research, as well as some problems;

(e)   finally, to offer some suggestions as to where we
      ought to go from here in basic and applied research
      on work stress, social support and health.


## 2   THE NATURE OF SOCIAL SUPPORT AND ITS EFFECTS

What is social support and how does it operate to affect work
stress and health?  I define social support (13, pp. 13-40) as a
flow of one or more of four things between people (Table 1):   (a)
emotional concern (empathy, caring, concern); (b) instrumental aid
(giving money, assistance); (c) information (advice, suggestions,
directions); and/or (d) appraisal (feedback or social comparison

Table 1.  Potential Forms of Social Support.

| Content of supportive acts | Source of Support | | | | | | | | |
|---|---|---|---|---|---|---|---|---|---|
| | (1) Spouse or partner | (2) Other rela- tive(s) | (3) Friend(s) | (4) Neigh- bor(s) | (5) Work super- visor | (6) Coworker(s) | (7) Service or care giver(s) | (8) "Self-help" group(s) | (9) Health/Welfare professional(s) |
| 1. *Emotional Support* (esteem, affect, trust, concern, listening) | | | | | | | | | |
| 2. *Appraisal Support* (affirmation, feedback, social comparison) | | | | | | | | | |
| 3. *Informational Support* (advice, suggestion, directives, information) | | | | | | | | | |
| 4. *Instrumental Support* (aid in kind, money, labor, time, modifying environment) | | | | | | | | | |

Within this matrix of types of social support, each can be:

(a) *general versus problem-focused*
(b) *objective versus subjective*

relevant to a person's self-evaluation). This definition identifies a minimal set of behaviors or characteristics of relationships that are potentially supportive. It encompasses the major ideas in most other major definitions of support (4, 6, 9, 18), while being more comprehensive than any one of these definitions yet still reasonably parsimonious. We do not yet understand the relations among these different types of support and the degree to which they have different effects. It is hard to observe one type in isolation from the others. Emotional support, however, appears to be the most important of the four types both intuitively and in theoretical discussion and empirical research.

This definition of support is embodied in the rows of Table 1. This table suggests several other things which are important to recognize about social support. First, support can come from many sources (spouse, friends, work supervisors, coworkers, psychotherapists). We need to distinguish among sources of support as well as types of support, because they have, or can reasonably be expected to have, different effects on stress and health. Second, we need to recognize that social support, and measures thereof, may be either subjective or objective, that is, either based on the perceptions and reports of the people with whose level of support we wish to assess or derive from independent observation and assessment of the person's social relationships by another party. Neither the objective nor the subjective versions are necessarily better. Rather, as I will reiterate in my conclusion, we need to understand the relation of the objective situations, relationships and interactions that people experience, to their subjective perceptions of support, as well as the relation of both of these to health. Finally, concepts and measures of support may be either general or role- or problem-specific. For example, we can ask how supportive other people are in general, or how supportive they are with respect to work and work-related problems.

The conceptualization of support embodied in Table 1 assumes that specific concepts and measures of support need to be tailored to the specific scientific or applied problems. The research in which I have been involved, for example, has focused on measuring subjectively perceived emotional support from work supervisors, coworkers, and spouses in connection with work-related problems. This focus has been appropriate for our work to this point, but will not necessarily remain our focus in future work nor should it necessarily be the focus in other research. Table 1 attempts to provide a systematic framework for thinking about and developing new concepts and measures of support.

How is social support related to stress and health? Figure 1 graphically represents the three ways suggested above that social support can affect health. Generally, these effects are expected

162

to be positive or beneficial for health, though some forms of
support in some situations can have adverse effects. Two of these
effects can be referred to in statistical terms, as additive or
main effects. One of these is a direct effect of social support
on health (arrow c). That is, support may enhance health and
well-being because it directly meets important human needs for
security, affiliation, approval, and affection. If support
enhances health in this way, it may help to compensate for the
adverse health consequences of stress or any other threat to
health. The other main effect in Figure 1 involves a direct effect
of social support on stress, and hence an indirect effect of support
on health. In the work setting, for example, supportive supervisors
and coworkers are likely to reduce certain kinds of work stresses
such as role conflict and interpersonal tension (arrow a).
Reductions in these stresses can, in turn, have beneficial effects
on health (arrow d).

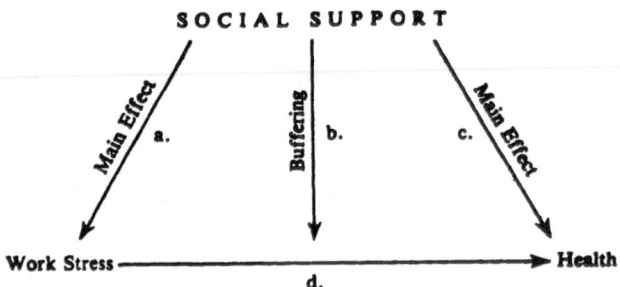

FIG. 1   *Potential effects of social support on work stress
and health*

Finally, social support may buffer the impact of work stress
on health (arrow b). The nature of this buffering effect has,
however,  not always been clearly understood in the literature.
Essentially, it involves a special kind of statistical interaction
between stress and support in predicting health outcomes. The
nature of this interaction is illustrated in the left-hand graphs
(a and c) of Figure 2; a deleterious impact of stress on health
is clearly manifest when social support is low, but this impact
decreases, and perhaps even disappears, as the level of social
support increases from low to high. This effect may occur with
(Figure 2c) or without (Figure 2a) other additive effects of support
on health. In contrast, although support has beneficial main or
additive effects on health in Figure 2b, there is no buffering
present in that case. The mechanisms through which buffering

operates are not fully understood at this point, but they appear
to involve effects of social support on the processes of appraisal
of and adaptation to stress. In the presence of social support,
we may perceive given objective conditions as less stressful or
respond to objective stressors or perceived stresses in more
adaptive ways, thus mitigating or obviating deleterious effects
on health.

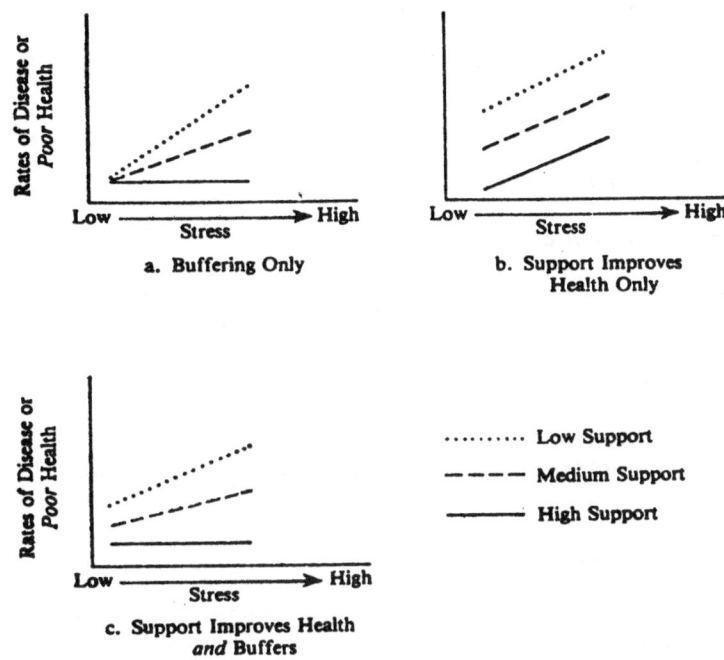

FIG. 2    *Different patterns of effects of social support and occupational
stress on health*

Figures 1 and 2 from James S. House, <u>Work Stress and Social Support</u>.
Mass.: Addison-Wesley, 1981.

Reading,

The formulation of social support embodied in Figures 1 and 2
and Table 1 has important methodological implications. First,
measures of social support should be as specific as possible regarding both types and sources of support, so that we can begin to better
understand <u>who</u> gets <u>how much</u> of <u>what kinds</u> of support <u>from whom</u>
regarding <u>which</u> problems of stress and health, and with <u>what effects</u>.
Second, empirical research needs to attend to several types of
effects of social support, the direct or additive effects of
support on stress and/or health and the buffering effects of
support on relationships between stress and health. Statistically,
this involves estimating the main effects of support on stress and
health and the specific type of interaction between stress and

support in predicting health status that is embodied in Figures
2a and 2c.  This estimation can be performed in a number of ways,
but the research reported in detail below uses OLS regression to
estimate equations of the following general type:

$$Y = a + b_1 S \qquad (1)$$

$$Y = a + b_1 X + b_2 S + b_3 SX \text{ where} \qquad (2)$$

Y = health or illness

X = a measure of work stress

S = a measure of social support

a = a constant

If the coefficient ($b_3$) associated with the SX term in equation
(1) is significant, and the full set of coefficients take on
appropriate values, we have evidence of buffering.  Otherwise,
the coefficients ($b_1$ and $b_2$) associated with the X and S terms of
equation (2) estimate the main or additive effects of stress and
support on health.  Similarly, the $b_1$ coefficient of equation (1)
estimates the additive effect of support on stress (13).


## 3  EMPIRICAL EVIDENCE

Given the conception of social support outlined above and its
effects, what is the evidence that social support can reduce work
stress, improve health, and buffer the impact of work stress on
health?  Evidence suggesting that social support can be a barrier
against the deleterious effects of work stress on health comes
from studies done outside of work settings as well as within them,
and from research done prior to the emergence of the concept of
social support as well as since then.  The evidence is quite
extensive from nonwork settings and from the period before the last
decade of analyses of support.  Space and time preclude more than
a cursory overview here, but numerous reviews are available (5,
13, 31).

### 3.1  Background

Experimental studies of both animals and humans have demonstrated that the presence of others, especially familiar others,
reduces the adverse effects of experimentally induced stressors
on psychological, physiological, and behavioral functioning (13).
A very recent study even suggests that supportive behavior by
humans can mitigate the arteriosclerotic effects of a high-fat

diet in rabbits (22). Studies of "social integration" by sociologists and social epidemiologists (8, 10, 11, 24) have consistently
found better physical and mental health and greater longevity
among the more socially integrated compared to the less integrated
(most notably, the married vs. unmarried). Two recent studies
(2, 15) show that a variety of indicators of social integration
(marriage, other intimate social relationships, and more formal
organizational and social activities) are predictive of mortality
in prospective studies of diverse community populations, even
with controls for a wide range of biomedical and health behavior
risk factors of mortality. Most of these studies document only
main effects of social integration on health. The few studies
that examine both buffering and main effects of support suggest
that the better physical and mental health of more socially
integrated people is due both to their lesser exposure to stress
and their lesser vulnerability to the deleterious effects of stress
on health (25).

Much theory and research on work organizations is also consistent with the idea that social support can reduce work stress,
improve health and buffer people against the unhealthy consequences
of occupational stress (13). All of this evidence, however, though
consistent with the theory of social support embodied in Figure 1
is also open to a variety of alternative interpretations, since
support has not been explicitly measured (and represents only one
of many ways in which the socially integrated, for example, may
differ from the more socially isolated), and since there is seldom
a comprehensive effort to test both the main effects of support on
stress and health and the potential buffering effect of support on
relations between stress and health.

The work in which I and my colleagues have been engaged these
past few years has attempted to provide more explicit measurement
of social support and direct tests of its main effects and buffering
effects in relation to occupational stress and health. I would
like to review in some detail two studies which applied similar
methods in different populations, arriving at generally consistent
conclusions with some interesting differences. At the end, I will
note some of the limitations of this work and important directions
for future basic and applied research.

## 3.2 Social Support, Stress and Health Among Factory Workers

The population for the first study was the hourly workforce
of a large tire, rubber, chemicals, and plastics manufacturing
plant. The measures of perceived stress, social support, and
health derive from self-administered questionnaires mailed to all
workers, with a response rate of 70% (N = 1,809) among white
males, the group used in the present analyses (there were too few

blacks and women for detailed analyses). Although the cross-
sectional and self-report nature of the data raises questions
about their validity and causal ordering which are dealt with
more extensively in previous reports (14, 32), the measures are
generally valid and reliable in comparison to any other questionnaire measures, and our results are most plausibly interpreted
as indicating that social support mitigates the effect of stress
on health. Analyses not reported here have showed the present
results to be unaffected by controls for age, smoking, and other
potential confounding variables (14).

We have examined how perceived social support from four
different sources (supervisors, coworkers, wives, and friends and
relatives) taken  singly and together in a measure of total
support conditions and buffers the relationship between self-
reported symptoms of five health outcomes (angina pectoris, ulcers,
itch and rash on skin, persistent cough and phlegm, and neurotic
symptoms) and seven indicators of perceived occupational stress:
job satisfaction and occupational self-esteem (lack of either is
stressful), workload, role conflict, responsibility, conflict
between job demands and non-job concerns, and quality concern or
worry over not being able to do one's work as well as one would
like. Items in the support measures are shown in Table 2 and the
intercorrelations of the variables are shown in Table 3. Most
notable in Table 3 is the lack of correlation between social
support and health except in the case of supervisor total support,
and the lack of correlation of support from wives and friends with
the occupational stress measures as well. On the basis solely of
these correlations, one might conclude that support from such
persons is irrelevant to the problem of occupational stress and
health, a quite erroneous conclusion in light of our further
analyses.

For each of the 35 possible combinations (Table 6) of seven
stress variables and five health outcomes, we used the regression
analysis methods described earlier (13, 16) to test whether each
of the four support measures as well as a  combined measure of
total support from all four sources conditions or buffers the
stress-health relationship in the manner depicted in Figure 2.
Results for the 35 tests involving total support are treated separately since they are clearly not independent of the 140 tests
involving support from supervisors, wives, coworkers, and friends
and relatives.

Our measure of total support reflects the cumulative amount
of support perceived from all four sources and approximates the
global support measure used in much previous research. Assuming
for heuristic purposes the 35 tests involving total support are
independent of each other, we would expect about 3-4 significant

Table 2.  Measures of Social Support Used by
House and Wells (16)

1. How much can each of these people be relied on when *things get tough
at work?*

| | Not at all | A little | Some- what | Very much | |
|---|---|---|---|---|---|
| A. Your immediate supervisor (boss) | 0 | 1 | 2 | 3 | |
| B. Other people at work | 0 | 1 | 2 | 3 | |
| C. Your wife (or husband) | 0 | 1 | 2 | 3 | Not Married |
| D. Your friends and relatives | 0 | 1 | 2 | 3 | |

2. How much is each of the following people *willing to listen to your work-
related problems?*

| | Not at all | A little | Some- what | Very much | |
|---|---|---|---|---|---|
| A. Your immediate supervisor (boss) | 0 | 1 | 2 | 3 | |
| B. Other people at work | 0 | 1 | 2 | 3 | |
| C. Your wife (or husband) | 0 | 1 | 2 | 3 | Not Married |
| D. Your friends and relatives | 0 | 1 | 2 | 3 | |

3. How much is each of the following people *helpful to you in getting your
job done?*

| | Not at all | A little | Some- what | Very much |
|---|---|---|---|---|
| A. Your immediate supervisor | 0 | 1 | 2 | 3 |
| B. Other people at work | 0 | 1 | 2 | 3 |

Please indicate *how true* each of the following statements is of your
*immediate supervisor.*

| | Not at all true | Not too true | Somewhat true | Very true |
|---|---|---|---|---|
| 7. My supervisor is *competent* in doing (his/her) job. | 0 | 1 | 2 | 3 |
| 8. My supervisor is very *concerned* about the welfare of those under him. | 0 | 1 | 2 | 3 |
| 9. My supervisor goes out of his way to *praise* good work | 0 | 1 | 2 | 3 |

(p = 0.10) results to occur by chance, and in only one or two of these cases should accord with the theoretically expected pattern of Figure 2. In fact, our test procedures yield significant results in 9 of the 35 tests, and the results accord with the buffering hypothesis expectation in all 9 of these cases, quite striking evidence that social support can indeed ameliorate the effects of occupational stress on self-reported symptoms of physical and mental health. Table 4 presents the regression coefficients for these analyses, along with predicted proportions of persons reporting marked symptoms of each health outcome at the highest and lowest levels of the stress variable within the highest vs. lowest levels of support. The last two columns of the table show that under maximum levels of social support, marked symptoms of self-reported ill health increase only slightly, if at all, as stress increases. In contrast, the two columns just to the left of these indicate that when social support is minimal, marked symptoms of ill health increase dramatically as stress increases.

Table 3. Correlations of Social Support Variables with Each Other, with Health Outcomes, and Work Stresses (13)

| | Supervisor Support | Coworker Support | Wife Support | Friend and Relative Support | Total Support |
|---|---|---|---|---|---|
| *Social Support* | | | | | |
| Supervisor Support | — | | | | |
| Coworker Support | .30 | — | | | |
| Wife Support | .11 | .29 | — | | |
| Friend & Relative Support | .16 | .32 | .62 | — | |
| Total Support | .78 | .62 | .58 | .64 | — |
| *Health Outcomes* | | | | | |
| Angina Pectoris | —.04 | — | — | — | — |
| Ulcers | —.06 | — | — | — | —.05 |
| Itch and Rash | —.10 | — | — | — | —.06 |
| Cough and Phlegm | —.05 | — | — | — | —.07 |
| Neurosis | —.07 | — | —.06 | — | —.10 |
| *Perceived Work Stresses* | | | | | |
| Job Satisfaction | .38 | .22 | .06 | .14 | .36 |
| Occupational Self-Esteem | .23 | .12 | — | — | .19 |
| Job-Nonjob Conflict | —.23 | —.10 | — | — | —.17 |
| Role Conflict | —.22 | —.10 | — | — | —.19 |
| Responsibility | —.13 | —.04 | — | — | —.11 |
| Quality Concern | —.39 | —.11 | — | — | —.29 |
| Workload | —.12 | —.08 | — | — | —.10 |

NOTE: Data are excerpted from Table 1 of House and Wells (1978). All coefficients are significant (p < .05, one-tailed). Nonsignificant coefficients are omitted and indicated by a "—."

It is noteworthy, however, that in almost every case where "total support" produced a conditioning effect, one of the four support measures composing it does also. Thus, the results for total support primarily reflect the impact of one or two particular sources of support, and it is critical to examine the results for each source of support as well, something which has seldom been done in studies using composite measures of support. Of the 140 tests of buffering effects of specific sources of support 24 yield statistically significant results, and 21 of these 24 accord with our predictions, four to five times as many as might occur by chance alone. Table 5 gives the same information for these 21 equations as Table 4 gave for those involving total support. Again, the last four columns indicate that perceived stress bears little or no relation to the health outcomes at the highest levels of support, but when social support is lowest self-reported symptoms of ill health rise sharply with stress.

Although 21 significant results out of 140 is in many ways a modest figure, it is important to note that these 21 effects are distributed over 18 different stress-health relationships. That is, over half of all the 35 stress-health relationships we have examined are significantly conditioned in the expected way by at least one form of social support. Table 6 summarizes the pattern of the results in Tables 4 and 5. Each of the 35 cells of the table represents a particular relationship between stress and health; within each cell are noted those measures of social support which significantly condition or buffer (in the predicted way) the impact of that stress on that health outcome.

Table 6 shows interesting patterns. First, as we expected, support from the most "significant" others is more effective in ameliorating effects of occupational stress on health. Of the 21 significant predicted conditioning effects of the four separate sources of support, nine occur with supervisor support and eight with wife support while only two occur with coworker support and two with friend and relative support. The potent effects of wives and supervisors and the weak effect of friends and relatives were as expected. However, the essentially chance level result for coworker support was somewhat surprising to us. We speculated that the organization of work in this plant (e.g., many individual and machine-bound jobs, tight management control of work scheduling and processes, high-noise levels) may make it unlikely that workers other than supervisors can do much to alleviate stress and/or its effects. Here the effects of coworker support might be greater in occupations or industries which inherently require greater coordination and communication. These speculations receive confirmation in the second study to be discussed shortly.

Table 4

REGRESSION EQUATIONS OF SIGNIFICANT, PREDICTED CONDITIONING EFFECTS OF TOTAL SOCIAL SUPPORT ON RELATIONSHIPS BETWEEN PERCEIVED STRESS AND HEALTH

| Health Outcome / Perceived Stress | Support Source | Inter-cept $a$ | Stress $b_1$ | Stress Support $b_2$ | Stress Support $b_3$ | Predicted Proportions with "Marked Symptoms" | | | |
|---|---|---|---|---|---|---|---|---|---|
| | | | | | | Lowest Support | | Highest Support | |
| | | | | | | Lowest Stress | Highest Stress | Lowest Stress | Highest Stress |
| **Angina Pectoris** | | | | | | | | | |
| None | None | — | — | — | — | — | — | — | — |
| **Ulcers** | | | | | | | | | |
| Job Satisfaction | Total Support | .3178* | -.0253* | -.0069* | .0009+ | .065 | .318 | .149 | .042 |
| Esteem | " | .4825* | -.0216+ | -.0124+ | .0007+ | .094 | .483 | .102 | (-.014) |
| Job-Nonjob Conflict | " | .0875+ | .0286+ | .0008 | -.0009+ | .088 | .431 | .120 | .031 |
| Role Conflict | " | .0656 | .0322+ | .0014 | -.0010+ | .066 | .452 | .122 | .028 |
| Workload | " | .0473 | .0209+ | .0032 | -.0008+ | .047 | .298 | .175 | .042 |
| **Itch/Rash** | | | | | | | | | |
| None | None | — | — | — | — | — | — | — | — |
| **Cough/Phlegm** | | | | | | | | | |
| Esteem | Total Support | .4124+ | -.0141o | -.0132+ | .0007o | .159 | .412 | (-.116) | .135 |
| **Neurosis** | | | | | | | | | |
| Esteem | Total Support | .5592* | -.0237* | -.0125* | .0006+ | .133 | .559 | .065 | .059 |
| Role Conflict | " | .0321 | .0545* | .0017 | -.0016* | .032 | .686 | .100 | (-.014) |
| Responsibility | " | .1129+ | .0291+ | -.0009 | -.0008o | .113 | .462 | .077 | .042 |

* p<.01   + p<.05   o p<.10

from James S. House and James A. Wells, "Occupational stress, social support, and health." In A. McLean, G. Black and M. Colligan (eds.), Reducing Occupational Stress: Proceedings of a Conference. DHEW(NIOSH) Publication No. 78-140. 8-29.

Table 5

REGRESSION EQUATIONS OF SIGNIFICANT, PREDICTED CONDITIONING EFFECTS OF TOTAL SOCIAL SUPPORT ON RELATIONSHIPS BETWEEN PERCEIVED STRESS AND HEALTH

| Health Outcome / Perceived Stress | Support Source | Inter-cept $a$ | Stress $b_1$ | Support $b_2$ | Stress Support $b_3$ | Predicted Proportions with "Marked Symptoms" | | | |
|---|---|---|---|---|---|---|---|---|---|
| | | | | | | Lowest Support | | Highest Support | |
| | | | | | | Lowest Stress | Highest Stress | Lowest Stress | Highest Stress |
| **Angina Pectoris** | | | | | | | | | |
| Job Satisfaction | Wife | .1211* | -.0088+ | -.0136* | .0018+ | .033 | .121 | .064 | .026 |
| Work Self-Esteem | Wife | .1412* | -.0051° | -.0195 | .0012+ | .049 | .141 | .064 | .005 |
| **Ulcers** | | | | | | | | | |
| Job Satisfaction | Supervisor | .2668* | -.0176+ | -.0104+ | .0012° | .091 | .267 | .117 | .080 |
| Esteem | Supervisor | .4919* | -.0232* | -.0294* | .0018* | .074 | .492 | .128 | (-.037) |
| Job-Nonjob Conflict | Supervisor | .0804* | .0261* | .0026 | -.0078+ | .080 | .394 | .127 | .052 |
| Job-Nonjob Conflict | Friend/Relative | .0924* | .0178+ | .0037 | -.0027° | .092 | .306 | .115 | .134 |
| Role Conflict | Supervisor | .0781* | .0246* | .0021 | -.0015+ | .078 | .466 | .208 | .180 |
| Workload | Coworker | .0302 | .0160+ | .0169* | -.0026+ | .030 | .222 | .132 | .136 |
| Workload | Friend/Relative | .0679° | .0119 | .0170 | -.0032 | .068 | .211 | .170 | .082 |
| **Itch/Rash** | | | | | | | | | |
| Job Satisfaction | Wife | .3829* | -.0340* | -.0216+ | .0032+ | .043 | .383 | .295 | .232 |
| Work Self-Esteem | Supervisor | .4705* | -.0168+ | -.0238+ | .0012+ | .168 | .471 | .042 | .129 |
| **Cough/Phlegm** | | | | | | | | | |
| Role Conflict | Supervisor | .0260 | .0324* | .0051 | -.0019* | .026 | .415 | .118 | .096 |
| Responsibility | Supervisor | .0537 | .0235* | .0042 | -.0016+ | .054 | .336 | .129 | .066 |
| Workload | Supervisor | .0007 | .0233* | .0064 | -.0014° | .001 | .280 | .116 | .093 |
| **Neurosis** | | | | | | | | | |
| Job Satisfaction | Wife | .4277* | -.0421* | -.0274* | .0035* | .000 | .428 | .060 | .236 |
| Work Self-Esteem | Coworker | .4698* | -.0218* | -.0335* | .0021+ | .077 | .470 | .103 | .269 |
| Role Conflict | Supervisor | .0166 | .0438* | .0053° | -.0024+ | .017 | .542 | .112 | .119 |
| Role Conflict | Wife | .0628* | .0358* | .0007 | -.0029+ | .063 | .492 | .068 | .254 |
| Quality Concern | Wife | .0578° | .0294* | .0003 | -.0023+ | .058 | .411 | .060 | .220 |
| Responsibility | Wife | .0774+ | .0267* | .0019 | -.0028+ | .077 | .398 | .091 | .176 |
| Workload | Wife | .0006 | .0287* | .0123 | -.0033* | .001 | .345 | .067 | .154 |

* $p<.01$  + $p<.05$  ° $p<.10$

from James S. House and James A. Wells, "Occupational stress, social support, and health." In A. McLean, G. Black and M. Colligan (eds.), Reducing Occupational Stress: Proceedings of a Conference. DHEW(NIOSH) Publication No. 78-140, 8-29.

Table 6. Summary of Significant Buffering Effects
of Social Support on Relationships Between
Perceived Stress and Health (13)

| PERCEIVED STRESS | HEALTH OUTCOME | | | | |
|---|---|---|---|---|---|
| | Angina Pectoris | Ulcers | Itching and Rash | Cough and Phlegm | Neurosis |
| Job Satisfaction | Wife | Supervisor<br>Total | Wife | | Wife |
| Work Self-Esteem | Wife | Supervisor<br>Total | Supervisor | Total | Coworker<br>Total |
| Job versus Nonjob Conflict | | Supervisor<br>Friend and Relative<br>Total | | | |
| Role Conflict | | Supervisor<br>Total | Supervisor | | Supervisor<br>Wife<br>Total |
| Quality Concern | | | | | Wife |
| Responsibility | | | | Supervisor | Wife<br>Total |
| Workload | | Coworker<br>Friend and Relative<br>Total | | Supervisor | Wife |

NOTE: Cell entries indicate measures of support that significantly buffer each health-stress relationship.

A second notable feature of Table 6 (also evident in Tables 4 and 5) is that support mitigates the effects of stress on ulcers and neurosis more than on other health outcomes. In fact, the results for the other health outcomes are not substantially greater than what might occur by chance. Again, this pattern is not unexpected in light of research which has especially emphasized the role of interpersonal processes in the etiology of ulcers (30) and neurosis (17). Support appears in these data, then, to buffer the effects of stress on some diseases (disorders) more than others.

## 3.3   Social Support, Stress and Health in 23 Occupations

The second study I want to discuss involved reanalyzing originally collected data by Caplan et al. (4) and analyzed by Pinneau
(26, 27) with respect to social support.  This study was based
primarily on questionnaire responses from male workers in 23 occupations ranging from physicians to assemblers and working in 67
different organizations or settings spread over the eastern, mid-
western, and southern United States.  Though hardly a probability
sample, the respondents in this study were more broadly representative of the total labor force than our earlier rubber workers
sample.  The analyses reported here are based on a subset of this
sample, which gives equal weight to each occupational group.
Measures of support closely parallel those in the House and Wells
(16) research, except that spouse and friend and relative support
were collapsed into a single measure of "home" support.  The
measures of perceived stress in the two studies are also similar,
while the health measures were comparable enough to allow some
replication, as well as extension of the earlier analyses (16).

Given the similarity of the studies, the failure of Pinneau
(26, 27) to replicate our buffering results was troubling and
perplexing.  Even more so since many of Pinneau's other findings
closely paralleled the House and Wells study.  His summary of the
main effects of support on work stresses and both job-related and
general psychological strains (indicative of poor mental health)
corresponds closely with the results seen in Table 3 except that
the effects of coworker support rival or exceed those of supervisor
support:

> Support from home had little effect on job stresses,
> while support from supervisor and from coworkers both
> had numerous effects on a variety of stress measures.
> The size of the correlations varied considerably from
> occupation to occupation, but the direction of signif-
> icant effects was almost always as predicted.  Men
> with high support from either supervisor or coworkers
> generally reported low role conflict, low role ambig-
> uity and low future ambiguity, high participation,
> and good utilization of their skills...  The magnitude
> of these correlations were often in the .30s and
> sometimes in the .40s...  social support predicted
> significantly to low levels of psychological strain in
> a number of instances...  home support correlated much
> less often with the job dissatisfaction measures than
> supervisor and coworker support.  Each of the general
> affective strains (i.e., depression, anxiety, and
> irritation) was, however, affected by both home and
> work support measures. (27, pp. 35-36)

Pinneau (26, 27) reported no more significant buffering effects in these data than might occur by chance. His analysis strategy for buffering effects, however, contained certain logical and technical flaws, most importantly failure to test for buffering unless support had main effects on stress and health. Reanalysis of these data by LaRocco, House and French (20), using methods comparable to those of House and Wells (16) discussed above, showed that support did indeed buffer the impact of stress on general psychological strains (e.g., anxiety, depression, somatic complaints). This analysis examined the impact of 9 measures of perceived work stress (see first 9 rows of Table 7) on 3 measures of general affects about the job (see last 3 rows of Table 7, e.g., boredom and dissatisfaction) and 4 general indicators of psychological strain (see columns of Table 7, i.e., anxiety, depression, irritation, and somatic complaints). The impact of job-related affects on general psychological strains were also examined.

These analyses revealed many more buffering effects than might occur by chance with respect to the general indicators of psychological strain, but only chance level results with respect to job-related affects, most notably job dissatisfaction. In almost all cases where impact of stress on psychological strain varied significantly across levels of support, the pattern of results indicated a pure buffering effect. For example, if social support from coworkers is low, somatic complaints increase as perceived stress increases; but if coworker support is high, perceived stress is not associated with increased somatic complaints. That is, in these data high social support can completely eliminate deleterious impact of stress on mental health.

The overall pattern of the results with respect to psychological strains is presented in Table 7. There are twelve measures of perceived stresses and job-related affects which can affect general psychological effects or strain. The first five perceived stress measures asked people directly whether they perceived aspects of the job as stressful or unpleasant. The last four were more experimental, constructed by taking the difference between people's reports of what their job was like and what they wished it to be like on four dimensions (workload, role ambiguity, etc.). For a number of reasons, the last three "fit" measures did not work well in most aspects of the larger study. Nor do they produce many positive results here.

If we exclude these last three "fit" measures from consideration, there are 36 relationships in Table 7 of the first five perceived stresses, workload fit and the three job-related affects to the four psychological strains. Of these 27 exhibit statistically significant and theoretically expected buffering effects from some form of social support. That is, 75% of the potential

deleterious effects on psychological strain are alleviated by
some form of social support, evidence quite consistent with the
House and Wells (16) study.

Table 7.  Significant Buffering Effects of Social Support
on Relationship of Perceived Stress and Job-
Related Affects to General Psychological Strain
(13)

| Perceived Stress/ Job-Related Affect | Psychological Strain | | | |
|---|---|---|---|---|
| | Depression | Irritation | Anxiety | Somatic Complaints |
| *Perceived Stresses* Role Conflict | Coworker Home | Supervisor Coworker Home | Coworker | Coworker Home |
| Future Ambiguity | Coworker | Supervisor | Supervisor | |
| Underutilization | Coworker | | | Coworker |
| Participation | Supervisor | Supervisor | | Coworker |
| Workload | Coworker | Supervisor Coworker | | Coworker |
| Workload Fit | Coworker Home | Coworker Home | Coworker Home | Coworker Home |
| Role Ambiguity Fit | | Coworker | | |
| Complexity Fit | | Supervisor Home | | |
| Responsibility Fit | | | | |
| *Job-Related Affects* Job Dissatisfaction | Supervisor Coworker | | Supervisor Coworker | |
| Boredom | Coworker Home | | Supervisor Coworker | Supervisor Coworker Home |
| Workload dis- satisfaction | Coworker Home | Coworker Home | Coworker | |

However, the relative importance of different sources of
social support is different in Table 7 than in the earlier study.
Of 36 relationships which might be buffered by a given source of
support, 9 are buffered by supervisor support, 12 by home support,
and 23 by coworker support.  Thus, supervisor and home support,
which were the most consequential forms of support in the House

and Wells study, remain important here, buffering between one-quarter and one-third of all stress-strain relationships. But coworker support emerges in these data as about twice as important, buffering almost two-thirds of the 36 possible stress-strain relationships.

Thus, these data further indicate that different sources, and perhaps types of support, are important in different contexts. In an earlier study by Cobb and Kasl of men losing their jobs, support from people outside of work, especially spouses, was critical because work-related sources of support were less available. House and Wells (16) speculated that coworkers were not very consequential sources of support in their data, because the organization of work in the factory study tended to isolate workers from each other, physically and socially. Thus, supervisors became the most available and important sources of support at work. The wider range of occupations studied by LaRocco et al. (20) included professional, managerial, supervisory, craft and service (e.g., police) workers, all of whom are often only nominally supervised and hence rely heavily on work peers and colleagues for support. Police officers get social support more from their patrol mates than from supervisors, too and die makers from their fellow craftsmen, and physicians, scientists, and engineers from their professional colleagues (to name just a few of the occupations in this study). In sum, we all can benefit from social support in relation to our particular occupational stresses, but who can give us the most effective support depends on the kind of work we do and the kind of stresses it imposes.

Another interesting consistency between these two studies is that neither found any evidence of support buffering of relations between perceived stress and job-related affects (i.e., job satisfaction, occupational self-esteem, boredom). This is part of the overall pattern of results in which support buffers some effects but not others. Support often has main effects on variables involved in relationships which are not buffered by support. Figuring out why some relations are buffered by some sources of support, but not others, and some relationships buffered by none is a major puzzle for further research. The existing knowledge suggests some possible reasons for not finding buffering effects.

In some cases buffering may be concealed in cross-sectional studies, especially using subjective measures of stress (13). However, the systematic nature of differences in relationships buffered suggests that something more than methodological artifact is involved. Specifically, the buffering effects of support may be mainly what my colleague John R. P. French, Jr. (personal communication) has termed "strain-responsive". That is, we offer support to others when we observe their manifesting symptoms which

we regard as pathological or undesirable and amenable to influence
by support. Thus we may regard anxiety, depression and ulcer
symptoms as serious enough to elicit our support, while job dissatisfaction and boredom are within normal range of experience,
elicit no special response. Thus we observe buffering effects of
support with respect to these health outcomes, but not the job-
related affects. Similarly, angina, respiratory and dermatological
symptoms may be serious, but many people may not see them or
especially stress-related or amenable to influence by support.


## 4   CONCLUSION

On balance, the available evidence suggests that social
support is a potent variable which both has main effects on stress
and health and buffers the relation between them. The evidence also
suggests, however, that all types of support are not equally effective in these regards and all types of stress and health are not
equally affected. Thus, it is probably time to stop simply trying
to debate or prove whether social support is related to stress and
health, and to begin more careful analysis of the conditions under
which support does or does not affect stress and health, and of
the mechanisms through which support operates. The work in which
we have been engaged has moved increasingly in this direction,
but much remains to be done.

We also need to begin paying greater attention to the causes
or determinants of social support as well as its effects or consequences (13). Social support is not a panacea for all problems
of work stress and health, but it can be one element of a larger
strategy for eventually reducing work stress and its deleterious
impact on health. Such application of our knowledge of social
support requires, however, that we understand the social structural,
interpersonal, and psychological variables which facilitate or
inhibit the development of supportive social relationships and a
felt sense of support. These variables constitute the levers of
change which must be used in any attempt to reduce stress or improve
health by enhancing levels of social support.

It is not premature to begin thinking about such efforts to
enhance levels of support as a means of reducing stress and improving
health (13). Initially, these efforts should be undertaken in the
form of field experiments, so that we can carefully evaluate our
ability to enhance social support and monitor its effects on stress
and health. The knowledge gained from such experiments can not only
improve future applied efforts, it can also help to resolve some
of the more difficult scientific problems in the study of social
support (e.g., is support really a cause of decreased stress,
improved health, or a lessened impact of stress on health?).

Social support has much to contribute to understanding and alleviating problems of work stress and health. Work organizations provide ideal contexts for efforts to enhance social support (e.g., from supervisors and/or coworkers) because channels of influence already exist and because more supportive supervisory and peer relationships are generally congruent with other goals of such organizations (e.g., increased productivity, reduced absenteeism, less turnover, higher morale). There is a strong tendency to emphasize individualistic strategies (e.g., biofeedback, individual counseling, exercise and relaxation) in existing programs of stress-reduction or management. Our knowledge of social support suggests a different strategy, placing greater emphasis on collective approaches to reducing and managing stress. Ultimately, each individual must learn to adapt to his or her particular work and life situation. But we all must recognize the importance of also seeking social and organizational responses to what are inherently social and organizational problems.

REFERENCES

1. Antonovsky, A. Health, Stress and Coping (San Francisco, Jossey-Bass, 1979).
2. Berkman, L.F. and S.L. Syme. Social Networks, Host Resistance, and Mortality: A Nine-Year Follow-Up Study of Alameda County Residents. American Journal of Epidemiology 100 (1979) 186-204.
3. Caplan, G. and M. Killilea. Support Systems and Mutual Help (New York, Grune and Stratton, 1976).
4. Caplan, R.D. et al. Job Demands and Worker Health (U.S. Department of Health, Education and Welfare, HEW Publication No. (NIOSH) 75-160, 1975).
5. Cassel, J. The Contribution of the Social Environment Host Resistance. American Journal of Epidemiology 102 (1976) 107-123.
6. Cobb, S. Social Support as a Moderator of Life Stress. Psychosomatic Medicine 38 (1976) 300-314.
7. Cohen, F. Personality, Stress, and the Development of Physical Disease. in G.C. Stone, F. Cohen, and N.E. Adler (eds.) Health Psychology (San Francisco, Jossey-Bass, 1978), pp. 77-111.
8. Durkheim, E. Suicide (New York, Free Press, 1951).
9. Gottlieb, B.H. The Development and Application of a Classification Scheme of Informal Helping Behaviours. Canadian Journal of Science 10 (1978) 105-115.
10. Gove, W.R. The Relationship Between Sex Roles, Marital Status and Mental Illness. Social Forces 51 (1972) 34-44.
11. Gove, W.R. Sex, Marital Status and Mortality. American Journal of Sociology 70 (1973) 45-67.

12. Heller, K. The Effects of Social Support: Prevention and Treatment Implications, in A.P. Goldstein and F.H. Kanfer (eds.) Maximizing Treatment Gains: Transfer Enhancement in Psychotherapy (New York, Academic Press, 1979) pp. 353-382.
13. House, J.S. Work Stress and Social Support (Reading, Mass., Addison-Wesley, 1981).
14. House, J.S. et al. Occupational Stress and Health Among Factory Workers. Journal of Health and Social Behavior 20 (1979) 139-160.
15. House, J.S., C. Robbins, and H.L. Metzner. The Association of Social Relationships and Activities with Mortality: Prospective Evidence from the Tecumseh Community Health Study (Unpublished manuscript, University of Michigan, 1981).
16. House, J.S. and J.A. Wells. Occupational Stress, Social Support, and Health, in A. McLean, G. Black and M. Colligan (eds.) Reducing Occupational Stress: Proceedings of a Conference (DHEW (NIOSH) Publication No. 78-140, 1978) pp. 8-29.
17. Jaco, E.G. Mental Illness in Response to Stress, in S. Levine and N.A. Scotch (eds.) Social Stress (Chicago, Aldine, 1970) pp. 210-217.
18. Kahn, R.L. and T.C. Antonucci. Convoys Over the Life Course: Attachment, Roles and Social Support, in P.B. Baltes and O. Brim (eds.) Life-Span Development and Behavior (Vol. 3), (New York, Academic Press, 1980) pp. 253-286.
19. Kaplan, B.H., J.C. Cassel and S. Gore. Social Support and Helath. Medical Care 25 (1977) 47-58.
20. LaRocco, J.M., J.S. House, and J.R.P. French, Jr. Social Support, Occupational Stress and Health. Journal of Health and Social Behavior 21 (1980) 202-218.
21. Lin, N. et al. Social Support, Stressful Life Events and Illness: A Model and an Empirical Test. Journal of Health and Social Behavior 20 (1979) 108-119.
22. Nerem, R.M., M.J. Lévesque, and J.F. Cornhill. Social environment as a Factor in Diet-Induced Atherosclerosis. Science 208 (1980) 1475-1476.
23. Nuckolls, K.B., J. Cassel, and B.H. Kaplan. Psychosocial Assets, Life Crisis and the Prognosis of Pregnancy. American Journal of Epidemiology 95 (1972) 431-441.
24. Ortmeyer, C.F. Variations in Mortality, Morbidity, and Health Care by Marital Status, in C.E. Erhardt, J.E. Berlin (eds.) Mortality and Morbidity in the United States (Cambridge, Harvard University Press, 1974).
25. Pearlin, L. and J. Johnson. Marital Status, Life Strains, and Depression. American Sociological Review 42 (1977) 704-715.
26. Pinneau, S.R. Effects of Social Support on Psychological and Physiological Stress. (Unpublished doctoral dissertation, University of Michigan, 1975).
27. Pinneau, S.R. Effects of Social Support on Occupational Stresses and Strains. (Paper presented at American Psychological Association, Washington D.C., 1976).

28. President's Commission on Mental Health. Report to the President. Vols. I-IV. (Washington D.C., Government Printing Office, 1978).
29. Selye, H. Forty Years of Stress Research: Principal Remaining Problems and Misconceptions. CMA Journal 115 (1976) 53-56.
30. Susser, M. Causes of Peptic Ulcer. Journal of Chronic Disease 20 (1967) 435-456.
31. Wallston, B.S. et al. Social Support and Physical Health. (Unpublished manuscript, Peabody College, 1981).
32. Wells, J. Social Support a Buffer of Stressful Job Conditions. (Unpublished doctoral dissertation, Duke University, 1978).

BARRIERS TO WORK STRESS:  II.  THE HARDY PERSONALITY

Suzanne C. Kobasa

Department of Behavioral Sciences
University of Chicago
Chicago, Illinois

Business executives, lawyers, and U.S. Army officers have at least three things in common:  (a) they are subjected to significant numbers of stressful life events in their work, (b) many members of each occupational group remain mentally and physically healthy in the face of even high stress levels, and (c) their health is explained, in part, by their characteristic personality styles which interact with other stress-resistance resources to buffer the negative impact of stressful life events. These are the general conclusions of a series of stress studies conducted on different occupational groups.  All were guided by the question:  How is it that some persons do not get sick following their encounter with frequent and serious life stresses? Each professional group provided a complementary but slightly different answer emphasizing personality.

In this paper, I would first like to consider the stress-resistance of business executives, U.S. Army officers, and lawyers in turn.  Because they were the first group to be studied, and the group chosen for longitudinal and prospective investigation, business executives are discussed most extensively.  But the lawyers and Army officers should be recognized as more than mere opportun-ities for replication of the executive results.  By the final section of this paper, both similarities and differences across the professional groups should be apparent.  The differences require the reconceptualization of profession or occupational context as itself a stress-resistance resource.  This broader view of stress-resistance, which encompasses both the psychological dimension of personality and the sociocultural dimension of occupation, allows a better understanding of how it is that persons stay healthy under work stress, and some suggestions for stress intervention within the work setting.

## 1 EXECUTIVE STUDY I

A study of business executives (24) was chosen as the best
place to start. At the time of its initiation, the investigation
into how people stay healthy under stress necessarily stood out
as a reaction to ongoing research in the stress area. In 1975,
the emphasis was still on how people stay healthy under stress.
Literally thousands of studies had been done which reported a low
but significant correlation between the occurrence of stressful
life events and the onset of physical and mental illness (cf. 10).
Using easy to administer and score instruments like the Schedule
of Recent Life Events and the Social Readjustment Survey (19),
many investigators appeared preoccupied with simply counting the
number of events subjects checked off as having happened to them,
weighing each event in terms of its consensually defined stressfulness weight, and summing across them to obtain a total stress
score which could then be associated with some indicator of
illness like number of physical symptoms reported, amount of medication requested, or length of hospital stay. These observed
stress and illness links, interpreted in the framework of Hans
Selye's general adaptation syndrome, led investigators to conclude
that stressful life events evoke "adaptive efforts by the human
organism that are faulty in kind or duration, lower 'bodily
resistance' and enhance the probability of disease occurrence"
(18, p. 68). This research was quickly taken up and elaborated
on by the popular media. Magazine and newspaper articles and
radio and television shows announced: Stress causes illness;
avoid stressful life events if you want to stay healthy (47).

In the face of this simple and pessimistic proclamation
about stress and illness, a question about the psychological
variables which might serve to weaken the positive correlation or
to buffer the effects of stress appeared unusually and unnecessarily
complex. To make it viable as well as provacative, it was
essential to ask the question of persons likely to be undergoing
high degrees of stressful life events, and with some chance of
proving to do well under them. Given the common assumption about
the responsibilities, pressures, and hectic pace of their lives,
and the fact that the marketplace and economy of the U.S.A. are
still reasonably successful, businessmen were selected as likely
candidates for placement in the high stressful life events/low
illness category.

The specific nature of the company in which all of these
executives worked was also relevant to the purposes of the
intended study. Although a public utility, and thereby not
generally thought to be as stressful a place to work in as is

a more market-determined company like Chrysler, Illinois Bell
Telephone provided a good context for observing both stress
and stress-resistance. The initiation of the study coincided
with the beginning of what are now clearly seen as drastic
changes in the Bell System, as the company prepares for being
a deregulated and competitive organization. The majority of the
middle and upper level executives who served as subjects did
indeed begin working in the company when it was still a very
secure and predictable organization, more like a Type Z than a
Type A company (cf. 35). But at the time of the stress data
collection, their company had become a shifting environment in
which an individual executive's career path could no longer be
so easily plotted. For example, many of the stressful life events
observed in the first year of the study were results of new
programs instituted by the utility like a job reevaluation
program through which many executives were promoted and many more
demoted. At the same time, increases in stress levels could also
be attributed to sources external to the company. Most stress-
inducing were changes brought on by affirmative action demands,
and government actions aimed at curbing the utility's so-called
monopolistic practices.

In spite of the switch to a more stressful environment,
the medical director of Illinois Bell Telephone, Dr. Robert
R. J. Hilker, maintained that there were many executives who
showed no signs of strain, i.e., the physical and mental debilitation typically associated with stress reactions. Further,
he pointed out that a significant number of those executives
at the top, whom he judged to be subject to the most serious and
frequent stressful life events in the current company situation,
were among the healthiest employees in the organization.

The first study attempted an empirical demonstration and
explanation of Dr. Hilker's remarks. The general proposition
was that there would be in the company both executives who
experienced high degrees of stressful life events and became
ill (high stress/high illness executives), and executives who
remained healthy under comparably high stress (high stress/
low illness executives), and that one could distinguish between
the two groups by referring to personality style. Personality
"hardiness" was hypothesized to be significantly greater in
executives who stayed healthy than it was in those debilitated
by stress. By personality hardiness was meant the constellation
of three distinct but interacting personality characteristics:
commitment, control, and challenge.

## 1.1 Conceptual Framework

Before presenting the specific hypothesis associated with each
of these personality characteristics, it would be helpful to review

the general theoretical orientation with which I was working.
Part of my reaction to the then current emphasis in stress research
was a reaction to the insistence by some stress researchers on a
fundamentally passive and reactive view of human behavior.  I
saw persons portrayed as mere victims of their environments in
those studies which predicted the likelihood of a subject's
falling ill solely on the basis of his stressful life event score
(e.g., a score of 300 or above on the Holmes and Rahe scale was
associated with an 80% chance of getting sick in the near future).
Left out of these formulations was Selye's notion that there
are organisms so constituted as to seek out stress without danger
of illness.

I chose to approach the stress question armed with a very
different view of human nature, one which emphasized human
initiative and resilliency rather than passivity and vulnerability.
There are several roots for my more optimistic orientation
from those philosopher/psychologists represented by William
James on the strenuous mood, Erich Fromm on the productive,
Gordon Allport on propriate striving, and Robert White on
competence, to the contemporary social psychologists like
Albert Bandura on self-efficacy and Jack Brehm on reactance.
All of these theorists assume that persons create as well as
react to the stressful life events in their lives, and thrive
on as well as tolerate stressful situations.  But it was within
existential personality theory (26) that I found the particular
notion of hardiness, and the most comprehensive model for
understanding how personality might interact with stressful life
events to promote health.  Existentialism portrays life as
always changing, and thereby, stressful.  The crucial problem
for both existential philosophers and psychologists has been
the elucidation of how persons best confront, utilize, and
transform this changing life.  Existential theory offers a
definition of personality as healthy or ideal when it consists
of characteristic interests, motivations, and values which
influence the successful perception and interpretation of and coping
with stressful life events.

The first hypothesis involved commitment: Among persons under
stress, those who feel committed to the various areas of their
lives will remain healthier than those who are without commitment,
or alienated.  Commitment is defined as the ability to believe in
the truth, importance, and interest value of who one is and what
one is doing.  With this comes a tendency to fully involve oneself
in the many situations of life, including work, family, social
institutions, and interpersonal relationships.  Commitment to
self allows one to recognize one's distinctive goals and
priorities, and to value the ability to make decisions. This
kind of self-assessment supports the internal structure and
strength that White and other theorists deem essential for the

handling of any life situation. Further, with this kind of overall sense of purpose, the committed person is prevented from being overwhelmed by the threat of any given life event.

Commitment to others also serves as a generalized resistance resource against the impact of stress (2). Committed persons benefit from both the knowledge that they can turn to others in stressful times if they need to, and a sense of accountability, or the recognition that others are counting on their not giving up easily under pressure. Committed persons have an ability and reason to cope successfully with stress.

The second hypothesis involved control: Among persons under stress, those who have a greater sense of control over what occurs in their lives will remain healthier than those who feel powerless in the face of external realities. Control is defined as the tendency to believe and act as if one has influence over the course of life's events. Persons with control seek explanations for why something happened not simply in terms of others' actions or fate, but rather with an emphasis on their own responsibility. The efficacy of control in warding off the harmful effects of stress has been suggested in a wide range of laboratory and field studies (3, 15, 29, 40, 43). Control allows persons to perceive many stressful life events as predictable consequences of their own activity, and thereby, as subject to their own future direction and transformation. The executive who appreciates the role he has had in bringing about his recent job transfer also recognizes the influence he will continue to have over its effects on his work and family life. But even those events which a person is not likely to have caused, e.g., death of a parent, are also best confronted with a spirit of control. Control involves the possession of a wide and varied coping repertoire (3). In the face of any stressful life event, persons in control should benefit from a sense of generalized autonomy and efficacy.

The third hypothesis involved challenge: Among persons under stress, those who view change as a challenge will remain healthier than those who view it as a threat. Challenge is defined as the tendency to value the change and unpredictability necessarily involved in living. The person who has a sense of challenge can perceive much of the disruption associated with the occurrence of a stressful life event as an opportunity and incentive for personal growth. The event is thereby not a threat. Challenge also leads persons to be catalysts in their environments, and to practice responding to the unexpected. Because of the value of the new and interesting experiences, persons who welcome challenge have explored their surroundings and know where to turn for resources to aid them in coping with stress. Further, they are characterized by an openness or cognitive flexibility and a tolerance of ambiguity. This allows them to integrate and

effectively appraise even the most unexpected of stressful
life events (34).

## 1.2 Procedure

The first procedural task was the identification of high
stress/low illness and high stress/high illness executive groups.
To this end, all of the middle and upper level executives ($\bar{n}$ = 837)
at the telephone company were asked to complete a stressful life
events and illness questionnaire. Those 670 executives who
responded checked off those events and illnesses which they had
experienced in the preceding $3\frac{1}{2}$ years indicating exact month and
year of each occurrence.

The measure of stressful life events was an adaptation of the
familiar Holmes and Rahe (19) Schedule of Recent Life Events.
Like the original, the executives' questionnaire was a list of
positive (e.g., job promotion), negative (e.g., illness of a
family member), common (e.g., traffic violation), and rare
(e.g., death of a child) occurrences. Adaptations of the
original included the specification of ambiguous items, and the
addition of stressful events peculiar to the distinctive population
under study. An example of the latter was the replacement of the
item "change in financial state" with two items: "improvement
in financial state" and "worsening of financial condition."
Fifteen new life events were added on the basis of a pilot
administration of the questionnaire with management personnel
of the utility not subsequently used as subjects. Additions
included "loss of a mentor" and "government ruling which disrupts
my office." Executives' total stress scores were computed using
the standard Holmes and Rahe procedure: each event checked
was multiplied by its consensual stressfulness weight, and all
products were summed. This provided a score indicating how
stressful an executive's life would be perceived to be by an
average person in our culture. Some stress investigators (22)
have advocated replacing the consensual stressfulness weights
for events with idiosyncratic or subjective weights provided
by the subjects themselves. I have not followed this suggestion.
As Dohrenwend, Krasnoff, Askenasy, and Dohrenwend (11) have
pointed out, subjective weights represent the confusing combination of the effects of environmental changes, the stressed
individual's personality and other predispositions, and his
or her evaluation of the consequences of the stressful event.
It was more appropriate, for the purposes of this study, to
determine the effects of consensually-defined stressfulness of
events separately from the effects of personality dispositions
on health and illness, and thereby obtain independent personal and
environmental effects.

The measure of illness was the Seriousness of Illness Survey (48), a self-report check list of 126 commonly recognized physical and mental diseases. In the development of this instrument, a general severity weight for each disorder was obtained by asking large samples of physicians and lay persons to rate each of them. Their ratings reflect prognosis, threat to life, duration, and degree of disability and discomfort. A highly significant mean rank order correlation was obtained between the various samples of judges, and a system of weights was accordingly constructed.

Both the Wyler et al. illness scale and the Schedule of Recent Life Events have been frequent tools in stress studies. They have, in fact, provided much of the basis for the claim by the popular media that stress causes illness. But these two scales have also provided extremely variable stress and illness scores with standard deviations as large as 8 times the size of the mean. The range of correlations between stress and illness scores has also been very wide, with the majority of correlations falling below .30, and frequently around .12 (38). These results suggest some association between stressful life events and illness onset. But they also indicate that there are subjects with high stress scores who are not getting sick, and they provoke questions about what other sorts of variables explain illness variance.

Subjects reporting high stress levels but little illness were indeed identified in the executive group. One hundred and twenty-six executives who scored above the median on total stress, and below the median score for total illness made up the high stress/low illness group. High stress/high illness executives were those 200 men who showed scores above the median for both stress and illness. These were the two groups that I was interested in. Before sending them a questionnaire designed to identify the differences between them, membership in both groups was reduced. Removed from the high stress/high illness group were 40 cases whose peak illness scores preceded rather than followed their peak stress score. At the request of the company that not all executives be involved in this state of personality testing, 100 cases were randomly selected from each of the two groups for administration of the personality hardiness questionnaire.

Included in the composite personality questionnaire were several standardized instruments thought to be appropriate for a test of the 3 hardiness hypotheses. Included were the Personality Research Form (21), the Internal-External Locus of Control Scale (41), the Alienation vs. Commitment Test (31), the California Life Goals Evaluation Schedules (17), and an adaptation of the Self-Consistency Test (14). Each of these instruments has been described at length elsewhere (24).

Executives were also asked in this second questionnaire about some possibly discriminating demographics, including age, job level, and time spent at current job level. It was already known at this point in the study that on other demographics there was remarkable homogeneity both within and across the two groups. Both high stress/low illness and high stress/high illness group had the following modal characteristics: White, male, married with two children, college-educated, and Protestant.

## 1.3 Results

Both executive groups had experienced, on the average, sufficient change and demands for readjustment in their lives, particularly work lives, to constitute major life stress. One group, the high stress/high illness executives, also reported a significant amount of illness during the same three-year period with average scores representing threat to life and discomfort comparable to suffering from both ulcers and high blood pressure in the same year. The other group, the high stress/low illness executives, showed only minor illnesses during the testing period.

Discriminant function analysis established that high stress/ low illness executives are significantly different in hardiness from high stress/high illness subjects. Taking into account those variables that make the greatest contribution to the discriminant equation and that produce significant mean differences between the groups, the high stress/low illness executives are distinguished by their commitment to self, their control as represented in a higher internal locus of control and a greater sense of meaningfulness, and their challenge expressed in a stronger vigorousness. The intercorrelations among these variables are significant and in the expected direction, supporting the conceptualization of hardiness as a style of interlocking parts. Demographic characteristics, even age, failed to provide any discrimination between the two groups. For a fuller discussion of these results, the status of other variables, and the use of "holdout" cases to test the generalizability of findings, see Kobasa (24).

## 2  U.S. ARMY OFFICER STUDY

A group of U.S. Army officers provided the second test of the stress-resistance power of personality hardiness. One hundred and five captains and majors, all preparing for their first assignments as R.O.T.C. instructors, completed stressful life events, illness, and personality questionnaires similar to those filled out by executives. Subjects were again all male, and the majority were white, married with two children, between the ages of 30 and 39, Protestant, college-educated, and members of the infantry branch with 10 to 15 years of service behind them.

When compared with normative data, officers' scores were, on the average, in the moderate range for illness and the high range for stressful life events. It was officers' correlation between stressful life events and illness, however, that established their distinctiveness. A Pearson product moment correlation of .56 (p = .001) was obtained between the Schedule of Recent Life Events Scale modified for a military sample and the Wyler et al. illness scale. This figure expresses a significantly stronger relationship between stress and illness than that typically found in research studies.

In the face of this strong explanatory power of stress, hardiness was placed to a real test. In regression analysis, it emerged as up to the task. The hardiness components of commitment, control, and challenge all made significant contributions to the explanation of illness variance, beyond that provided by stress. Like in the executive study, commitment and control lower symptom-atology. Challenge, however, was found to increase illness.

Although all forms of commitment are important in this group, one specific kind was found to matter most: commitment to other persons and interpersonal relationships. It is a sense of involvement with and responsibility to others that allows Army officers to do especially well under stress. Army officers confirm Antonovsky's (2) notion that a sense of coherence and community form the most fundamental resource for successful coping. That literature which portrays the soldier as a member of a primary group (44) may be relevant to an explanation of the crucial role of interpersonal commitment. The importance of "buddies" and of Army cohorts which function as family groups which has been elaborated with particular regard to the wartime situation appears to extend to peace time.

A personal sense of control over what occurs also lowers general illness scores, but emerges as more important for mental than for physical health among officers. In a regression analysis, powerlessness (or the lack of personal control) is a more powerful predictor of psychiatric symptomatology, including obsessive-compulsiveness and depression, than are stressful life event levels. The direct link between control and mental health may have to do with the nature of the Army as an organization. In a totalistic institution in which many decisions about one's career are made by others, one may especially need to maintain what Averill (3) calls cognitive control, or the ability to interpret, appraise, and incorporate the unexpected and unplanned for into an ongoing life plan. This should serve to curb unneces-sary worrying and anxiety while one waits for one's next orders.

Although not predicted, the health-damaging influence of the personality characteristic of challenge for officers can be explained through our general model of personality and stress-resistance. Personality is assumed to "work" to keep persons healthy under stress because it facilitates optimistic perception of and effective coping with stress, which in turn prevents that mental and physical activation or arousal that debilitates the organism, and makes it vulnerable to disease. In a peace-time Army situation, challenge may not do this. Many of the stressful life events currently confronted by our officers are those consistent with their new roles as scientifically-informed managers. These events, like the installation of a new computer system and gaining an organizational effectiveness supervisor, are quite different from the stressful life events these officers confronted when our country was at war (most of the subjects had done several tours of duty in Viet Nam). A sense of challenge might evoke memories of those formerly frequent events like the planning of troop movements or the disciplining of frightened young soldiers which often had to be met by a sense of risk-taking and adventure. To face the current stresses as a daring hero, as challenge could lead one to do, rather than as a careful bureaucrat would probably not constitute effective coping. In the new Army context, challenge promotes a subjectively perceived job orientation which conflicts sharply with the objective role definition prescribed by the organization. This subjective/objective conflict in the work setting is a well-documented facilitator of the illness-provoking effects of stressful life events (23).

## 3  THE LAWYER STUDY

Canadian lawyers participated in the third study of work stress, hardiness, and health (25). The 157 lawyers who participated in the study were involved in general practice, that kind of law which has been characterized in studies of coronary heart disease among lawyers as most conducive to stress-induced illness (42). The modal demographic characteristics of the subjects who completed the questionnaire were (a) male gender, (b) 40 years of age, (c) married with 2 children, and (d) living in a major metropolitan area. Like the officers, lawyers completed stressful life event, illness, and commitment and control questionnaires similar to those used in the original executive study. In addition, lawyers filled out a check list of strain symptoms and a questionnaire aimed at other stress-resistance resources. Most notable among the latter were lawyers' characteristic coping behaviors.

The strain measure was a list of 16 mental and physical symptoms commonly associated with stress reactions (e.g., difficulty concentrating, palpitations, intestinal spasms, and trouble sleeping). The research literature (9) has depicted strain as a reaction to stressful life events which is more immediate than is diagnosable illness which is thought to take from 6 months to 2 years to appear after the occurence of a stressful life event. Strain figured in two hypotheses in this study. In the first, personality and other stress-resistance resources were hypothesized to lower strain reports in conditions of high stressful life events. Like illness, strain was conceived to be a sign of that adaptational exhaustion or debilitation which personality hardiness should mitigate.

In the second hypothesis, strain was hypothesized to correlate significantly more strongly with stressful life events than diagnosable illness would for lawyers. This second proposition was based on the notion that lawyers would be more likely to both realize and admit to strain symptoms under stress than actual disease syndromes. According to Rahe (39), many individuals suffer strain, but only some of them go on to become diagnosably ill. For Rahe, being diagnosed requires that the individual be preoccupied and alarmed by body symptoms, and interpret them as requiring medical counsel. The lawyer is not so likely to take this psychological step from strain to illness. There is a myth surrounding lawyers, shared by those in and out of the profession, that lawyers thrive in stressful conditions. There are countless anecdotes about lawyers living long lives without ever retiring from work, and about lawyers actually creating stressful conditions for themselves because they believe that they work better under pressure. This professional mythology or ideology should lead lawyers, in times of stress, to postpone reporting actual illness for as long as possible, and even to avoid interpreting some strain symptoms as precursors of illness.

The second sort of measurement initiated in the study of lawyers involved specific coping behaviors. Lawyers were asked to complete a test which assessed the degree to which they typically engage in negative or regressive coping. From the perspective of existential personality theory, regressive coping was conceptualized to be that style of coping relied on by the uncommitted or alienated lawyer. It was thought to consist of attempts to deny, minimize, or run away from the situation characterized by stressful life events. All items on the test were designed to represent specific behavioral manifestations of alienation (vs. commitment), as well as to clarify the link between the psychological state of alienation and negative physiological changes. Responses like "I drank more under stress" were interpreted to be behavioral specifications of apathy and powerlessness, as well as actions directly detrimental to health.

Results from the lawyer study also contain some new elements. Between their high stressful life event scores and their moderate illness scores, lawyers show no significant correlation. Lawyers fail to replicate the stress and illness life event scores are, however, significantly associated with strain reports (r = .29, p = .0003). When lawyers report stress, they also tend to report not being able to sleep, having stomach problems, feeling nervous and other such symptoms; even though they do not report illnesses like peptic ulcer and high blood pressure.

These stress correlations support the hypothesis that the relationship between stress and strain would be stronger than that between stress and diagnosable illness, but they also render meaningless the question of stress-resistance posed in terms of illness syndromes. There is no association between stressful life events and diagnosable illness for personality and coping to mitigate.

Stress-resistance for this group of lawyers is only a matter of what reduces their strain scores during a period of stressful life events. Through regression analysis, high personality hardiness and the avoidance of regressive coping were found to do just that. A significant $R^2$ of .47 was obtained by regressing strain symptoms of stressful life events, the commitment and control dimensions of hardiness, and regressive coping.

The failure of lawyers to show the usual stress and illness correlation might be explained on methodological grounds. All data were collected at one point in time and covered only the past 12 months of a lawyer's experience. It may be that there was not enough passage of time for the measured stresses and strains to have the kind of impact on the organism that results in reports of diagnosable illness. But there may also be a psychological explanations based on the psychological distinctiveness of lawyers as a group. Lawyers may indeed participate in perpetuating the myth that portrays them as thriving in stressful situations, and are thereby reluctant to interpret their strain symptoms as deserving the attention of a medical specialist, and to cut down on their activities in a way that goes with being sick. Lawyers may be following a kind of professional norm that says they stay healthy under stress: lawyers are allowed to have a few sleepless nights or heartburn, but ulcers and hypertension in response to a stressor are violations of how they are expected to act.

But how is it that lawyers are able to act according to such a norm? Their personality scores, in the form of high commitment and control, are indeed stronger than those observed in both executives and Army officers. It may be that hardiness is a potent and widespread enough phenomenon among these Canadian laywers to buffer completely the illness-provoking effects of

stress. Although it can only be raised as a speculation at this
point, one could develop a case for viewing law school as
socialization for hardiness. Law school has been described in
the research literature (4, 37) as a difficult initiation period
in which much anxiety and stress are undergone for the sake of
gaining the right amount of toughness and agility for later
professional competence. For the law student with the "right"
personality predispositions, this tough initiation might serve
as the opportunity for learning the value of commitment and
control.


## 4  EXECUTIVE STUDIES II AND III

The two most recent projects involving IBT executives,
completed in 1977 and 1980, offered both methodological and
conceptual clarification of the stress, personality, and health
story.

### 4.1 Executive Study II

Two crucial questions pertaining to method remained at
the end of the first or retrospective executive study: (a) Does
hardiness actually promote successful stress perception and
coping, or does it merely result from having been healthy in
the face of stress? and (b) Are hardy executives really healthier
than non-hardy executives, or do they just say that they are?

The first question raises the possibility that an executive
might be so impressed by his ability to live $3\frac{1}{2}$ years worth of
stressful life events without getting sick that he now presents
himself as committed, in control, and interested in challenge.
Even more likely, the executive who has gone through the same
years with high stress and high illness has suffered a blow to
his self-understanding which leads him to fill out a questionnaire in a manner taken to indicate lack of hardiness, but which
is really better understood as a statement of his current
disappointment. This alternative interpretation throws into
question my basic assumption that personality hardiness (or
lack of it) was there before and while the executive confronted
and reacted to the stressful life events in the way that he did.

Executive Study II, a prospective extension of Study I,
achieved a partial, but significant, answer to this charge by
collecting stress and illness reports for 2 years following
the measurement of hardiness (28). Two hundred and fifty-
nine executives who had participated in the 1975 data collection
provided reports of stressful life events and health and illness
status for each of the next 24 months. Using the total illness
score for the final 2 years as dependent variable, an analysis

of covariance was run.  The hardiness composite measured in the
original study and stressful life event reports obtained later,
or from the time period concurrent with that of illness, were
entered as independent variables.  Executives' illness scores
from the retrospective study, covering 1972-1975, served as the
covariate.  This had the effect of controlling for prior illness,
and hardiness was thereby put to the test of predicting changes
in executives' stress-provoking illness scores.

Through this analysis, our prior understanding of stress-
resistance was confirmed and extended.  Even with prior illness
controlled for, stressful life events are linked with an increase,
and hardiness with a decrease in recent illness reports.  There
is also a significant interaction involving stressful life events
and hardiness, demonstrating that it is especially crucial for
one's health to be hardy when one is undergoing an intensely
stressful time.  Most important in these results is that hardiness,
as it exists prior to the encounter with stressful life events
and its consequences, is associated with staying healthy.

The second methodological question confronted in Executive
Study II, "Are hardy executives really healthier than non-hardy
executives?" raises doubts about the validity of self-reports of
health and illness, those indicators relied on in the first
executive study.  Some investigators notably Mechanic (32), have
pointed out that individuals differ in their inclination to play
the role of a sick person.  This social psychological predisposition
has been observed to influence the degree to which one will actually
report physical and mental illness.  It results in some cases in
an exaggeration of what are really minor symptoms, and in others,
in a minimizing of serious problems.  In other words, the self-
report version of illness may be very different from what one
might conclude about a subject's health status by looking at
actual physiological or biological indicators like tissue damage
or increased white cell count in the blood.

One form of support for the biological or physiological
validity of executives' reports of their health status is based
on the kinds of illnesses that they check off.  Mild and vague
symptoms like indigestion and headache might indeed be overlooked
by hardy executives.  But it is unlikely that definite illnesses
requiring medical diagnosis and care, such as heart attack, cancer,
detached retina, and even hypertension, would be erroneously
reported.

Another finding from Executive Study II gave me even more
confidence.  Forty-eight executives were randomly selected for
additional illness observation.  The records of medical examin-
ations conducted on these men in the telephone company's medical
department were scrutinized.  Illnesses recorded in the charts

were noted and compared with those reported on questionnaires for
the same time period.  Complaints of the 12 minor illnesses noted
on the self-report instrument (e.g., sore throat) could not be
validated against the medical files.  But with regard to the 114
more serious illnesses (e.g., psoriasis, high blood pressure,
peptic ulcer), agreement between self-report and physician's
diagnosis ranged from 82% to 93%, with a mean of 89%.   These
levels of agreement suggest that our non-hardy executives who are
reporting symptoms in the face of stress are not simply playing
a sick role.

## 4.2 Executive Study III

The most important issue addressed by the third stage of
the work with executives was how personality interacts with other
stress-resistance resources.  Although personality has been
emphasized in the research presented, it was never assumed that it
was the only factor keeping executives healthy under stress.  A
number of biological, social, cultural, and other psychological
variables have been identified as facilitating or hindering the
debilitating effects of stressful life events.  Among those
found to reduce illness likelihood are:  need for sensation
seeking (45), absence of Type A behavior pattern (13), person-
environment fit at work (12), coping strategies (8), supportive
relationships (16), high income (30), immunological mechanisms
(5), health practices (1), and absence of certain disease in
one's blood relatives (46).  Given what we knew already about
the independent effectiveness of these and other stress-resistance
resources, it seemed appropriate to ask about the power of
additive effects and interactions between some of them.  Recent
work with executives has focused on the role of personality and
each of the following:  constitutional predisposition, exercise,
and social support.  I would like to discuss each of these pairs
briefly.

4.2.1. Personality and constitutional predisposition.  Those
physiological and biological structures and processes which
link stressful life events and illness onset have remained
within the black box in many social science studies of stress.
But most investigators assume that a person's basic constitution
acts somewhat like a filter that shapes both the initial
organismic response to stresses, and the eventful physical breakdown in the aftermath of stress (39).  This basic constitution is
thought to be, itself, a very complex entity, involving mechanisms
like the immunological system, and being the result of at least
a person's own illness history and his genetic predisposition for
illness inherited  from blood relatives (46).

In spite of its complexity, constitutional predisposition
appeared to be the best variable with which to initiate a question

about the interaction between personality and basic physiological or biological status (27). The medical records of executives were searched for information about family medical history. In 157 cases, executives had filled out a standardized check list of illnesses thought to have a genetic basis (peptic ulcer, essential hypertension, various allergic reactions). In every instance, these check lists were completed with references to executives' natural parents. A constitutional predisposition score was formulated by simply counting the number of illnesses checked, and dividing the total by ages of parents at the time that the questionnaire was taken. The constitutional score was examined for its influence on 24 months of illness reports. But it was evaluated alongside of personality hardiness and stressful life event occurrences for the three preceding years. The three independent variable (constitution, personality, stress) were found to be independent of each other, yet each predictive of illness. Conforming to our hypotheses, both stressful life events and constitutional predisposition increase illness, whereas hardiness decreases it. Because only the main effects, and not the interaction terms, in the analysis of variance are significant, it would appear that hardiness, constitution, and stress have an additive impact on symptomatology.

4.2.2. Personality and exercise. From these results on constitution, it appears that the kind of body one inherits influences adulthood illness experience. Research also supports the notion that the kind of body one develops makes a difference. Working with cardiovascular disorders, investigators (36) appear to agree that exercise decreased the likelihood of heart attacks by increasing the efficacy of cardiac action, slowing the heart, and regularizing rhythm. The evidence that exercise protects against other illnesses is less clear, though it has been found to show some positive effect (20, 46).

To check out its benefit for our subjects, executives were asked whether they engaged in organized sports and/or non-sports exercise, how many hours a week they do it, and how strenuous their sports and non-sports exercises are. It was hypothesized that exercise would add to the stress-buffering effect of hardiness, so that the hardy executives who exercise would be the healthiest of all subjects. Results show this to be the case. Executives who are low in hardiness and who fall in the lower range of the exercise composite show significantly higher mean illness scores, and significantly higher stress/illness correlations than the other executives (i.e., those who fall in the other three groups formed by splitting the executives at the median on both hardiness and exercise). Executives who are high on both, who are hardy and who exercise, show the lowest mean illness and lowest stress/ illness correlation.

4.2.3 Personality and social support. Some non-altogether-unexpected surprises emerged as I looked at the joint effects of personality and social support.

Social support is the variable to which researchers interested in stress-resistance have paid the most attention (6). Working with stressful life events as different as job loss, pregnancy, and hospitalization of a child, investigators have argued for the buffering effect of support from others. Its effectiveness has been said to lessen the likelihood or seriousness of at least the following illnesses: tuberculosis, schizophrenia, elevated cholesterol, and alcoholism. This popularity, however, has not provided clear and consistent formulation of hypotheses or interpretation of results. There are marked differences in the literature about how social support should be defined, how it should be operationalized, and how its stress-resistance effects should be conceptualized. The only point about which the majority of social support researchers appear to agree is that social support is a good thing for persons under stress.

But even this last point struck me as somewhat questionable. The social support literature provoked in me the same concern that the early stress and illness research elicited. Again, individuals were apparently being portrayed as passive victims of their stressful environments, without the capability of dealing with the situation on their own. Social support studies, using operationalizations of support as varied as the number of persons available to the subject for conversation and the amount of money a subject has in the bank, appeared to be offering a way of understanding how a person might not fall ill in the face of stress, but a way dependent on and determined by other persons and things. From the pure social support perspective, one could stay healthy under stress as long as one had other persons to take care of him or her, or sufficiently middle-class credentials. There appeared to be little room or need in this position for individuals' exercise of control, personal sense of commitment, or an autonomous pursuit of challenge. In fact, one might be concerned that some of the aspects of social support which are thought to be helpful (like the care of worried others) might actually hinder the exercise of hardiness among executives.

To answer some of these concerns, executives were asked about social support at home and at work in the most recent data collection. Along with the usual stressful life event, illness, and hardiness measures, executives completed the Work Environment and Family Environment Scales (33). Most relevant for the social support question were the peer cohesion and staff support work scales, and the cohesion and expressiveness family scales. The peer cohesion scale measures the degree to which co-workers are seen as friendly and supportive to each other; staff support indicates the extent to which one's superiors in the comapny are perceived as supportive; family cohesion refers to the degree to which family members are concerned about and committed to the family, as well as helpful and supportive to each other; and finally, the expressiveness scale assesses the degree to which family members are allowed and encouraged to act openly and directly express their feelings.

Three-way analyses of variance with stressful life events for 1977-1980, each of the environmental perception scales, and personality hardiness as independent variables (with illness for 1977-1980 as dependent) present a much more complicated picture of the function of social support than that suggested in the research literature. Two of these analyses, one involving a composite family environment measure (cohesion plus expressiveness) and the other, the work staff support scale, are most provocative.

In the three-way analysis with perceived family support, main effects on illness are found for only stressful life events and hardiness, and not for social support. But there are interaction effects. A significant two-way interaction between hardiness and family support establishes that being low in hardiness and at the same time perceiving high cohesiveness and expressiveness in one's family increases an executive's illness score. The executives who report the most symptomatology are those scoring high on family cohesiveness and expressiveness, high on stressful life events, and low on hardiness. From these results, one is justified in claiming that family support is positively related to health only when one is commenting on executives who are hardy.

The three-way analysis of variance involving perceived staff support at work presents social support as less dependent on personality for its role in stress-resistance, but still only equivocally protective of health. Again, only stressful life events and hardiness have main effects on illness. Social support at work emerges as significant only in a two-way interaction between it and stressful life events. When stressful life events are high for executives, regardless of their hardiness scores, perceiving support from superiors or top management reduces symptomatology.

Although social support at work provided positive stress-resistance, social support from the family confirmed some of my suspicions about its potentially detrimental impact. Executives without hardiness are put at greater risk for illness under stress by a supportive family. It may be that to feel alienated, without personal control, and threatened by change directly and severely limits how successfully one can cope, but to also perceive one's family as cohesive and expressive lessens the likelihood that one will even try to cope. An executive who is low on hardiness and finds his family situation unified, warm, and open, faces the strong temptation to give up the demands of his job situation, stay home, and let his family take care of him.

## 5   OCCUPATION AS A STRESS-RESISTANCE RESOURCE

A good deal of research has been reviewed in this paper, covering various findings from several different studies.  I apologize for creating the possibility of confusion and boredom, but have to admit that the broad sweep and specification of varied details were quite intended.  It is important for the paper to provoke thoughts about both the similarities and differences in the personality and stress-resistance process across different contexts.

The most important similarity is that personality always serves to lower illness scores.  Sometimes, it is only the characteristics of commitment and control that do this, and not all three dimensions of hardiness.  Sometimes it is only the link between stressful life events and mental (rather than general) illness that is being mediated.  But in all cases, personality deserves the title of stress-resistance resources.

But some differences also need to be underlined.  Army officers report a stress and illness relationship for personality to mediate that is much stronger than that found in any other group.  Army officers are also distinctive in showing the personality characteristic of challenge to have negative, rather than the predicted positive, effects on health.  Lawyers provoke special interest because of their failure to show the typical stress and illness score, and their unusually high hardiness scores.

A conceptual challenge to stress and personality researchers lies in these differences.  One potentially fruitful way of explaining them requires the consideration of occupation as itself a stress-resistance resource.  It has been commonly thought that occupations might be differentiated and ranked in terms of simple stressfulness levels.  On such lists, air traffic controllers and policemen are usually near the top.  But a further kind of distinction is being suggested here.  Occupations may differ from one another in how they influence their members' perceptions and interpretations of stressful life events, and coping.  At least three mechanisms by which occupations might have this influence have been suggested in this paper:  (a) occupational stress mythology, (b) fit between individual and organizational role expectations, and (c) socialization for the occupation.

The first mechanism, or stress mythology, was best exemplified in the lawyer sample. Both lawyers and the public share the belief that lawyers thrive under stressful conditions. This view of stress tolerance is quite different from that stress mythology which appears to surround many contemporary executives. It is the executive who is typically written about as the classic stress victim in popular stress articles, and for whom cardiac rescue units are being built in corporate headquarters. The notion being proposed here is that these vague and general mythologies shape lawyers' and executives' perception of stressful events. The lawyers' profession encourages a view of stress as a challenge to be overcome, whereas the executives' mythological context appears to foster some worrying in the face of stresses.

The second mechanism, fit between individual and organizational role definitions, was best demonstrated in the Army officers. Both the unpredicted positive association between challenge and illness, and the unusually high stress/illness correlation suggest the importance of how an organization prescribes hardiness character- istics. It was speculated that in today's peacetime Army, oriented towards organizational effectiveness and other business practices, there may actually be a discouragement of at least one dimension of hardiness (i.e., challenge). There is at least an indication that some manifestations of hardiness lead to a conflict between how an individual enacts his role and what is expected of him. This conflict has been found to promote ineffective coping with stress.

The third possible mechanism, socialization, refers to the organization's role in promoting the development of hardiness, and thereby, effective stress perception and coping. This point was evoked by lawyers' distinctiveness. It was suggested that law school might be a training center for commitment, control, and challenge. The well-documented stresses and strains of this educational experience may well prepare the young lawyers for later confrontations with the environment. The business world and today's Army do not appear to provide comparable socialization experiences.

These occupational mechanisms should not be seen as replace- ments for personality's role in maintaining health. In every instance, their effectiveness has been understood in interaction with personality characteristics. Their value lies in both elaborating stress resistance to include a sociocultural as well as psychological dimension, and in suggesting some inroads for intervention.

An existential view forces a conceptualization of personality as continuously capable of change. It also emphasizes the understanding of personality as that <u>in</u> situation or environment, rather than personality as a collection if internal traits. To change personality, or more specifically, to increase personality hardiness, one has to confront it as it expresses itself in work and other life areas. The stress (management) therapist needs to understand both the individual and the occupation that he or she is part of. Only with this understanding can one seek to transform outlooks and actions in such a way that clients become aware of and able to influence the stressful life events of their experience.

## REFERENCES

1. Altekruse, E.G. and J.H. Wilmore. Changes in Blood Chemistries Following a Controlled Exercise Program. Journal of Occupational Medicine 15 (1973) 110-113.
2. Antonovsky, A. Health, Stress, and Coping. (Washington, Jossey-Bass, 1979).
3. Averill, J.R. Personal Control Over Adversive Stimuli and Its Relationship to Stress. Psychological Bulletin 80 286-303.
4. Barry, K.H. and P.A. Connelly. Research on Law Students: An Annotated Bibliography. American Bar Foundation Research Journal 4 (1978) 751-804.
5. Burnet, M. Genes, Dreams, and Realities. (New York, Basic Books, 1971).
6. Cobb, S. Social Support as a Moderator of Life Stress. Psychosomatic Medicine 38 (1976) 300-314.
7. Coehlo, G.V., D.A. Hamburg, and J.F. Adams (Eds.). Coping and Adaptation. (New York, Basic Books, 1974)
8. Cohen, F. and R.S. Lazarus. Coping with the Stresses of Illness. In G. Ston, F. Cohen, N.E. Adler & Associates. (Eds.) Health Psychology: A Handbook. (Washington, Jossey-Bass, 1979).
9. Dohrenwend, B.P. Stressful Life Events and Psychopathology: Some Issues of Theory and Method. In J.E. Barrett et al. (Eds.). Stress and Mental Disorder. (New York, Raven Press, 1979).
10. Dohrenwend, B.S. & B.P. Dohrenwend (Eds.) Stressful Life Events: Their Nature and Effects. (New York, Wiley & Sons, 1974).
11. Dohrenwend, B.S., A.R. Krasnoff, A.R. Askenasy and B.P. Dohrenwend. Exemplification of a Method for Scaling Life Events: The PERI Life-Events Scale. Journal of Health and Social Behavior 19 (1978) 205-229.

12. French, J.R.P., Jr. Person Role Fit. Occupational Mental Health 3 (1973) 15-20.
13. Friedman, M., R.H. Roseman and V. Carroll. Changes in the Serum Cholesterol and Blood Clotting Time in Men Subjected to Cyclic Variation of Occupational Stress. Circulation 17 (1958) 852-861.
14. Gergen, K.J. and S. Morse. Self-consistency: Measurement and Validation. Proceedings of the 75th Annual Convention of the American Psychological Association 2 (1967) 207-208.
15. Glass, D.C., J.E. Singer, L.N. Friedman. Psychic Cost of Adaptation to an Environment Stressor. Journal of Personality and Social Psychology 12 (1969) 200-210.
16. Gore, S. The effect of Social Support in Moderating the health Consequences of Unemployment. Journal of Health and Social Behavior 19 (1978) 157-165.
17. Hahn, M.E. California Life Goals Evaluation Schedule. (Palo Alto, Western Psychological Services, 1966).
18. Holmes, T.H. and M. Asuda. Life Change and Illness Susceptibility. In B.S. Dohrenwend & B.P. Dohrenwend (Eds.) Stressful Life Events: Their Nature and Effects. (New York, Wiley & Sons, 1974).
19. Holmes, T.H. and R.H. Rahe. The Social Readjustment Rating Scale. Journal of Psychosomatic Research 11 (1967) 213-218.
20. Insull, W. (Ed.) Coronary Risk Handboo. (New York, American Heart Association, 1973)
21. Jackson, D.N. Personality Research Form Manual. (Goshen, New York, Research Psychologists Press, 1974).
22. Johnson, J.H. and I.G. Sarason. Life Stress, Depression, and Anxiety: Internal-External Control as a Moderator Variable. Journal of Psychosomatic Research 22 (1978) 205-208.
23. Katz, D. and R.L. Kahn (Eds.). The Social Psychology of Organizations (New York, Wiley & Sons, 1978).
24. Kobasa, S.C. Stress Life Events, Personality, and Health: An Inquiry into Hardiness. Journal of Personality and Social Psychology, 37 (1979) 1-11.
25. Kobasa, S.C. Commitment and Coping in Stress Resistance Among Lawyers. Journal of Personality and Social Psychology (1981) in press.
26. Kobasa, S.C. and S.R. Maddi. Existential Personality Theory: In R. Corsini (Ed.) Current personality theories. Itasca, Illinois, Peacock Publishers, 1977).
27. Kobasa, S.C., S.R. Maddi and S. Courington. Personality and Constitution as Medicators in the Stress-Illness Relationship.
28. Kobasa, S.C., S.R. Maddi and S. Kahn. Hardiness and Health: A Prospective Study. Journal of Personality and Social Psychology (1981) in press.

29. Lefcourt, H.M.  Locus of Control:  Current Trends in Theory and Research.  (Hillsdale, New Jersey, Lawrence Erlbaum, 1978).
30. Luborsky, L., T.C. Todd, and A.H. Katchen.  A Self-Administered Social Assets Scale for Predicting Physical and Psychological Illness and Health.  Journal of Psychosomatic Research 17 (1973) 109-120.
31. Maddi, S.R., S.C. Kobasa, and M. Hoover.  An Alienation Test. Journal of Humanistic Psychology 19 (1979) 73-76.
32. Mechanic, D and E. Volkart.  Stress, Illness Behavior, and Sick Role.  American Sociological Review 26 (1961) 51-58.
33. Moos, R.H., P.M. Insel, and B. Humphrey.  Family, Work, and Group Environment Scales Manual.  (Palo Alto, California, Consulting Psychologists Press, 1974).
34. Moss, G.E. Illness, Immunity, and Social Interaction. (New York, Wiley & Sons, 1973).
35. Ouchi, W.  Theory Z: How American Business Can Meet the Japanese Challenge.  (New York, Addison-Wesley, 1981).
36. Paffenberger, R.S., Jr., Wing, A.L. and R.T. Hyde.  Physical Activity as an Index of Heart Attack Risk in College Alumni. American Journal of Epidemiology 108 (1978) 161-175.
37. Pipkin, R.M.  Legal Education:  The Consumers' Perspective. American Bar Foundation Research Journal 4 (1976) 1161-1192.
38. Rabkin, J.G. and E.L. Struening.  Life Events, Stress, and Illness.  Science 194 (1976) 1013-1020.
39. Rahe, R.H.  The Pathway Between Subjects' Recent Life Changes and the Near-Future Illness Reports.  In B.S. Dohrenwend and B.P. Dohrenwend (Eds.) Stressful Life events:  Their Nature and Effects.  (New York, Wiley & Sons, 1974).
40. Rodin, J. and E.J. Langer.  The Effects of Choice and Enhance Personal Responsibility for the Aged:  A Field Experiment in an Institutional Setting.  Journal of Personality and Social Psychology 34 (1976) 191-198.
41. Rotter, J.B., M. Seeman and S. Liverant.  Internal vs. External Locus of Control of Reinforcement:  A Major Variable in Behavior Therapy.  In N.R. Washburne (Ed.) Decisions, Values and Groups.  (London, Pergamon, 1962).
42. Russek, H.J.  Emotional Stress and Coronary Heart Disease in American Physicians.  American Journal of Medicine and Science 243 (1962) 716-721.
43. Seligman, M.E.P.  Helplessness.  (San Francisco: Freeman, 1975).
44. Shils, E. and M. Janowitz.  Cohesion and Disintegration in the Wehrmacht in World Ware II.  Public Opinion Quarterly 12 (1948) 280-315.
45. Smith, R.E., J.H. Johnson, and I.G. Sarason.  Life Change, the Sensation Seeking Motive, and Psychological Distress. Journal of Consulting and Clinical Psychology 46 (1978) 348-349.
46. Weiner, H. Psychobiology & human Diease.(N.Y., Elsevier,1977).

204

47. Wolfe, S.W.  Avoid Sickness -- How Life Changes Affect
    Your Health.  Family Circle.  May (1972) pp. 30; 166-170.
48. Wyler, A.R., M. Masuda and T.H. Holmes.  Seriousness of
    Illness Rating Scale.  Journal of Psychosomatic Research
    11 (1968) 363-375.

ANGER MANAGEMENT AND WORK STRESS: HEALTHY AND UNHEALTHY
STYLES


W. Doyle Gentry

Department of Behavioral Medicine
and Psychiatry
University of Virginia
Charlottesville, Virginia (USA)

## 1 INTRODUCTION

Two conclusions that are inescapable as one digests
the extant literature on work stress and health are:
(a) Little is known about the affective or emotional
mediators or strains that link psychosocial stressors
in the work environment to various illness outcomes;
and, (b) Little or no research attention has been given
to the role of anger, as contrasted for example with
anxiety or depression, and anger-coping styles per se
as they mediate relationships between work stress and
health.  In this chapter, we ask and then attempt to
answer several questions relevant to this two conclusions.


## 2 WHAT IS THE ROLE OF ANGER IN WORK STRESS-ILLNESS RELATIONSHIPS?

In his excellent book "From Stressors to Strains,"
van Dijkhuizen provides a comprehensive, longitudinal
analysis of stress-strain relationships in a sample of
578 workers, including sub-samples of: middle managers,
superiors of middle managers, supervisors, workers, and
technical staff specialists.  In doing so, he explains
the "critical path," linking occupational stressors to
what he calls general psychological affects, including
irritation (which here is seen as synonymous with anger),
and in turn to behavioral and physiological strains.
The latter include a variety of end-points (e.g., blood

pressure, cholesterol level, heart rate, obesity, and cigarette smoking), all of which have major import for coronary heart disease.

Van Dijkhuizen (1) shows rather convincingly that self-reported irritation on the part of the employee, no matter what their respective level in the organizational hierarchy, results from stressors such as: role conflict, lack of supervisor support, excessive workload, interpersonal tension in relations with co-workers and other departments in the organization, and job-related threat (i.e., uncertainty about how one is doing as regards either the expectations of superiors and colleagues or his/her ability to meet the demands of the job). This finding is consistent across all categories of workers and/or age groups. Also, irritation appears certainly related to elevated cholesterol levels, if not as clearly to other strain variables, e.g., blood pressure, smoking, obesity, and absenteeism. However, his analyses leave perhaps more questions unanswered than answered. For example: Why are the links between work stressors and behavioral/physiological strains more evident for affects such as depression and anxiety than irritation? Why does one reach the "end of the line" so often with irritation, whereas anxiety goes on to link up with numerous strains? What is the relationship among the various strains, e.g., depression and irritation, the former often seen clinically as resulting from "anger turned inward"? And, finally, is it possible that the sequential links between irritation and strain(s) would be more evident if one took into account obvious differences in how individual employees managed or coped with such feelings?

A large-scale epidemiologic study of 10,000 Israeli male civil service employees, reported by Kahn et al. (2), in part answers such questions. That is, these investigators conducted a prospective study, aimed at determining those biomedical and/or psychosocial factors which predisposed workers to essential hypertension. They collected data on some 90 separate variables on this large sample, including such information as: density of current living arrangements (number of persons living together); diet; smoking patterns; history of CHD, ulcer, and diabetes; cholesterol level; financial problems; and, information about current emotional state and ways of resolving interpersonal conflict. Interestingly, only 9 of the 90 predictor variables appeared to be statistically significant in predicting the 5-year incidence of hypertension. Two of these predictor variables

had to do with the way workers handled anger in the work
setting. That is, employees who indicated that they
tended to brood when hurt by a superior at work and/or
restrain retaliation when hurt by a superior at work
were more apt to develop essential hypertension over
time. In similar fashion, there was a near-significant
tendency for employees who reported a tendency to brood
when hurt by co-workers to eventually develop high blood
pressure. Also of interest was the fact that work
problems per se or negative emotional state (anxiety)
associated with same did not predict incidence of hypertension. This finding suggests (a) that how one handles
irritation or anger in the workplace is the primary
determining factor in whether or not they are at risk
for illness and (b) that anger-coping styles are more
important in determining risk for illness than other,
more conventional socioeconomic or biomedical markers.
Brooding and restraining retaliation (aggression) here
reflect a tendency on the employee's part to inhibit
anger, rather than expressing it in some direct manner,
e.g., at the supervisor or co-worker who provoked such
feelings.

In our own research, we (3) noted a similar mediating effect of anger expression on the relationship
between job strain and illness potential. In a study
of 431 working men, we assessed habitual anger-coping
styles (i.e., tendency to inhibit or express anger across
5 different hypothetical situations involving anger
provocation), level of job strain (dissatisfaction), and
diastolic blood pressure. The measures of anger expression and job strain were obtained via an extensive
public health questionnaire administered to respondents
in their own home, while blood pressure (a mean of 3
consecutive readings) was measured directly during that
same home interview. Job strain scores were derived
from answers to questions such as the following: How
much chance do you have to earn more money at work?, How
much chance do you have to learn new skills at work?,
How much chance do you have for advancement at work?,
and How much chance to you have to work with friendly
people? In each instance, respondents could answer on
a 5-point scale, ranging from "not good at all" to
"very good". Figure 1 shows the relationship that emerged
between these three variables. Those workers experiencing
high levels of job strain who were able to openly express
their anger (presumably associated with same) had diastolic pressure levels comparable to respondents experiencing low job strain. However, those who experienced

208

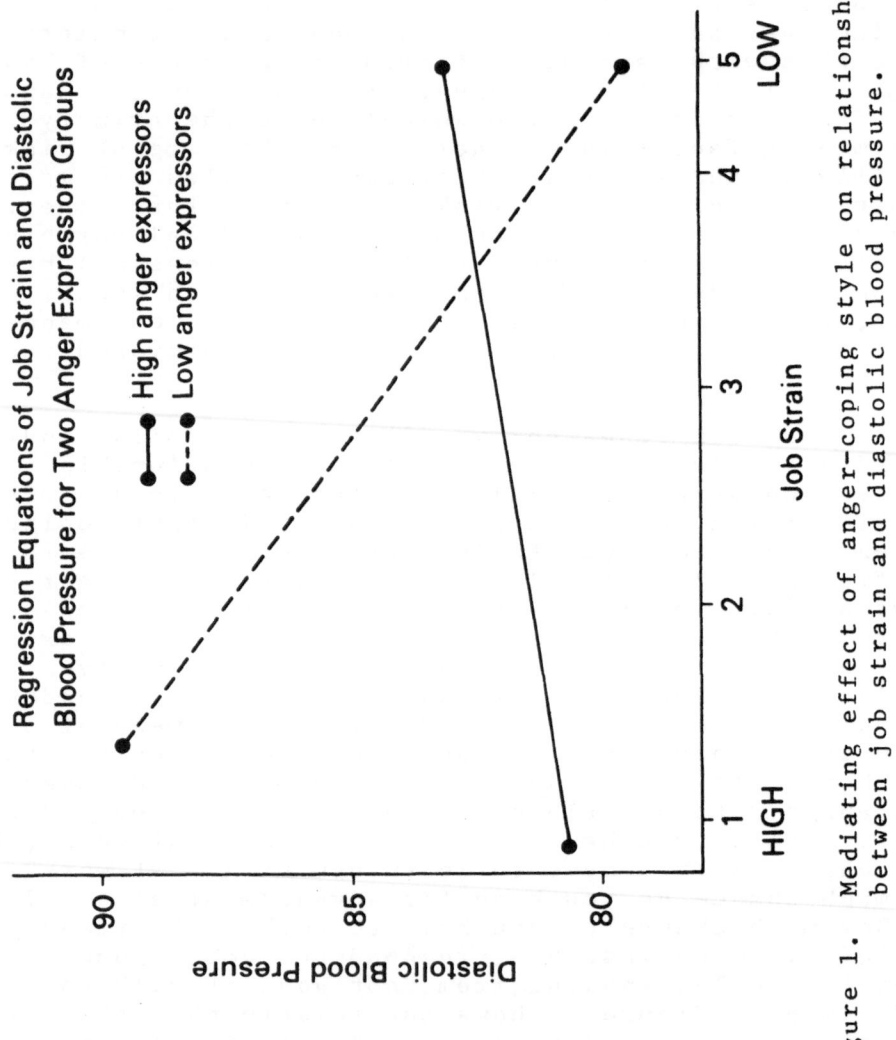

Figure 1.   Mediating effect of anger-coping style on relationship
between job strain and diastolic blood pressure.

high job strain but generally did not openly express anger when provoked had mean DBP levels approximately 10 mm Hg higher. This difference is indeed noteworthy when one considers that a difference of 5 mm Hg in blood pressure is associated with a 20% differential in CHD mortality (4).

In this study, we found a similar relationship between family strain, anger-coping styles, and diastolic pressure. Family strain reflected self-reported failure to: spend time with spouse; make decisions with spouse; have good sex with spouse; receive appreciation from spouse; and, spend time with children and be a good parent. Figure 2, as can be seen, is virtually identical to Figure 1; that is, those employees who reported high levels of family strain and who inhibited expression of anger had the highest mean level of DBP, in this case approximately 14 mm Hg greater pressure than that noted for their counterparts who experienced high family strain but expressed their anger openly. Kahn et al. (2) also noted that a tendency to keep marital conflict to self was predictive of essential hypertension.

Our observations at this point suggest that individuals tend to experience comparable levels of strain (high vs. low) in both work and non-work (family) settings and also that they tend to handle angry feelings much the same in both types of situations.

## 2 WHAT TYPE(S) OF INDIVIDUALS ARE LIKELY TO EVIDENCE UNHEALTHY ANGER-COPING BEHAVIOR IN THE WORK SETTING?

In a recently published report, we (5) noted that black American males were significantly more likely to evidence an "anger in" coping style, as compared to black females or white men and women. In our study of 1,006 respondents, we found that 23% of black men habitually tended to inhibit expression of angry feelings; black women showed this same tendency 18% of the time, white men 14% of the time, and white women 19%, respectively. We also noted that residents of high socioecological stress areas (high density housing, high crime rates, low education and income levels) were more likely to inhibit anger expression than were persons living in low stress areas. The common thread in this research seems to be the "minority status" of those individuals who employ unhealthy anger-coping styles. Elsewhere, Averill (6) points out that the commonly held notion that women are more likely to sup-

210

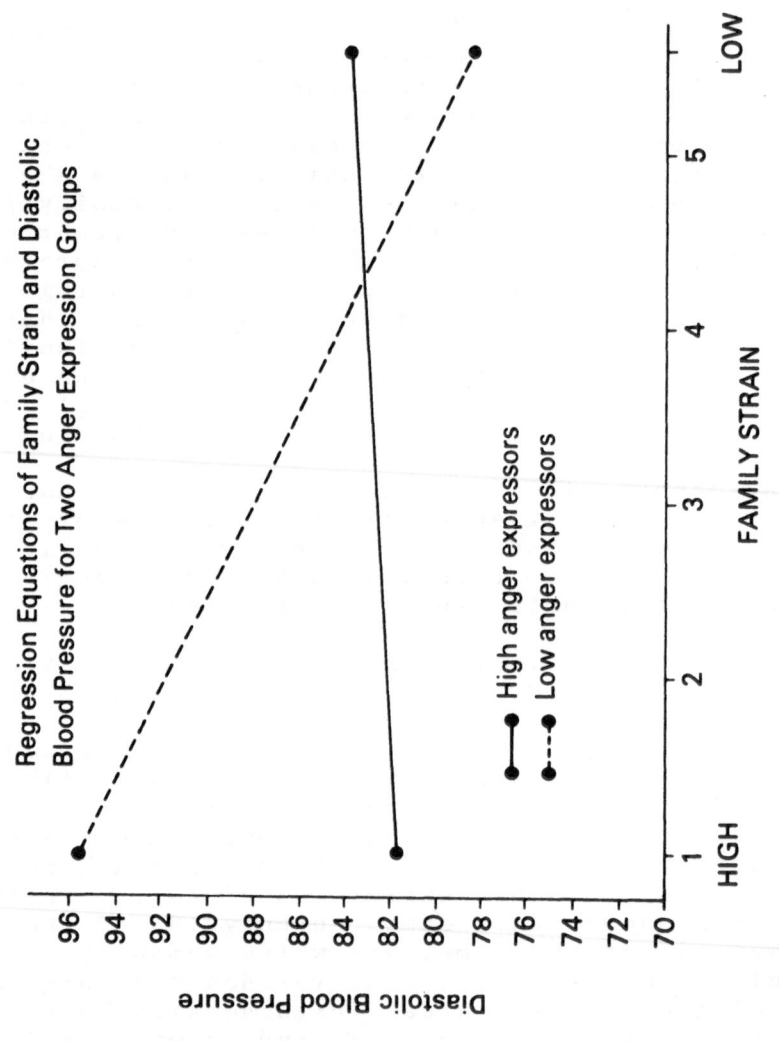

Figure 2.  Mediating effect of anger-coping style on relationship between family strain and diastolic blood pressure.

press anger lacks scientific support. In our research (5), we also failed to find any baserate differences in anger-coping styles for men and women.

Harburg, Blakelock, and Roeper (7), however, noted that working women and middle-class workers were more likely to <u>reflective</u> anger coping in dealing with an angry boss than were their male or lower-class counterparts. The latter two categories (men and working-class persons) were more likely to manifest <u>resentful</u> anger coping in response to anger provocation at work. An example of the reflective mode of anger expression was: "Try to reason with him at the time." or "Talk to him about it after he has cooled down." Resentful anger expression, on the other hand, included both <u>anger in</u> ("Just walk away from the situation.") and <u>anger out</u> ("Report him to the union.") responses on the part of the employee. Some 56.4% of female workers vs. 44.0% of male workers showed the reflective anger coping style. Interestingly, workers using the resentful anger-coping style had higher levels of diastolic blood pressure, as well as a higher proportion of hypertensives, than did workers using the reflective style.

Kets de Vries (8) has also noted that the <u>entrepreneurial personality</u> pattern, so often seen in the work setting, is in large part characterized by "controlled rage, hostility, and guilt," an observation also noted for <u>Type A</u> pattern individuals (9) who evidence extremes of aggressiveness (sometimes stringently repressed). As McClelland (10) points out, it appears to be the common thread of "the inhibited power motive" that puts such individuals at risk for high blood pressure, i.e., men who try to keep deep-seated hostility and resentment controlled or under cover in interpersonal (work) situations.

3   HOW DOES ONE ALTER UNHEALTHY ANGER-COPING STYLES IN THE WORK SETTING?

Before one can embark on any type of intervention program aimed at altering unhealthy anger-coping behavior in employees, one must first select out, screen, or target those workers who are "at risk" because of such behavior. This is no easy task since little is currently available in terms of basic methodology for determining how individuals express anger in various situations. Measures such as the Navoco Anger Scale (11) and the Spielberger State-Trait Anger Scale (12) are designed to

estimate how angry a person generally is, rather than
how he/she expresses such feelings. While these are
useful tools in defining "high anger" individuals, i.e.,
persons who are likely to have trouble dealing with
anger on a day-to-day basis simply because they experience it so much of the time, they do not provide needed
information as regards, for example, differences in
"reflective" versus "resentful" anger expression. At
this point, we know of no scale that does provide this
information; thus, we have chosen to select hypothetical
situations identical or similar to those offered by
Harburg and co-workers (13-15) and used elsewhere by
Haynes et al. (16), which distinguish between persons
who are either (a) resentful vs. reflective, (b) anger
in vs. anger out, or (c)aggression guilty vs. not guilty.

Having selected employees out that fit one or the
other unhealthy anger-coping styles, we then present these
individuals with an anger management training program,
the essence of which includes:

## 3.1  Defining Anger and Related Concepts

Here, se simply use the distinctions offered by
Buss (17) as regards basic differences between anger
(an emotion), hostility (an attitude of ill will), and
aggression (behavior, verbal or physical, aimed at harm-
ing another person). We also educate persons as to how
these three interrelate, e.g., hostility may evoke anger
which in turn leads to aggressive behavior. It is important to point out, though, that these relationships
are not universal or fixed, i.e., one can learn to
experience anger without becoming aggressive; this, in
fact, is the essence of assertive training.

## 3.2  Defining the Positive, Adaptive Functions of Anger

Here, we refer to the work of Novaco (18), emphasizing that anger can lead adaptive coping in that it:
(a) energizes behavior; (b) provides an impetus for new
types of interpersonal communication with intimates;
(c) reduces feelings of anxiety and vulnerability; and,
(d) fosters a sense of mastery or control over one's
immediate environment. As we have noted elsewhere (19),
expressed anger can even lead to a reduction in conflict
behavior or aggressiveness. This, we hope, will provide
a new incentive for acquiring healthier styles of anger
expression.

## 3.3 Defining the Undesirable, Unhealthy Consequences of Resentful Anger-Coping Patterns

Here, as we have done earlier in this chapter, we point out the adverse consequences of inhibited anger expression or aggressive, anger-out behavior. These include, but certainly are not limited to: disturbances in perception, cognitive inefficiency, interpersonal tension, a heightened probability for extreme forms of violence (homocide, suicide), depression, various psychosomatic disorders, as well as major threats to one's physical health status (hypertension, CHD, cancer). We also point out the short- (avoiding conflict) versus long-term (illness) consequences of resentful anger-in coping behavior.

## 3.4 Defining Strategies for Healthier Management of Anger

Finally, we offer the subject a range of options for dealing with anger provocation in those situations where he/she is most vulnerable. We have found the Novaco Scale (11) useful in defining specific "trigger situations, persons, or events" which tend to elicit feelings of frustration and anger on a consistent basis. First, one can simply avoid those situations, people, or events that anger them on a day-to-day basis. Second, one can try and change their attitudes or perceptions of events or situations which trigger anger, using the concepts and techniques offered by Burns (20). To a large extent, this means learning not to personalize every encounter one has with the organization or other employees that involves some type of frustration of one's needs or abilities, not to assign malevolent intentions to others who cause one frustration (e.g., a supervisor who advises one that they have to work overtime), etc. Third, we teach individuals to confront anger-provocation head on in terms of assertive behavior, feeling-cause language (19), and "I" statement (e.g., I feel angry or uncomfortable....). Other strategies for dealing with anger on a day-to-day basis include: learning relaxation techniques, regular physical exercise, catharsis which can come via some type of supportive, counseling relationship, or simply buying time (e.g., by counting to 10).

We find the schema presented by Carlson (21) is the most useful as regards anger management training in the work setting. Step 1 involves identifying the negative feelings (hurt, anger) and evaluating their intensity. Step 2 suggests that no action be taken until the angered person has had time to think through the anger-provoking situation and is in full control of their own words and actions. Step 3 involves identifying the true cause of the negative feelings. Step 4 is an evaluation of their legitimacy, e.g., are the supervisor's criticisms valid or unjustified? Step 5 gives the angered person a full range of options for dealing constructively with the angry feelings; these include, but are certainly not limited to: direct verbal confrontation (sharing "I feel" messages); establishing limits with consequences; getting counsel; catharsis; compromise; and, simply passing over the issue. Step 6 involves forgiving and forgetting, i.e., preventing a build-up of hostility.

## 4 WHAT IS ORGANIZATION'S ROLE IN ANGER MANAGEMENT IN THE WORK SETTING?

We believe the organization can play an active role as regards both primary and secondary prevention of anger-related illness (strain) in the work setting. First every attempt should be made to minimize sources of anger provocation in the work environment, e.g., providing supervisor support, adapting the demands of the organization to fit the abilities of the individual employee, being clear about what is expected of given workers and providing precise feedback as regards their perforamnce in meeting these expectations; and, if at all possible, avoiding frequent or chronic overwork or underutilization - all of which lead to feelings of irritation and anger (1). Second, the organization can attempt to screen out those employees who are showing signs of anger-related illness and provide them with a program of anger management training similar to that described elsewhere in this Volume by Collings. It is noteworthy that Japanese industry some years ago provided employees at all levels of the organizational hierarchy with a means of catharsis (letting off steam) during the work day; they established "tension control rooms" in the work situation in which all employees were free for limited periods of time to beat inflated life-like dolls with sticks to release their pent-up anger and frustration. Their goal here was both to minimize a pathologic build-up of aggressive energy (anger), but also to insure maximal performance (efficiency) on the part of their workers at all times during the work day. As we noted earlier in this chapter, inhibited anger also leads to cognitive inefficiency and interpersonal tension.

Third, the organization can promote (and, if necessary, provide training for) better relations between supervisors and line employees. As Argyris (22) noted over 20 years ago, supervisors tend to "blow up" at employees under their charge in ways that are perceived as arbitrary and which lead inevitably to anger; this accounts for the fact that a significant proportion of workers report either "blowing their stack" or "feeling low or blue" while at work following exchanges with their supervisors (23).

REFERENCES

1.    van Dijkhuizen, N. From Stressors to Strains. Lisse, Swets and Zeitlinger B.V., 1980).

2.    Kahn, H.A., J.H. Medalie, H.N. Neufeld, E. Riss, and U. Goldbourt. The Incidence of Hypertension and Associated Factors: The Israel Ischemic Heart Disease Study. American Heart Journal 84 (1972) 171-182.

3.    Chesney, A.P., W.D. Gentry, H.E. Gary, C. Kennedy, and E. Harburg. Anger-Coping Style as a Mediator in the Relationship Between Life Strain and Blood Pressure. Unpublished manuscript (1984).

4.    Kaplan, N.M. The Control of Hypertension: A Therapeutic Breakthrough. American Scientist 68 (1980) 537-545.

5.    Gentry, W.D., A.P. Chesney, C.D. Kennedy, R.P. Hall, H.E. Gary, and E. Harburg. The Relation of Demographic Attributes and Habitual Anger-Coping Styles. Journal of Social Psychology 121 (1983) 45-50.

6.    Averill, J.R. Studies on Anger and Aggression: Implications for Theories of Emotion. American Psychologist 38 (1983) 1145-1160.

7.    Harburg, E., E.H. Blakelock, and P.J. Roeper. Resentful and Reflective Coping with Arbitrary Authority and Blood Pressure: Detroit. Psychosomatic Medicine 41 (1979) 189-202.

8.    Kets de Vries, M.F.R. Stress and the Entrepreneur. In C.L. Cooper and R. Payne (Eds.) Current Concepts in Occupational Stress. (New York, Wiley, 1980).

9.    Jenkins, C.D. The Coronary-Prone Personality. In W.D. Gentry and R.B. Williams (Eds.) Psychological Aspects of Myocardial Infarction and Coronary Care. (St. Louis, C.V. Mosby, 1975).

10. McClelland, D.C. Inhibited Power Motivation and High Blood Pressure in Men. Journal of Abnormal Psychology 88 (1979) 182-190.

11. Novaco, R.W. Anger and Coping with Stress: Cognitive Behavioral Interventions. In J.P. Foreyt and D.P. Rathjen (Eds.) Cognitive Behavior Therapy. New York, Plenum, 1978).

12. Spielberger, C.D., G.A. Jacobs, S. Russell, and R.S. Crane. Assessment of Anger: The State-Trait Anger Scale. In J.N. Butcher and C.D. Spielberger (Eds.) Advances in Personality Assessment, Volume 2. (Hillsdale, N.J., LEA, 1982).

13. Gentry, W.D., A.P. Chesney, H.E. Gary, R.P. Hall, E. Harburg, and C.D. Kennedy. Behavioral Medicine and the Risk for Essential Hypertension. International Review of Applied Psychology 32 (1983) 85-94.

14. Gentry, W.D., A.P. Chesney, H.E. Gary, R.P. Hall, and E. Harburg. Habitual Anger-Coping Styles: I. Effect on Mean Blood Pressure and Risk for Essential Hyptertension. Psychosomatic Medicine 44 (1982) 195-202.

15. Gentry, W.D., E. Harburg, and L. Hauenstein. Effects of Anger Expression/Inhibition and Guilt on Elevated Diastolic Blood Pressure in High/Low Stress and Black/White Females. Proceedings of the American Psychological Association (1973) 115-116.

16. Haynes, S.G., M. Feinleib, and W.B. Kannel. The Relationship of Psychosocial Factors in Coronary Heart Disease in the Framingham Study: III. Eight-Year Incidence of Coronary Heart Disease. American Journal of Epidemiology 109 (1980) 37-58.

17. Buss, A.H. The Psychology of Aggression. (New York, Wiley, 1961).

18. Novaco, R.W. The Functions and Regulation of the Arousal of Anger. American Journal of Psychiatry 133 (1976) 1124-1128.

19. Gaines, T., P.M. Kirwin, and W.D. Gentry. The Effect of Descriptive Anger Expression, Insult, and No Feedback on Interpersonal Aggression, Hostility, and Empathy Motivation. Genetic Psychology Monographs 95 (1977) 349-367.

20. Burns, D.D. Feeling Good: The New Mood Therapy. (New York, Morrow, 1980).

21. Carlson, D.L. Overcoming Hurts and Anger. (Eugene, Oregon, Harvest House, 1981).

22. Argyris, C. Interpersonal Competence and Organizational Effectiveness. (Homewood, Illinois, Dorsey,

1962).
23. Warren, D.I. Neighborhood and Community Contexts in
       Help Seeking, Problem Coping, and Mental Health:
       Data Analysis Monograph. Program in Community
       Effectiveness. Unpublished manuscript (1976).

# REDUCING CORONARY RISK IN OCCUPATIONALLY SUCCESSFUL TYPE A MEN

Ethel Roskies

University of Montreal
Montreal, Canada

In seeking to develop a treatment program that would reduce the coronary risk associated with being type A in occupationally successful, apparently healthy, middle-aged men, two distinct types of problems are encountered: clinical and conceptual-methodological. The clinical issues in type A intervention are those common to all treatment programs, such as formulating a therapy and motivating individuals to accept the treatment preferred. The conceptual-methodological issues are more complex and more idiosyncratic since, contrary to obesity, smoking and hypertension where treatment goals and outcome measures are at least clearly defined, for type A there is considerable ambiguity concerning what specific behaviors in the global pattern lead to increased coronary risk and what changes indicate reduction in this risk (35,36). Thus, before the would-be therapist can embark on treatment he or she must first delineate the goals of treatment, as well as the measures used to evaluate treatment effects. In this chapter we shall trace the efforts of my colleagues and myself to develop a type A intervention program for healthy men, focusing both on the clinical and the methodological aspects of our treatment studies.

More basic than these clinical and conceptual concerns, however, is the ethical issue of whether treatment is justified at all, particularly for occupationally successful individuals who do not yet show signs of heart disease. The type A pattern has been associated not only with increased coronary risk,

but also with superior occupational achievement.   If
modifying type A behavior improved future physical
health but, at the same time, reduces current
occupational productivity or success, then how much
change can a person be expected to risk, or legitimately
be advised to risk?   If type A behavior does indeed
make the wheels of industry go round, then how much
intervention can our society afford to support?   This
potential for conflict between work and health values
in type A intervention is often mentioned, but has not
been subjected to any detailed scrutiny.   A forum on
"Work, Stress and Health" is an appropriate opportunity
for opening discussion on this issue.   Before embarking
on the account of our personal experiences in devising
treatment programs, therefore, we shall first survey
the general type A literature for its bearing on the
relationship between type A behavior and work performance.

## 1 TYPE A AND OCCUPATIONAL ACHIEVEMENT

Most studies that have gathered occupational data
have found a positive association with type A scores.
For example, in the Western Collaborative Group Study,
higher occupational levels were associated with
increased percentages of men classified as A (32).
Shekelle, in the Chicago Detection in Industry Study,
also found that type A scores were positively
correlated with occupation in each of the four sex and
race groups studied (44).   Outside the United States,
Kornitzer has recently reported similar findings for
a large Belgian sample, composed both of Flemish and
French speaking individuals (20).   In a study of white
collar middle class males from five different work
organizations in Buffalo, Mettlin also found the type As
attain their higher status and income at a younger age,
suggesting that they are likely to receive faster as
well as more promotions (28).   Thus, the popular belief
that type As have above-average success in the work
world is amply supported by the research data.

Though there is no evidence that the occupational
advancement of As results from higher innate intelli-
gence, it may result, at least in part, from earlier
success at school.   As for occupation, the findings
point to a positive correlation between type A behavior
and educational attainment (28, 32, 44, 49).   According
to the testimony of As themselves, however, it is
primarily work habits and attitudes that distinguish

them from Bs.

In two separate Canadian studies, of prison administrators and senior corporate officers respectively (4, 17), extreme As claimed to put in the longest work weeks, work more discretionary hours per week, travel more days per year, and supervise larger numbers of people. They were keenly aware of the time expended on work, reporting that work encroached substantially on their leisure, their home life and their relationships. Nevertheless, they perceived their jobs as requiring such effort, describing them in terms of intense competition, heavy work loads, conflicting demands, and multiple responsibilities. To offset these stresses, however, there was the gratification provided by the opportunity to utilize skills and influence the course of events. In fact, Burke et al. (4) conclude that the psychological gratification and tangible rewards which extreme type A individuals obtain from the work experience far outweigh whatever stress they experience.

The picture of the type A manager that emerges from the reports is of an individual who holds a particularly demanding job, responds to its pressures by working very hard and, in turn, is rewarded by advancement to jobs with even greater responsibilities. Since most of this portrait comes from the self-reports of As themselves, it is important to distinguish how much of this is reality and how much is myth. Are the jobs held by As more demanding than those held by Bs? Will an employee who does not manifest A characteristics reduce his or her chances for advancement?

There is no definite answer to the question of possible differences in the job characteristics of As, compared to Bs, because most of the studies on occupational differences have focused on job rewards (e.g., income, prestige), but have ignored job demands. The best available data comes from a study conducted by the Institute for Social Research, relating job demands to worker health (6). To provide a wide range of job characteristics, the sample was selected from 23 occupational groups working in 67 different sites; the 2010 males queried held jobs as diverse as physician, policeman, air traffic controller, forklift driver and machine tender. The results of this study were equivocal. Individuals in the specific high pressure jobs of physician and administrator did have the highest mean scores by far on a type A questionnaire, but even in these job classifications some individuals could be classified as Bs. Thus, while there may be a tendency for As to select themselves for high pressured jobs, or alternatively, for these jobs to stimulate A behavior, there is no evidence that any job is so demanding as to require type A workaholism. In fact, the current President of the United States is a prime example of the fact that it is possible to retain type B work habits and attitudes even in the most demanding position.

The second justification for type A work habits is that it supposedly improves work performance. To the best of our knowledge, there are no studies comparing the performance of As and Bs in the actual work situation. The data that do exist come from a series of laboratory experiments in which As and Bs were asked to perform various tasks (e.g., mental arithmetic, puzzles) in order to measure their respective autonomic and endocrine responses to stress. While As typically show greater elevations in blood pressure, heart rate and catecholamine levels, this greater arousal does not lead to improved performance. On the contrary, eight recent experiments reported no performance differences between As and Bs, one reported superior A performance, but only under a high distraction condition, and two actually reported inferior A performance when As were required to delay their responses (Table 1). The finding that type A characteristics can hinder rather than help performance is supported by a recent investigation of Streufert et al. (46). In this study different degrees of time pressure were experimentally induced for the purpose of examining resulting variations in performance on a simulated complex managerial task. Based on the deterioration in performance that occurred under time-urgent conditions, the authors conclude that managerial activities which require complex decision making and long-term future planning are impeded rather than aided by type A time urgency.

It is possible, of course, that type As perform better in the real world because their frenetic drive leads them to increase the quantity of tasks undertaken though this remains to be shown. For quality of performance, in contrast, where we do have some empirical data, the evidence suggests that As usually perform no better than Bs and under some conditions actually do worse. Given the fact that As show greater autonomic and endocrine arousal when performing these laboratory tasks, they are expending more energy to

Table 1

Differences in Performance of As and Bs
on Laboratory Tasks

| Authors | Task | Performance differences As vs Bs |
|---|---|---|
| Abrahams and Birren (1973). | Reaction time tasks. | Decreased type A as opposed to type B performance in long waiting condition. |
| Burnam, Pennebaker, Glass (1976). | Arithmetic test. | No difference in no. of errors. |
| Carver, Coleman, Glass (1976). | Balke test (treadmill test). | No difference in time spent on treadmill. |
| Dembroski, MacDougall, Shields, Petito, Lushene (1978). | Perceptual motor-task involving cognitive skills. | No differences. |
| Dembroski, MacDougall, Herd, Shields (1979). | Choice reaction time. | No difference in speed of reaction. |
| Glass, Snyder, Hollis (1974). | DRL (Task requiring a low rate of response for reinforcement). | Type A's were reliably less successful than type B's in the "long" condition. No differences were observed between type A's and type B's in the "short" condition. |
| Lundberg, Forsman (1979). | Vigilance task for understimulation condition. Stroop Color-word task for overstimulation. | No differences. No differences. |
| Manuck, Craft, Gold (1978). | Feldman – Drasgow Visual Verbal Test. | No differences in number of correct solutions, sum of earnings. |
| Manuck, Garland (1979). | Feldman – Drasgow Visual Verbal Test. | No incentive condition: (received no instructions concerning performance-contingent rewards). Type As performed better than B's. Incentive condition: (10 ¢ for each correctly solved test item). No differences. |
| Matthews, Brunson (1979) | Stroop color task. | Distractor condition: As performed better than B's. No distractor condition: No difference. |
| Williams, Lane, White, Kuhn, Shanberg (1981). | Mental arithmetic (Serial subtraction). | No difference. |

achieve the same results. In this respect, type As are inefficient workers.

Even if type As do not actually produce more than Bs, it is possible that the workstyle of As causes them to be <u>perceived</u> as more effective and hence more likely to be promoted. The converse of the type A's successful image would be the type B employee who, regardless of performance, is perceived as stagnant, lacking ambition and motivation, and is thus barred from advancement. The positive correlation described earlier between type A and occupational status would seem to confirm the desirability of the type A image. However, once again it should be pointed out that no study has found high occupational status to be exclusively reserved for As; even among the most senior officers of the fastest growing of the largest corporations in Canada, fully one-third (34%) were classified as clear-cut Bs (18). The image of type A may facilitate promotion, but is obviously not a necessary requirement for it.

The relationship between type A behavior and occupational success is complex and much still remains to be discovered. We do know enough now, however, to develop some guidelines for the treatments we can ethically recommend. To the degree that Bs can and do succeed in the work world, we can legitimately reassure potential clients that participating in type A modification is not incompatible with occupational achievement. Moreover, the fact that As experience more physiological wear and tear to achieve the same results justifies treating A hyperreactivity, at least in part, as a problem of individual functioning. On the other hand, the fact remains that as a group As do achieve more and faster promotions, possibly because their behavior style is congruent with the North American emphasis on individualism, competition and quick results. For this reason, it behooves us to be cautious in advocating indiscriminate lifestyle change. In summary, therapeutic intervention is ethically justified, but the goal is a therapy that will produce a maximum reduction in coronary risk for a minimum amount of behavior change.

## 2 THE INITIAL TREATMENT PROGRAM: RELAXATION VS. PSYCHOTHERAPY

Although it is only five years ago that my colleagues and I began our work in type A intervention,

most of the knowledge we now have about the behavior
pattern was not then available.  In the summer of 1976
the emphasis was still on showing an association
between type A and heart disease, and the final report
of the WCGS, the first prospective epidemiological
investigation, had just been published (31, 32).
Laboratory investigation of the situational determinants
of type A behavior, of behavioral and physiological
differences between As and Bs, and exploration of
physiological mechanisms linking A behavior to CHD
were only beginning (7, 13, 16).  There were no
summaries of the type A literature such as those
provided subsequently by Glass' book (14), the Forum
on Coronary Prone Behavior (8) and the Review Panel
on Coronary-Prone Behavior (29).  Most important of
all, the only published report of an intervention
attempt was a Letter to the Editor describing a pilot
program with 10 subjects (48).  This report was of
limited usefulness for our purposes since subjects were
post coronary patients and had not been formally
classified as As.

The attempt to develop an intervention program
for healthy type As, therefore, constituted an
exploration into virgin terrain.  The first decision
was to focus our efforts on type As with specific
demographic characteristics:  middle-aged male managers
and professionals.  We chose to work with middle-aged
males because this group is at greatest risk for premature coronary heart disease, and because the best
data linking type A to heart disease comes from the
Western Collaborative Group Study which used a sample
with these demographic characteristics (31).  We chose
to work with managers and professionals both because
type A is most prevalent at this occupational level
(51), and because this group is likely to experience
most acutely the conflict between the physical cost of
type A vs. its social benefits.

The next step was to formulate a theoretical
rationale for treatment.  At that time, the only
explanatory model of type A behavior existant was
that formulated by David Glass (16).  According to
his view, type A behavior is essentially a coping
response used to counter the threat of actual or
potential loss of control.  In contrast to individuals
who are unable or willing to adapt to social norms,
type A individuals have internalized thoroughly
Western society's emphasis on the ability to control
one's environment.  The positive side of this mastery

orientation is enhanced self-esteem and increased social reinforcement. The negative side of this adaptive pattern, in contrast, is the threat experienced in any situation in which the individual cannot be sure of complete control. When signs of possible loss of control do occur, as inevitably they must, the initial response is an increased effort to regain control, involving greater mental and physical exertion, stepped up pace, heightened competitiveness, and so on (14, 15). Even in situations where control is not attainable, type A subjects tend to avoid recognition of this fact and continue actively struggling. Only when the cues signifying absence of control are highly salient will the type A individual lapse into a state of learned helplessness (14, 21). Thus, the usual coping style of the type A person is one of psychological and physio-logical hyper-responsiveness interspersed with periods of helplessness and hypo-responsiveness.

Assuming this pattern of functioning in type A individuals, it should be possible to leave the basic need for mastery untouched, but, instead, to focus on the behavior that the individual uses to cope with threat. A series of muscular and breathing relaxation exercises, common techniques in behavior therapy, could be used as a substitute coping strategy for the usual pattern of frantic activity. Once he had learned the basic techniques, the type A individual could be given instructions in monitoring his level of tension during his daily activities and in using relaxation to reduce tension whenever necessary. Even if he could not control the situation, the type A individual could control his reactions to it.

The advantage of this treatment approach was its potential appeal to healthy, occupationally successful, type A managers and professionals. Rather than repeating the same tired arguments concerning the physical harm-fulness of their hyper-active lifestyle, we would approach the men in an area where they were unused to reproach and, therefore, highly vulnerable: Type A behavior was an ineffective way of coping with the stresses of daily life. The individual who responded to all stress situations with an automatic four-alarm mobilization was clearly showing his inability to exert control, as well as placing a great deal of wear and tear on his coronary arteries.

Our solution to this hyper-reactivity was, once again, very different from the usual advice to "take it easy". Instead, we suggested that a more healthful coping pattern involved active effort, but effort directed as much toward control of self as toward control of the outside world. By following our treatment program, type As would be trained to become aware of their level of muscular tension and to attribute importance to bodily cues of loss of self-control (i.e., heightened tension). When confronted with a challenging situation (a tense business meeting, a difficult project with a tight deadline), the usual coping pattern of frenzied activity could be replaced, or at least supplemented, by efforts at tension regulation. In this way the previous stereotyped response would be replaced by a more differentiated one, and the person would probably be able to accomplish more with less strain.

To test the feasibility and utility of tension regulation for healthy type A men, we decided to recruit 30 type A individuals. Criteria for entry into the program were stringent: extreme type A characteristics (type A-1), ages 39-59, non-smoker, full-time managerial or professional position, salary $25,000+, commitment to attend at least 12 of the 14 treatment sessions, and willingness to deposit $100 as a guarantee of attendance. The method of recruitment was via a newspaper article describing the program and the criteria for entry. The nature of the recruitment appeal and/or the stringent criteria for entry obviously appealed to the type of sample we wished to attract for we were deluged by over 150 applicants.

The Structured Interview was used to screen for type A characteristics (30). This interview yields four classifications: fully developed A (A-1), somewhat A (A-2), uncertain (X) and non-A (B). All individuals selected for the pilot program were fully developed As (type A-1).

Of the 27 individuals who passed the physical examination (6 of the 33 men initially selected as A-1 were later placed in a separate group because of cardiac abnormalities revealed on an exercise ECG), 13 were randomly assigned to a 14-week tension regulation program. In this program individuals were first taught how to quantify their level of tension using a 1-10 scale and then instructed for a period of a week to record hourly the activity currently in progress and the level of tension experienced. This self-observation permitted participants to become more aware of variations in their level of arousal, and the situations associated with these changes. At the same time, a sequence of relaxation exercises designed to foster physiological self-control was introduced. A fifteen minute modified version of Jacobsonian muscle relaxation (19) was presented and participants were asked to practice this exercise twice daily following recorded instructions and noting tension levels before and after each practice session. After a few weeks of this regime, the muscle relaxation exercise was shortened to five minutes and specific neck and shoulder and breathing exercises were added.

Eventually, participants reached a level of proficiency where they could both detect early warning signs of physical tension and relax upon command. The task now became one of using these skills to maintain a comfortably low level of tension. Regularly occurring events in the daily routine (e.g., shaving, opening one's agenda book, driving the car) became signals to check tension level and adjust it if necessary. Even when unexpected or strong arousal did occur (e.g., a discourteous driver cutting in, an argument with one's superior), relaxation techniques could be used to lower the tension level.

Although we had previously rejected the possibility of psychotherapy for non-clinical subjects, the necessity of finding a control condition that would be credible to these type A men led us to turn to the psychotherapy unit of the hospital in which the program was carried out. But instead of simply serving as an attention-placebo condition, the therapists concerned, experienced and enthusiastic practitioners of brief psychotherapy utilized their 14 sessions to run an active treatment program. Based on their view of type A behavior as an initially useful solution to a conflictual family constellation in childhood, the aim of therapy became one of showing these men how their childhood perceptions and responses distorted their current behavior. The assumption here was at once the individual understood why he was behaving in a certain way then he would be free to change this automatic pattern. While there was no explicit instruction in behavior change, the male and female cotherapists did serve as role models for a more relaxed, less competitive, behavior style.

The weakest part of this pilot study was the evaluation procedures used. There is no self-evident criterion for measuring clinically significant change

in the type A pattern. Neither of the two methods
currently in use for diagnosing the presence of the
pattern, the Structured Interview and the questionnaire
Jenkins Activity Survey, is sufficiently accurate to
measure intra-individual change over time. While
reduction in cardiac morbidity and mortality constitute
acceptable substitute criteria from the clinical
standpoint, these indices are only likely to show
significant change when very large or very high risk
samples are followed over long periods of time. For
the purposes of the pilot study, therefore, we simply
measured change in standard physiological and psychological risk factors.

The results of this study were encouraging in that
without apparent change of their diet or exercise
habits, and while continuing to work the same hours
per week and to carry the same type of responsibility,
men in the behavior therapy group showed significant
decreases on physiological (serum cholesterol, systolic
blood pressure) and psychological (time pressure, life
dissatisfaction) risk factors (40). Even more
important, six months later most of these changes had
been maintained (41). However, contrary to our
expectations, men in the psychotherapy group showed
almost as good treatment effects immediately after
treatment; although the drop in serum cholesterol was
larger and more consistent for the relaxation group,
differences between the two treatment conditions were
not statistically significant. They only became so
at the follow-up (41).

3 THE SECOND TREATMENT PROGRAM: A COGNITIVE-
  BEHAVIORAL APPROACH

The fact that participants in the pilot program
were motivated to stay in treatment and seemed to
derive benefits from it encouraged us to attempt a
more ambitious intervention effort. For this new,
improved version, significant changes were made in
sample constitution, program content and evaluation
procedures. In terms of sample, we wanted to see if
the results obtained with a very select group of
extreme type As could be broadened to a less carefully
chosen, but probably more representative, group of
managers. With the cooperation of medical and personnel
officers of three large Canadian companies, letters
were sent to all men at a designated middle-management
level inviting them to participate in a research stress

management program. Entry criteria were much less
stringent than for the previous program: All men at
the designated occupational level who did not manifest
overt signs of heart disease would be accepted. The
degree to which participants had to commit themselves
to the program was also considerably less. In contrast
to the first study, there was no deposit and both the
initial screening interview and the treatment program
were held at the worksite.

Sixty-six men volunteered during the two week
recruitment period in December 1978. Unlike the men
in the first sample, all of whom had been English-
speaking, 44% of this group was Francophone. Because
these men were chosen at the middle-manager level,
rather than the senior managers and professionals of
the first study, they were also considerably younger
($\bar{x}$ = 41.33 vs. $\bar{x}$ = 47.60). In this study smokers were
not excluded and, in fact, 30% of the sample were
currently smokers. Most important of all, however, was
the difference in type A status. In contrast to the
first study where all participants had been classified
as extreme type As (A-1), here only 47% of the sample
(31 men) were placed in that category. An additional
40% were less extreme As, while 13% were classified
as non-As (B and X).

Forty of these sixty-six men were randomly assigned
to a 13 week immediate treatment program, while 26
constituted a waiting list control. The men in the
immediate treatment condition met weekly in groups of
10 (there were 2 Anglophone and 2 Francophone groups)
for thirteen 1½ hours sessions between February and
June 1979. Participants in the waiting list control
condition were offered the same treatment between
October 1979 and February 1980.

For this second project, we also made major changes
in the treatment program (37, 38). Rather than simply
seeking to modify the physiological response to a given
stressor, we wanted to change as well the mental set
with which the person approached a potential stress
situation and the ways in which he sought to manage both
the tension and the situation (39). For this purpose,
we increased the number of coping strategies taught to
include muscle relaxation (2), rational-emotive thinking
(12, 26), communication skills training (47), problem-
solving (11) and, in a special role, an adaptation of
stress inoculation (27).

The third change was in the measures used to evaluate outcome. Based on our belief that it was the frequency, intensity and duration of sympathetic arousal that constituted the pathogenic elements in the type A pattern, we attempted to measure change by charting a number of indices of this arousal, both in a laboratory and a field situation (34). Prior to and immediately following the intervention, all participants were exposed to a standard stress situation in the laboratory and fluctuations in systolic blood pressure, diastolic blood pressure, and heart rate, plasma epinephrine and plasma norepinephrine before, during and after the task were recorded.

In the field situation, one working day every fortnight during the course of the project was designated as a monitoring day (nine days in all). During this day four types of measures were tracked: psychological state, blood pressure, urinary catecholamines, and serum cholesterol and testosterone. Participants were asked to record hourly levels of muscular tension, irritability, time pressure and performance (using a 0-10 scale) and follow this by a blood pressure reading using an electronic machine - Labtronix 4000 - designed for home use. Urine for analysis of catecholamine levels was collected for 24 hrs. divided into three time periods: the night before the working day, the working day itself, and the evening after.

The results for this second project were mixed. While not quite as high as for the initial project, attendance continued to be good (29 of the 40 men in the initial treatment group attended at least 8 of the 13 sessions) and only 5 men completely abandoned the program. Moreover, the major reason for missing sessions was business trips outside the city; these middle managers simply did not have the same control over their schedules as did the more senior professionals and executives of the first study. From the motivational point of view, therefore, this study could be judged successful in that we had managed once again to recruit healthy, occupationally successful type A participants and keep them in treatment.

In terms of treatment benefits, the major changes were psychological. Participants in the treatment program, compared to the controls, showed significantly increased life satisfaction ($p = .01$) and a borderline significant decrease in psychological symptoms ($p = .06$).

Moreover, the change in global life satisfaction was
due to significant improvement in two dimensions
particularly relevant to treatment content: health
and ability to control one's life. On the other hand,
the treatment group did not show significantly greater
reduction in self-rating of Type A (Jenkins Activity
Survey, Thurstone) than did the control group. The
psychological benefits of treatment, therefore, were
directed more to general stress reduction, rather than
to specific type A modification (43).

More disappointing was the failure to show changes
in physiological reactivity resulting from treatment.
Most physiological measures did show a significant
decline over time, but the changes were not significantly
different for men in the treatment condition than for
the controls (3, 43). Since we had previously designated
reduced physiological hyperreactivity as the criterion
of treatment – as well as strongly affirming the
importance of delineating a priori specific criteria
for evaluating treatment (34, 36) - we can only conclude
that this intervention failed to achieve its goals.

One obvious explanation for this failure is the
ineffectiveness of the treatment program itself. It is
possible that in adding a panoply of coping strategies
to the basic relaxation approach (38) we had subjected
the men to sensory overload and inadvertently diluted
the strength of the therapy. The therapeutic message
may have been further weakened by the heterogeneity of
the group to which it was addressed. In contrast to
the exclusively A-1 sample of the first study, this
effort included less extreme and even some uncertain As.
Therapeutic leverage was thereby reduced since it was
possible for participants to claim that specific
problems being discussed did not really apply to them.

Before placing the onus for failure completely on
the treatment program, however, there are reasons for
subjecting both our data collection and our sample
selection procedures to critical scrutiny. The
complexity of the measures we sought, coupled with
deficiencies in equipment and personnel, led to considerable missing and/or invalid data, particularly
in the measures taken in the field (3). For instance,
we were unable to include in the statistical analyses
the urinary catecholamine data of more than half the
sample, either because a given day's collection was
incomplete, or there was an insufficient number of
measuring days (we required a minimum of six for analysis,

two at the beginning of treatment, two in the middle,
and two at the end), or because of problems in transportation, storage and handling. Blood pressure measures
during the working day had the additional handicap of
invasiveness, i.e., the fact that the subject had to
pull out his apparatus to measure his blood pressure
meant that he was unlikely to do so at the moments of
greatest upset, precisely those time periods we most
wished to record.

There were fewer missing data in the laboratory
stress situations, since participants only had to
attend two sessions, but a major methodological hurdle
encountered here was the unexpectedly strong effects of
habituation. We had allowed a half-hour for habituation
before beginning baseline screening, but this time
period obviously was not long enough to overcome the
novelty of surroundings and procedure (particularly
the venipunctures!). As a result, all participants
showed such a marked drop in heart rate, catecholamine
excretion and blood pressure in the post treatment
session that it completely drowned but any changes that
might have resulted from the treatment itself (43).

A final unanticipated problem was the heterogeneity
of the sample in terms of the principal dependent
measures-physiological reactivity. Type As as a group
are more reactive than type Bs, but not all type As are
reactive. (Not all type As have heart attacks either,
and it is possible that physiological reactivity is
one of the discriminating indices). As a result, we
found ourselves in the position of seeking to lower
values that for some participants were not very high
to begin with.

4 FUTURE PROSPECTS FOR TYPE A INTERVENTION

To draw up a balance sheet of the successes and
failures of our efforts to reduce the coronary risk
associated with being type A in healthy, occupationally
successful, middle-aged men, there are two significant
pluses and one crucial minus. The pluses are in the
areas of conceptualization and motivation, the minus
in the area of experimental methodology. Since our
first tentative efforts in 1976, we have come a long
way in delineating who and what we are seeking to treat
and how treatment effects can be evaluated (cf. 34, 35,
36, 37). Equally as important, the treatment approach
developed appears to be acceptable to the population

towards which it is directed. Where we have failed is in showing that treatment produces the kind of physiological changes we consider to be significant. Furthermore, deficiencies in study design make it impossible to ascertain whether it is the treatment itself, or the way that change was measured, that account for the failure to observe physiological treatment benefits.

This failure to produce the wishes for results has left us disappointed, but not discouraged. Given the complexity of the phenomena involved, it is probably unrealistic to have expected to solve all the conceptual, motivational and methodological problems in one fell swoop. Thus, our intentions for the future are to mount another intervention study, using the benefit of hindsight to improve the methodology. Because we believe that reducing the frequency, intensity and duration of sympathetic arousal is, in the current state of our knowledge, the most viable therapeutic target for type A intervention (36), we shall continue to pursue this goal. This time, however, we shall attempt to increase our chances of therapeutic success by improving both the sampling and the measuring procedures (42). Only when we have subjected our therapeutic hypothesis to a valid test, can we decide whether to pursue this line of investigation, or search for a different approach.

REFERENCES

1. Abraham, J.P. and J. E. Birren. Reaction Time as a Function of Age and Behavioral Predisposition to Coronary Heart Disease. Journal of Gerontology 28 (1973) 471-478.
2. Bernstein, C.A. and T. D. Borkovec. Progressive Relaxation Training: A Manual for the Helping Professions. (Champaign, Research Press, 1973).
3. Brochocka, J. Evaluation d'un Traitement Chez les Sujets de Type A Dans le Milieu de Travail. Unpublished master's thesis in psychology. University of Montreal (1981).
4. Burke, R.J. and T. Weir. The Type A Experience: Occupational and Life Demands, Satisfaction, and Well-Being. Journal of Human Stress 6 (1980), 28-38.

5. Burnam, M.A., J.W. Pennebaker and D.C. Glass. Time
   Consciousness, Achievement Striving, and the
   Type A Coronary-Prone Behaviora Pattern. Journal
   of Abnormal Psychology 84 (1975) 76-79.
6. Caplan, R.D., S. Cobbs, J.R.P. French, R.V. Harrison
   and S. R. Pinneau. Job Demands and Worker Health.
   (Washington, D.C. Department of Health, Education
   and Welfare, Publication No. (N1OS-H) (1975) 75-
   160.
7. Carver, C.S., A.E. Coleman and D.C. Glass. The
   Coronary-Prone Behavior Pattern and the Suppression
   of Fatigue on a Treadmill Test. Journal of
   Personality and Social Psychology 33 (1976)
   460-466.
8. Dembroski, T.M., M. Feinleib, S.G. Haynes, J.L. Shields
   and S. M. Wiess (Eds.) Proceedings of the Forum
   on Coronary-Prone Behavior. (Washington, D.C.
   Department of Health, Education, and Welfare,
   Publication No. (NIH) 78-1451, 1977).
9. Dembroski, T.M., J.M. MacDougall, J.L. Shields,
   J. Pettito and R. Lushene. Components of the
   Type A Coronary-Prone Behavior Pattern and
   Cardiovascular Responses to Psychomotor Performance
   Challenge. Journal of Behavioral Medicine 1 (1978)
   159-176.
10. Dembroski, T.M., J.M. MacDougall, J.A. Herd and
    J.L. Shields. Effects of Level of Challenge on
    Pressor and Heart Rate Responses in Type A and
    B Subjects. Journal of Applied Psychology 9
    (1979) 209-228.
11. D'Zurilla, T.J. and M.R. Goldfried. Problem Solving
    and Behavior Modification. Journal of Abnormal
    Psychology 78 (1971) 107-126.
12. Ellis, A. and R. Grieger (Eds.) Handbook of Rational
    Emotive Therapy. (New York, Springer, 1977).
13. Friedman, M., S.O. Byers, J. Diamant and R.H. Rosenman.
    Plasma Catecholamine Response of Coronary-Prone
    Subjects (Type A) to a Specific Challenge.
    Metabolism 24 (1975) 205-210.
14. Glass, D.C. Behavior Patterns, Stress, and Coronar
    Disease. (Hillsdale, New Jersey, Lawrence
    Erlbaum Associates, 1977).
15. Glass, D.C. and S.C. Carver. Environmental Stress
    and the Type A Response. In A. Baum and J.E. Singer
    (Eds.). Advances in Environmental Psychology.
    (Hillsdale, New Jersey, Lawrence Erlbaum
    Associates, 1980).

16. Glass, D.C., M.L. Snyder and J.F. Hollis.  Time
    Urgency and the Type A Coronary-Prone Behavior
    Pattern.  Journal of Applied Social Psychology
    4 (1974) 125-140.
17. Howard, J.H., D.A. Cunningham and P.A. Rechnitzer.
    Health Patterns Associated with Type A Behavior:
    A Managerial Population. Journal of Human Stress
    2 (1976) 24-33.
18. Howard, J.H. D.A. Cunningham and P.A. Rechnitzer.
    Work Patterns Associated with Type A Behavior:
    A Managerial Population.  Human Relations 30
    (1977) 825-836.
19. Jacobson, E.  Progressive Relaxation. (Chicago,
    University of Chicago Press, 1938.
20. Kornitzer, M. Type A Behavior Pattern.(Paper
    presented at the NATO Advanced Study Institute
    on "Behavioral Medicine: Work, Stress and Health",
    Castera-Verduzan, France, August, 1981).
21. Krantz, D.S., D.C. Glass and M.L. Snyder.
    Helplessness, Stress Level, and the Coronary-Prone
    Behavior Pattern.  Journal of Experimental Social
    Psychology 19 (1974) 284-300.
22. Lundberg, U. and L. Forsman. Adrenal-Medullary and
    Adrenal-Cortical Responses to Understimulation
    and Overstimulation: Comparison Between Type A
    and Type B Persons.  Biological Psychology 9
    (1979) 79-89.
23. Manuck, S.B. and F.N. Garland.  Coronary-Prone
    Behavior Pattern, Task Inventive, and Cardio-
    vascular Response.  Psychophysiology 16 (1979)
    136-142.
24. Manuck, S.B., S.A. Craft and K.J. Gold.  Coronary-
    Prone Behavior Pattern and Cardiovascular Response.
    Psychophygiology 15 (1978) 403-411.
25. Matthews, K.A. and B.I. Brunson. Allocation of
    Attention and the Type A Coronary-Prone Behavior
    Pattern.  Journal of Personality and Social
    Psychology  37 (1979) 2081-2090.
26. Maultsby, M. and A. Ellis.  Techniques for Using
    Rational-Emotive Imagery.  In A. Ellis and
    E. Abraham (Eds.) Brief Psychotherapy in Medical
    and Health Practice (New York, Springer, 1978).
27. Meichenbaum, D. Cognitive Behavior Modification:
    An Integrative Approach. (New York, Plenum,
    1977).
28. Mettlin, C. Occupational Careers and the Prevention
    of Coronary-Prone Behavior. Social Science and
    Medicine 10 (1976) 367-373.

29. Review Panel on Coronary-Prone Behavior and Coronary Heart Disease. Coronary-Prone Behavior and Coronary Heart Disease: A Critical Review. Circulation 63 (1981) 1201-1215.

30. Rosenman, R.H. The Interview Method of Assessment of the Coronary-Prone Behavior Pattern. In T.M. Dembroski, M. Feinleib, S.G. Haynes, J.L. Shields and S.M. Weiss (Eds.) Proceedings of the Forum on Coronary-Prone Behavior. (Washington, D.C., Department of Health Education and Welfare, Publication No. (NIH) 78-1451, 1977).

31. Rosenman, R.H., M. Friedman, et al. A Predictive Study of Coronary Heart Disease: The Western Collaborative Group Study. Journal of the American Medical Association 189 (1964) 15-22.

32. Rosenman, R.H., R.J. Brand, et al. Coronary Heart Disease in the Western Collaborative Group Study: Final Follow-up Experience of 8½ Years. Journal of the American Medical Association 233 (1975) 872-877.

33. Rosenman, R.H., R.J. Brand, R.I. Sholtz and M. Friedman. Multivariate Prediction of Coronary Heart Disease During 8.5 Year Follow-up in the Western Collaborative Group Study. American Journal of Cardiology 37 (1976) 902-910.

34. Roskies, E. Evaluating improvement in the Coronary-Prone (Type A) Behavior Pattern. In D.J. Osborne, M.M. Gruneberg and J.R. Esser (Eds.) Research in Psychology and Medicine. (New York, Academic Press, 1979).

35. Roskies, E. Considerations in Developing a Treatment Program for the Coronary-Prone (Type A) Behavior Pattern. In P. Davidson and S.M. Davidson (Eds.) Behavioral Medicine: Changing Health Lifestyle. (New York, Brunner/Mazel, 1980).

36. Roskies, E. Type A Intervention: Finding a Disease to fit the cures. (Paper presented at the NATO Symposium on Behavioral Medicine, Port Carras, Greece, June 1981).

37. Roskies, E. Stress Management for Type A Individuals In D. Meichenbaum and M. Jaremko (Eds.) Stress, Prevention and Management: A Cognitive-Behavioral Approach. (New York, Plenum, in press).

38. Roskies, E., and J. Avard. Teaching Healthy Managers to Control Their Coronary-Prone (Type A) Behavior. In K. Blankstein and J. Polivy (Eds.) Self-Control and Self-Modification of Emotional Behaviors. (New York, Plenum, in press).

39.Roskies, E. and R. S. Lazarus. Coping Theory and
    Teaching of Coping Skills. In P.O. Davidson and
    S.M. Davidson (Eds.) Behavioral Medicine:
    Changing Health Lifestyles. (New York, Brunner/
    Mazel, 1980).
40.Roskies, E., et al. Changing the Coronary-Prone
    (Type A) Behavior Pattern in a Non-Clinical
    Population. Journal of Behavioral Medicine 1
    (1978) 201-215.
41.Roskies, E., et al. Generalizability and durability
    of treatment effects in an intervention program
    for Coronary-Prone (Type A) Managers. Journal
    of Behavioral Medicine 2 (1979) 195-207.
42.Roskies, E., P. Seraganian, and R. Oseasohn. Changing
    Type A in a Non-Clinical Population: Project III.
    (Research proposal submitted to Department of
    Health and Welfare, Ottawa, July 1981).
43.Sarrasin, S.  Evaluation des Effets d'un Traitement
    Visant la Reduction du Risque Coronarien chez
    des Sujets de Type A. (Unpublished master's thesis
    in psychology.  University of Montreal, August
    1981).
44.Shekelle, R.B., J.A. Schoenberger, and J. Stamler.
    Correlates of the JAS Type A Behavior Pattern
    Score.  Journal of Chronic Diseases 29 (1976)
    381-394.
45.Snow, B.  Level of Aspiration in Coronary-Prone and
    Non-Coronary-prone Adults.  Personality and Social
    Psychology Bulletin 4 (1978) 416-419.
46.Streufert, S., S.C. Streufert and D.M. Gorson.
    Time Urgency and Coronary-Prone Behavior: The
    Effectiveness of a behavior Pattern.  Journal of
    Experimental and Applied Social Psychology, in
    press.
47.Stuart, R.B. (Paper presented at the annual meeting
    of the Association des Specialistes en Modification
    du Comportement.  Moncton, New Brunswick, June
    1974).
48.Suinn, R.M., L. Brock, and C.A. Edie.  Letters to
    the Editor:  Behavioral Therapy for Type A Patients.
    American Journal of Cardiology 36 (1975) 269.
49.Waldron, I., et al. Coronary-Prone Behavior Pattern
    in Employed Men and Women.  Journal of Human
    Stress 3 (1977) 2-19.
50.Williams, R.B., Jr., et al. Type A Behavior Pattern
    and Neuro-Endocrine Response During Mental Work.
    Psychosomatic Medicine 43 (1981) 92.

51. Zyzanski, S.J.  Associations of the Coronary-Prone
    Behavior Pattern.  In T.M. Dembroski, M. Feinleib,
    S.G. Haynes, J.L. Shields and S.M. Weiss (Eds.)
    Proceedings of the Forum on Coronary-Prone Behavior.
    (Washington, D.C., Department of Health, Education,
    and Welfare, Publication No. (NIH) 78-1451, 1977).

# STRESS INTERVENTION AT THE ORGANIZATIONAL LEVEL

Charles J. de Wolff

Workgroup on Psychology of Work
and Organization
University of Nijmegen
Nijmegen, the Netherlands

## 1  INTRODUCTION

There is now ample evidence that psychosocial stressors have considerable impact (strain) on the health and well-being of individuals operating within an organizational context. Given this reality, one might well ask: Can remedial action be taken either to prevent individual workers from experiencing strain and/or to help them recover from same? Of course, one might argue that the state-of-the-art knowledge about relationships between psychosocial stressors and strains, as well as about the processes linking to two, is still insufficient to justify action at this point, that such efforts would be premature. Then again, one might equally argue that experimental intervention is warranted even while research on such relationships continues, since the level(s) of strain evidenced in the normal workplace is on the rise and obviously affecting increasing numbers of workers as time goes on. Of course, one would also want to monitor any adverse effects of such experimental remedial efforts towards alleviating strain, thus gaining knowledge which might increase our present understanding of stress-strain relationships in the work setting.

It is important, as one approaches the question of remedial intervention, to realize that knowledge about how to proceed with remedial action need not stem from stress research alone. In fact, there is much relevant information available which comes to us from other

sources, e.g., when role ambiguity and future uncertainty
turn out to be important stressors, an industrial-
organizational psychologist will immediately refer to
literature about other organizational problems where
ambiguity is involved (organizational change, performance
appraisal interviews, management by objectives, etc.).

In this chapter, I will restrict myself to interventions at the organizational level, particularly to
those related to personnel practices. This does not
imply that these are the only types of action that one
might attempt; there are other interventions which are
targeted at the level of the individual which clearly
have merit as regards stress management, e.g., biofeedback, transcendental meditation, and various
relaxation therapies (see chapters by Benson and Collings
in this Volume). I do, however, want to make the case
that the organization per se can be an important venue
for stress intervention.

## 2    INTERVENTION APPROACHES

In the literature, we find a number of approaches
which lend themselves to organizational intervention:
person-environment fit, social support, reducing ambiguity, and improving individual coping behavior. Each
of these has roots in other theories as well (e.g.,
leadership, personnel selection, organizational effectiveness), and has been applied in other contexts.

### 2.1  Person-Environment Fit

In several theories, it is stressed that there should
be correspondence between the abilities and needs of the
individual and the demands and rewards of the organization. A good example of such a theory is given by
Lofquist and Dawis (6) in their work adjustment theory.
Figure 1 presents their model as it relates to personnel selection, but the model is useful for stress as
well. Lack of correspondence between abilities-demands
or needs-rewards is an important stressor. Lack of
correspondence between needs and rewards means that the
individual feels frustrated. Lack of correspondence
between abilities and demands means that the individual
is not able to cope. Correspondence is not a static
concept. Both the individual and the environment change,
sometimes slowly and sometimes fast. So correspondence
is a dynamic concept; it has to be maintained over time.
Continuous effort is needed to perserve it. Several

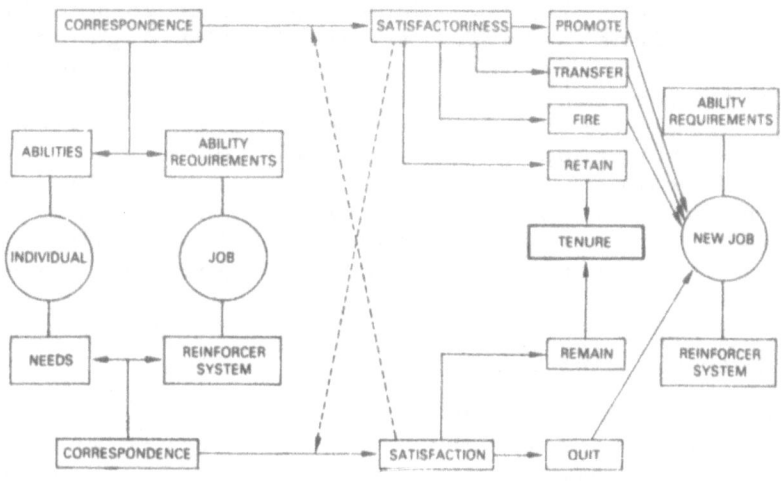

Figure 1.    The work adjustment model offered by Lofquist
             and Dawis.

activities might contribute to establishing and maintaining person-environment correspondence; these include
staffing procedures, supervisory practices, the way the
organization handles organizational change, etc.    Each
of these activities will be discussed in turn later on
in this chapter.

## 2.2   Social Support

Several studies show that social support is an
important variable for reducing psychosocial strain(s).
Individuals who report high levels of support from co-
workers and supervisors experience less impact from
stressors, and thus lower levels of strain.    Evidently
support acts as a kind of buffer.    Support has been an
important concept in many study (e.g., on leadership)
and much research has concentrated on how superiors can
behave in a supportive manner.    Interventions have to
do with supervisory practices, including performance
appraisal and managing ineffective performance (see
below).

## 2.3   Reducing Ambiguity

In a number of studies, role ambiguity is the variable having the most negative (strain) consequences.
In other studies, it has become clear that there is
much ambiguity in organizations, particularly at the

middle management level. Many employees do not know
what expectations relevant people in the organization
have of them as regards their performance. They often
do not know what opinion(s) their superior has of them.
And, many feel insecure about the extent to which they
can rely on the support of superiors when they encounter
problems at work. Interventions aimed at reducing ambiguity have to do with structuring the organization,
supervisory activities (including goal setting, work
planning, performance appraisal) and job and career
planning.

## 2.4   Improving Coping Behavior

People confronted with difficult situations at
work, as well as elsewhere, differ in their ability to
cope with problems. Coping behavior is learned and,
in principle, it is possible to teach individuals how
to cope with threatening situations. A particular
problem might be a challenge to an experienced person,
but be frightening for an inexperienced individual.
Most people learn by trial-and-error, i.e., from accumulated successes and failures. But it is possible
to learn in a more systematic way. There is a vast
literature on training, such as behavioral modeling,
which can be used to enlarge an employee's coping repertoire. This can be used for management training,
but also for specific groups who are exposed to certain
types of stressors.

## 3   TYPES OF INTERVENTION

All together this leads us to a large, rather
diverse list of possible intervention strategies that
can be employed at the organizational level. These
include:

- job structuring
- structuring the organization
- staffing procedures
- supervisory practices
- management of ineffective performance
- career planning and guidance
- periodic medical check-up programs
- monitoring of absenteeism
- preparation for disability status
- introducing organizational change
- teaching coping skills

About all of these interventions, there is a considerable amount of relevant literature. In this chapter, it is not possible to describe this in detail; rather, we can only point out possible directions one might pursue. Most of these interventions are well developed; some need further refinement. This is not to say that all those listed are widely used; on the contrary, as we will note, some have only seen limited application.

## 3.1   Job Structuring

Many published works have emphasized that work content is very important (11). Applying Tayloristic principles has led to jobs which are unrewarding, and which induce psychosocial strain(s)(5). There is a long tradition aiming at improving the content of work. In a recent study in the Netherlands (1), where an improved measurement instrument was used, large correlations were found between job characteristics and a number of strains such as absenteeism, work satisfaction, health, and anxiety. Principles for job structuring have been formulated by psychologists from the Tavistock Institute (9) and by Hackman and Oldham (4). Relevant characteristics are task variety, autonomy, and challenge. Changing job content is a complex process; it is not only an attempt to make jobs more rewarding, but it is also a reorganization. The latter might increase ambiguity, and meet resistance from employees. So several authors have pleaded for a combination of job structuring and organizational change programs, in which employees participate in decision making processes. Others suggest that one should concentrate on system design, and give special attention to job content when the production system is still on the drawing board. There is a need for more knowledge about the relationship between production technologies and job characteristics. Studies about this have been done by the department of work psychology at Nijmegen (2).

## 3.2   Structuring the Organization

There is much classic work concentrating on job descriptions, procedures, accountability, responsibilities, organization maps, span of control, etc. All these activities contribute to clarification of work roles, and to the reduction of job ambiguity. Bureaucratic rules serve an important purpose in organizations. Many consultants specialize on these activities. It is likely that in well organized social systems, people suffer less from role ambiguity and role conflict, two major sources of psychosocial strain.

## 3.3   Staffing Procedures

In the model presented by Lofquist and Dawis (6), two matching processes are indicated:  demands and abilities and needs and rewards.  In selection proce- dures, psychologists have traditionally concentrated on only one of these;  demands vs. abilities.  Needs were essentially neglected.  But gradually attention has shifted and now several authors give more consideration to the staffing process (8,10).  Large organizations have often bureaucratized staffing procedures, having special departments looking after recruitment, selection, training, etc.  What is often missing is an integrating philosophy.  Many organizations have large turnover rates in the first half year after employment, much larger than in the period after that.  This reflects, we believe, a lack of correspondence between individual employee needs/abilities and organizational demands/ rewards.  Staffing should concentrate on establishing correspondence and making it clear how the organization tends to interact with the employee.  In effect, the way organizations structure their staffing procedures demonstrates how they see employees and what expectations they have about and for them within the work setting.

## 3.4   Supervisory Practices

Superiors can do very much when it comes to pre- vention and remedial action.  They can help to preserve correspondence between abilities-demands and/or needs- rewards.  They can provide much needed support.  They can reduce ambiguity.  And, they can teach employees how to cope with difficult problems at work.  Much has already been done as regards research on supervisory behavior and management training; however, there is still much that is misunderstood about leadership. Supervision requires that the supervisor, on the one hand, look after the interest of the organization (e.g., production targets, quality of products, meeting dead- lines) and, on the other hand, look after interests of employees (e.g., giving support, reducing ambiguity, etc.)  To be supportive requires more than being friendly; leadership must contribute to, or maintain, the employees' sense of personal worth and perceived importance.  It has to do with stimulation and help, but also the way one handles inadequate behavior such

tardiness, chronic absenteeism, and low quality performance. Research shows that supervisors often do not
know when and how to criticize employees working under
them (7,12). Supportive behavior can be learned; again,
behavioral modeling has proved to be effective in this
regard. This approach is now used by several large
American companies.

Maintaining correspondence is also the responsibility of the worker himself. When he/she cannot
achieve this objective, however, we believe the dis-
cordance should be resolved, if possible, by the
superior.

## 3.5 Management of Ineffective Performance

Ineffective performance reflects a lack of correspondence. It can be a matter of demands being greater
than abilities or a mismatch between needs and rewards.
In either case, the employee's motivation and performance is affected. This can obviously be a stressful
(at time threatening) situation for the worker. He/she
may eventually lose their job as a result. Often there
is reluctance on the part of the supervisor to act. One
is hesitant to criticize, either because it is difficult
to prove that the employee is not meeting demands, or
because the supervisor feels that he himself has failed.
So there is a tendency to wait and see, which tends to
lead to deterioration of the already problematic situation. Finally, when the problem can no longer be
neglected and others begin to complain, some corrective
action has to be taken. Often one tries to fire the
employee. When remedial action takes place as soon as
discorrespondence is noted, such drastic measures are
not necessary. Waiting makes the chances of finding
good (effective) solutions less possible.

It is important to make a good differential diagnosis of the problem(s). Periodic performance apparisal
may well contribute to early detection of discorrespondence leading to ineffective performance.

## 3.6 Career Planning and Guidance

In a career, one can distinguish several phases.
Problems of younger employees are different from those
of older ones. Younger employees might experience difficulties in building up a professional identity, while
older ones might have to cope with declining capabilities.

Others experience a mid-career crisis. So, in every
phase, there can be specific problems, causing lack
of correspondence, and eventually leading to strain.
As already stated above, the early detection of discorrespondence is vital. Here, both supervisory
staff and the personnel department can be of assistance,
e.g., in re-locating employees (job transfers) so as
to re-establish correspondence.

## 3.7  Periodic Medical Check-Up Programs

The medical check-up program may be an effective
means of detecting employees who suffer from organizational strain. Many companies now have regular check
ups for employees, particularly for older workers;
these may include both medical assessments (e.g., blood
pressure, cholesterol level) and psychological questionnaires (e.g., assessing Type A behavior pattern).
This combination of information makes it possible to
identify high risk individuals, e.g., an employee with
high blood pressure, psychosomatic complaints, a high
level of anxiety associated with role ambiguity, etc.

As a result of such check ups, employees may then
be referred for remedial action at the individual level
(see chapter by Collings).

## 3.8  Monitoring Absenteeism

Absenteeism might be a serious sign of lack of
correspondence on the employees part. In this respect,
there can be large differences across countries. In
the Netherlands, for example, where income is protected
since absent workers receive sickness benefits, someone
suffering from serious lack of correspondence might
stay home with illness. To some extent, this solves
the immediate problem; one is no longer forced to meet
demands or endure frustration. It is not likely that
this is a conscious choice. In the Dutch system, this
will eventually lead to work disability, since after
one year one almost automatically qualifies for disability benefits.

Interventions should take place as early as possible,
not later than 3 or 4 months after the onset of
absenteeism. Early intervention leads to a greater
probability of return to work; interventions attempted
after that time are more likely to fail. Interventions
turn out to be difficult. Being ill is generally seen

as incompatible with interventions from the organization. Many individuals feel that people suffering
from illness should rest, and only after they have recovered can they address problems of organizational
correspondence. Another problem is that control, to
prevent abuse of social insurance, is incompatible
with remedial action. To help individual to find solutions requires a supportive approach; but it is difficult
to be both supportive and controlling.

## 3.9 Preparation for Disability Status

In the Dutch situation, a year of absenteeism
precedes the moment when one officially acquires disability status. During the year, there is not much
interaction with the work organization. The chances
of becoming disabled increase rapidly during the first
months of absenteeism. After 6 weeks, the chances are
16% and after six months they increase to 64%. We
suspect that during this year most employees are more
preoccupied with what happened in the past than with
what will happen in the future. Unfortunately, there
is not much research on this subject. But, if our
suspicion is warranted, the new status will be a shock
for workers. Loss of work presents very difficult
problems, i.e., loss of identity, and will miss the
social support of co-workers. It is also possible that
they will feel guilty or ashamed, not having been able
to fulfill their job successfully. They may also suddenly be confronted with existential questions about
the meaningfulness of life, which may prove burdensome.
In this period when one needs the help of peers, the
loss of supportive relationships may be hard to endure.
This begs the question: Can organizations provide
necessary support for employees during prolonged absenteeism?

## 3.10 Introducing Organizational Change

Changes in organizations have an enormous impact
on person-environment fit, e.g., introducing a new
technology might lead to dramatic changes in job demands.
Merging two organizations might affect rewards to a
considerable extent. Workers might become redundant,
or might lose a position which has taken them years to
build up.

Change also leads to an increase in ambiguity. In
the stable organization, employees know more or less

what expectations are realistic, but reorganization
leads to uncertainty.

During reorganization, managers are overburdened
and do not have sufficient time to talk with individual
employees and clarify issues and concerns. This in
turn may lead to workers feeling less supported.

Thus, there are many arguments for providing
introduction and preparation for organizational change
(3) in an effort to minimize or prevent altogether
strain.

## 3.11   Teaching Coping Skills

In many occupations, one finds that job holders
are confronted with special problems. Many of these
problems are of a recurrent or chronic nature, e.g.,
managers have to criticize employees because they are
tardy or turn in products of insufficient quality. In
principle, it is possible to define these types of
problems in precise terms and to devise strategies for
alleviating them. Managers can be trained, as they are
in many American companies, to model correct (effective)
coping behaviors for employees under their charge;
use of video tapes and behavioral rehersal supplement
such efforts on the manager's part.

## 4   PROBLEMS WITH APPLICATIONS

The interventions listed above are only used in a
limited capacity at the organizational level to prevent or alleviate strain. Why is this? The knowledge
is available, yet it is not fully applied. Certainly
people at all levels of the organization are sensitive
to how serious the problem(s) can be; or are they?
Changes in health status occur gradually and are only
partially visible (e.g., hypertension); much of the
strain goes unnoticed! In addition, the knowledge that
is available is not accessible to those who would
actually do the intervention; in some cases, the theories
are not made operational so as to affect individual
employees. Thirdly, and unfortunately, often decision
makers in the organization (e.g., managers) are too
preoccupied with emergencies to pay sufficient attention
to such matters. Also, most interventions are thought
to require a lengthy period before results can be seen;
no short-term pay-offs are forthcoming. Remedial
efforts, when in evidence, are scattered and continuity
of effort is always a problem. Finally, compelling

cost-benefit analysis is lacking, often because it is
difficult to place a monetary value on psychosocial
end-points (strain). Unless such problems are resolved,
it is unlikely that we will witness any major change in
the stress-strain nature of modern day organizations.

REFERENCES

1. Algera, J.A., Kenmerken van werk. Leiden, doctoral
   thesis, 1980.

2. van Assen, A., Het rijke effect van semi autonome
   groepen. Management totaal, 1981, 44-46.

3. Bennis, W.G., Benne, K.D. & Chin, R., The planning
   of change. Holt, Rinehart & Winston, 1969.

4. Hackman, J.R. and Oldham, G.R., Motivation through
   the design of work: test of a theory, Organizational
   Behavior and Human Performance, 1976, 16, 250-279.

5. Kornhauser, A., Mental Health of the Industrial
   Worker. New York, Wiley, 1965.

6. Lofquist, L.H. and Dawis, R.V., Adjustment and Work.
   New York, Appleton, 1969.

7. Meyer, H.H., Key, E., and French, J.R.P., Split
   roles in performance appraisal. Harvard Business
   Review, 1965, 1, 123-129.

8. Schneider, B., Staffing Organizations, Pacific
   Pallisades: Goodyear, 1976.

9. Thorsrud, E.L., Job design in the wider context,
   in Davis, L.E., and Taylor, J.C., Design of jobs.
   London, Penguin books 1972.

10. de Wolff, Ch.J. en van de Bosch, G.,
    Personeelaanname, in Drenth, P.J.D., Thierry, H.,
    Willems, P.J., and de Wolff, Ch.J., Handboek
    Arbeid en Organizatie-psychologie. Deventer,
    van Loghum Slaterus, 1980.

11. Work in America, Report of a special task force to
    the Secretary of Health, Education and Welfare.
    Cambridge, MIT Press, 1973.

12.  Zander, A.F. (ed), <u>Performance Appraisals</u>.
     Ann Arbor, Foundation for the Research on Human
     Behavior, 1963.

STRESS MANAGEMENT AT WORK: THE NEW YORK TELEPHONE EXPERIMENT

Gilbeart H. Collings, Jr.

Corporate Medical Director
The New York Telephone Company
New York, New York

## 1   INTRODUCTION

It is commonly accepted that stress is a significant part of the modern world.  Whether we are subjected to greater stresses than our cavemen forebears or even our grandparents may be a matter of debate.  However, we all do have stress in our daily lives and it is also realistic to recognize that the stress levels wax and wane depending on life's circumstances and our responses to them over time.  It is unrealistic to assume that these stresses do not produce significant effects on the mental and physiological processes of the body and thereby either contribute to or cause outright disease.

In the world of today, the one constant characteristic is "change" and change is inherently stressful to the human organism. We are experiencing vast social changes in the structure and fabric of our society.  The increasing number of employed women has resulted in two working members in most families.  The changing role of both males and females and our rapidly altering moral and ethical values are striking down traditional sources of security while substituting new and unfamiliar relationships, and complex-ities.  Massive changes in technology, communications and trans-portation and many other equally significant developments are alter-ing the substance of the average lifestyle.  The working world is also undergoing revolutionary alterations.  For example, the change from predominantly blue-collar to predominantly white-collar work force and individual performance or craft skills are being replaced by team-oriented demands where relationships with others become of greater importance than physical output.  As corporations

grow with success or change with failure there are frequent internal
reorganizations and functional realignments, as well as mergers of
previously independent companies. This has extensive and serious
implications for the long-term employee. In such a world the
employee has a less secure future, greater anxieties about his/
her abilities to meet as yet unfaced demands, competitive pressures
and many other real or perceived stresses as a normal part of each
day's activity. It should not be surprising therefore to see these
influences reflected in the employee's performance on the job and
also in the employee's "performance" as to the occurrence of illness and disability.

In most industrial medical operations, it has long been recognized that probably 40% or more of all the patients who walk into
a medical facility are there either because of psychosomatic symptomatology alone or physical disease which has strong emotional/
situational overtones. In spite of this recognition, industrial
medicine has not been very effective in coping with these kinds of
cases. In fact, the general tendency is to treat the presenting
symptomatology and not delve into the true cause if it is not an
obviously organic one. In the New York Telephone Medical Department,
however, we had an early interest in trying to find answers to
these problems and over the course of the years have added psychi-
atrists to our staff; experimented with programs designed to improve
our total understanding of the patient; emphasized the constructive
role of the primary physician in helping patients to cope with
life's problems; and have maintained a healthy curiosity about
various esoteric and even unorthodox methods put forward as solutions
to these kinds of problems.

It was, therefore, natural for us to follow developments surrounding such modalities as meditation, biofeedback, progressive
muscular relaxation, and other similar forms of intervention. We
first became interested in meditation through the work of Dr.
Herbert Benson at Harvard and we engaged in a few preliminary trials
of Dr. Benson's relaxation method, currently referred to as the
Respiratory One Method (ROM). We used ROM in connection with the
clinical management of moderate hypertension and among employees
in our general working population who expressed an interest in
learning about meditation.

In these early trials, the common experience was an initial
high interest and enthusiasm on the part of employees, with large
numbers responding to the first invitation to join a group on meditation. However, over a period of months the dropout rate was
very high and our training in meditative techniques was not very
successful. By the end of six months or so we would find that only
a handful of individuals professed to be continuing in the medita-
ting process. We were impressed, however, by the fact that among

those who did, some lives were profoundly improved. We also observed that those people who seemed to benefit were, almost without exception, individuals who could be described as having been at high levels of stress at the time that they entered the meditation program.

Because it seemed that we were doing some good, at least for certain types of individuals and because of our observation that our training methods needed substantial improvement, we designed a major study to be devoted solely to intervention among individuals at higher than average levels of stress. The objectives were:

1. To field test more effective meditation training methods (preferably by semiautomated means), and

2. To study the comparative practical usefulness in the work setting of various techniques for relaxation.

The study was conducted and has been reported elsewhere (1). It explored the foregoing questions by comparing the effects of 3 leading meditation-relaxation techniques on symptoms of employee stress, measured over a five and a half month period. Stress levels were determined by the SCL-90-R questionnaire, a well validated multidimensional measure of distress developed by Derogatis (2) of Johns Hopkins University, and by the A-C questionnaire, an instrument developed by us to evaluate the perceived value of meditation/relaxation to the participant.

## 2  STUDY

Some 154 New York Telephone Company volunteers, self-selected on the basis of subjectively perceived stress and screened to eliminate persons with previous experience in meditation-relaxation were randomly assigned to one for four groups:  Clinically Standardized Meditation (CSM), Respiratory One Method Meditation (ROM), Progressive Muscle Relaxation (PMR), or served as waiting list controls.  Thirty-eight subjects were assigned to each of the three treatment groups and 40 subjects to the control group.

## 3  RESULTS

Compliance with meditation-relaxation practice was even higher than we had hoped for.  At the end of the study 81% of CSM subjects, 76% of ROM subjects and 63% of PMR subjects were still practicing their respective techniques.  As expected, the participants in these three groups taken as a whole showed symptom reduction over the five and a half months of observation (Figure 1).  The sur-

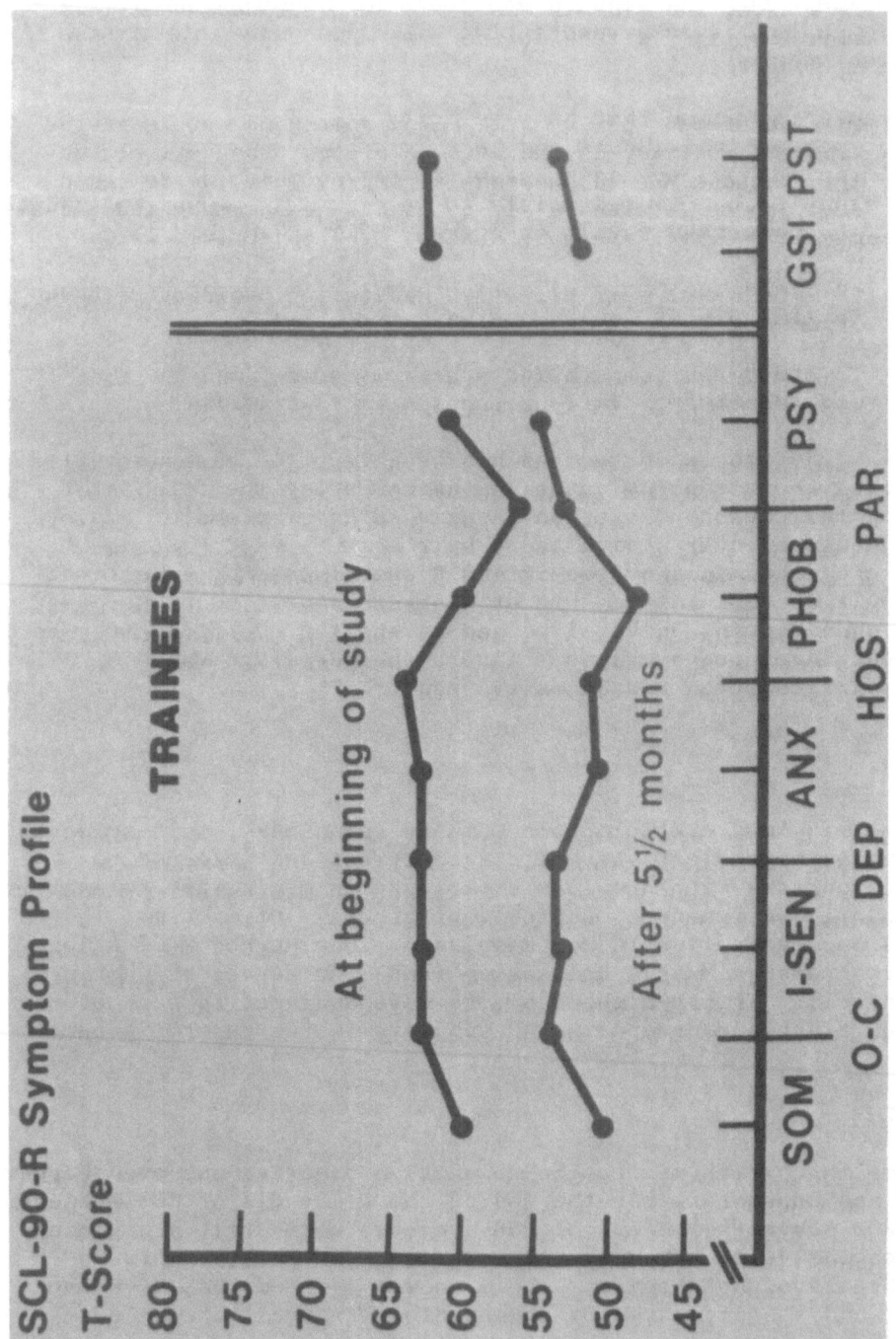

Figure 1.

257

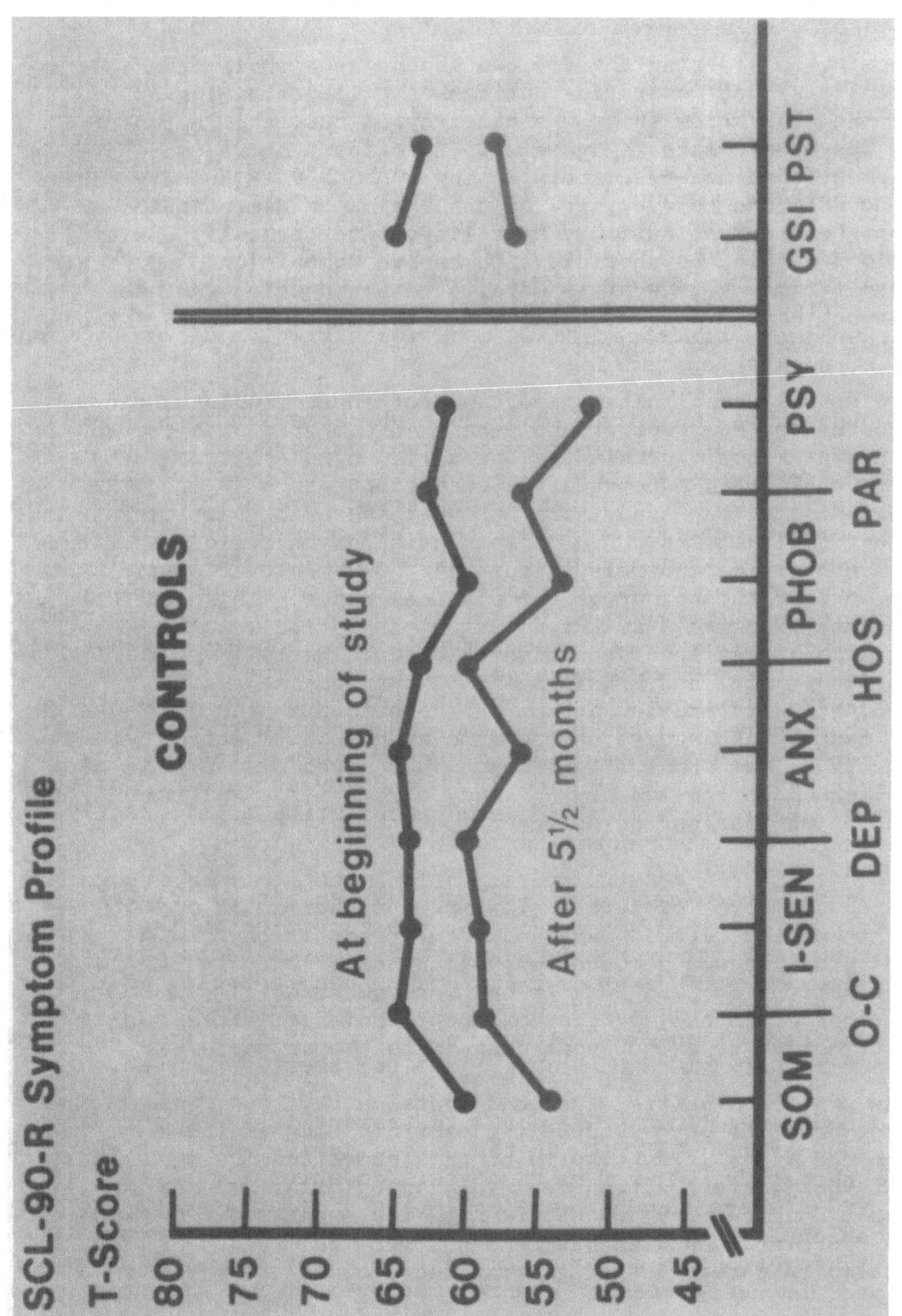

Figure 2.

prising finding was that controls also showed symptom reduction over that period (Figure 2). But subjects who received training, taken as a whole, showed significantly greater symptom reduction than controls as measured on the SCL-90-R.

Again, considering the trained groups as a whole (the meditators/relaxers) but separating out those still practicing at the end of the study from those who had dropped out, the therapeutic effect was even clearer (Figure 3). Practicers showed more symptom improvement than non-practicers on the two SCL-90-R summary indices (GSI and PST) and on every one of the 9 symptom dimensions (Somatization, Depression, Anxiety, Hostility, Interpersonal Sensitivity, Paranoid Ideation, Psychoticism, Obsessive Compulsion, and Phobic Anxiety) (Figure 4). What is more, stress reduction was seen whether subjects practiced their techniques frequently or infrequently - another unexpected finding.

To assess the clinical importance of these findings, the SCL-90-R scores for our four groups were then compared with the scores of groups previously studied by Derogatis, a non-patient normal group (N = 974) and a psychiatric outpatient group (N = 1,002). At the beginning of our study, the SCL-90-R scores of participants in our study fell between those of Derogatis' psychiatric outpatients and his non-patient normals (Figure 5). Our employee participants' scores were on the border of the clinical range. This confirmed the fact that our self-selected target population was indeed living with stress levels considerable above normal. At the end of the study, five and a half months later, the scores for those in the meditation-relaxation groups had come down to the middle of the normal range, with scores on one dimension (Somatization) now significantly below normal (Figure 6). In contrast, scores for the control group at the end of the study were still significantly above Derogatis' non-patient normal group.

When the three meditation-relaxation techniques were examined separately in terms of degree of symptom reduction in those practicing them, the methods were found to differ in their effectiveness. The PMR group showed no more improvement than controls. But the two meditation (CSM and ROM) groups were substantially and significantly better. Thus, meditation, not muscle relaxation, appeared to be effective as a therapeutic agent for these employees.

As mentioned before, a second instrument (the A-C questionnaire) covering benefits perceived by the participating employee was also used in the study. The results of this questionnaire agreed with the SCL-90-R where the two were exploring similar aspects but the A-C questionnaire provided opportunity for spontaneous comments as well. Ninety-two spontaneous comments were recorded. Of these, 42 related to categories of general improvement not measured by the

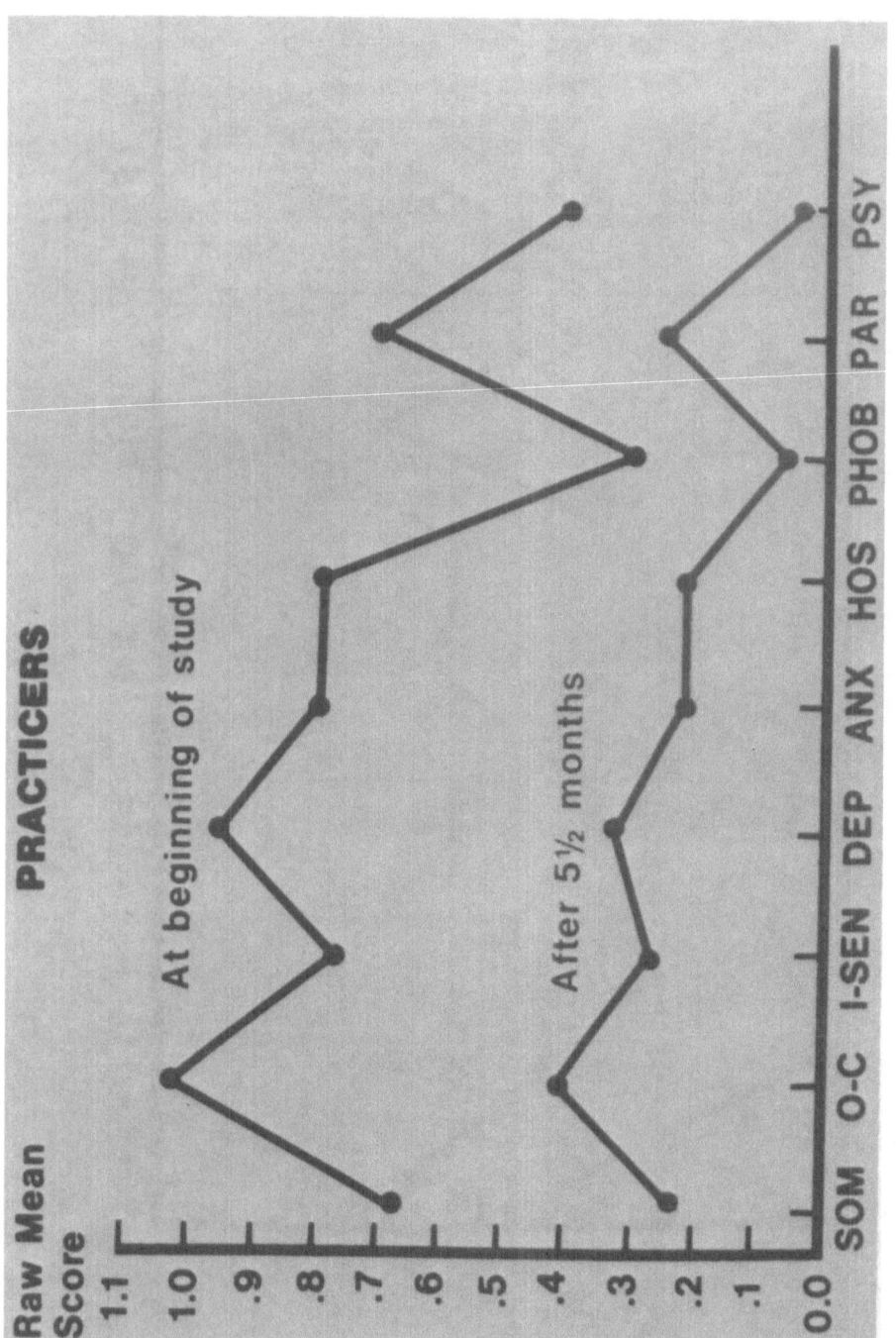

Figure 3.

260

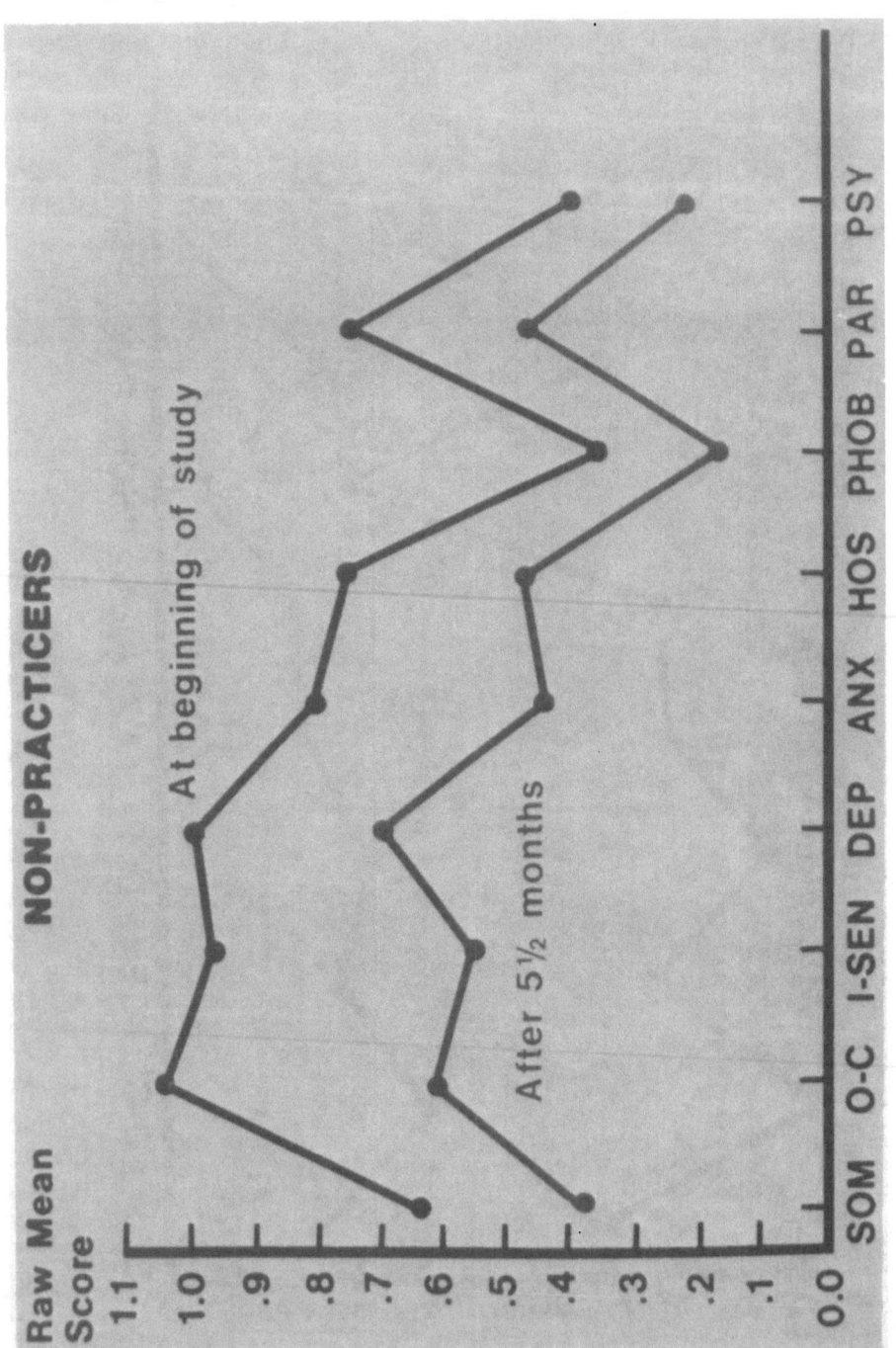

Figure 4.

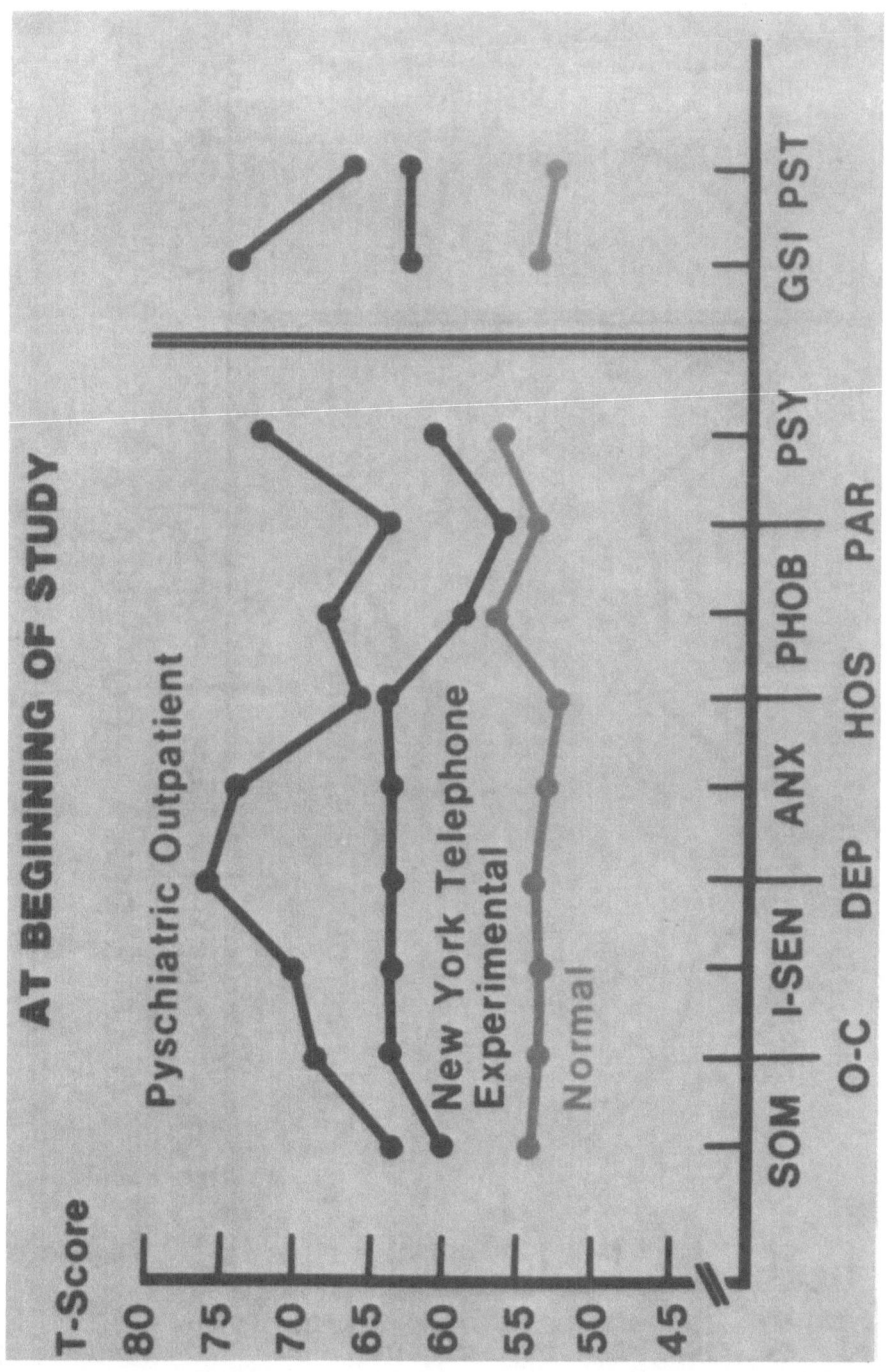

Figure 5.

262

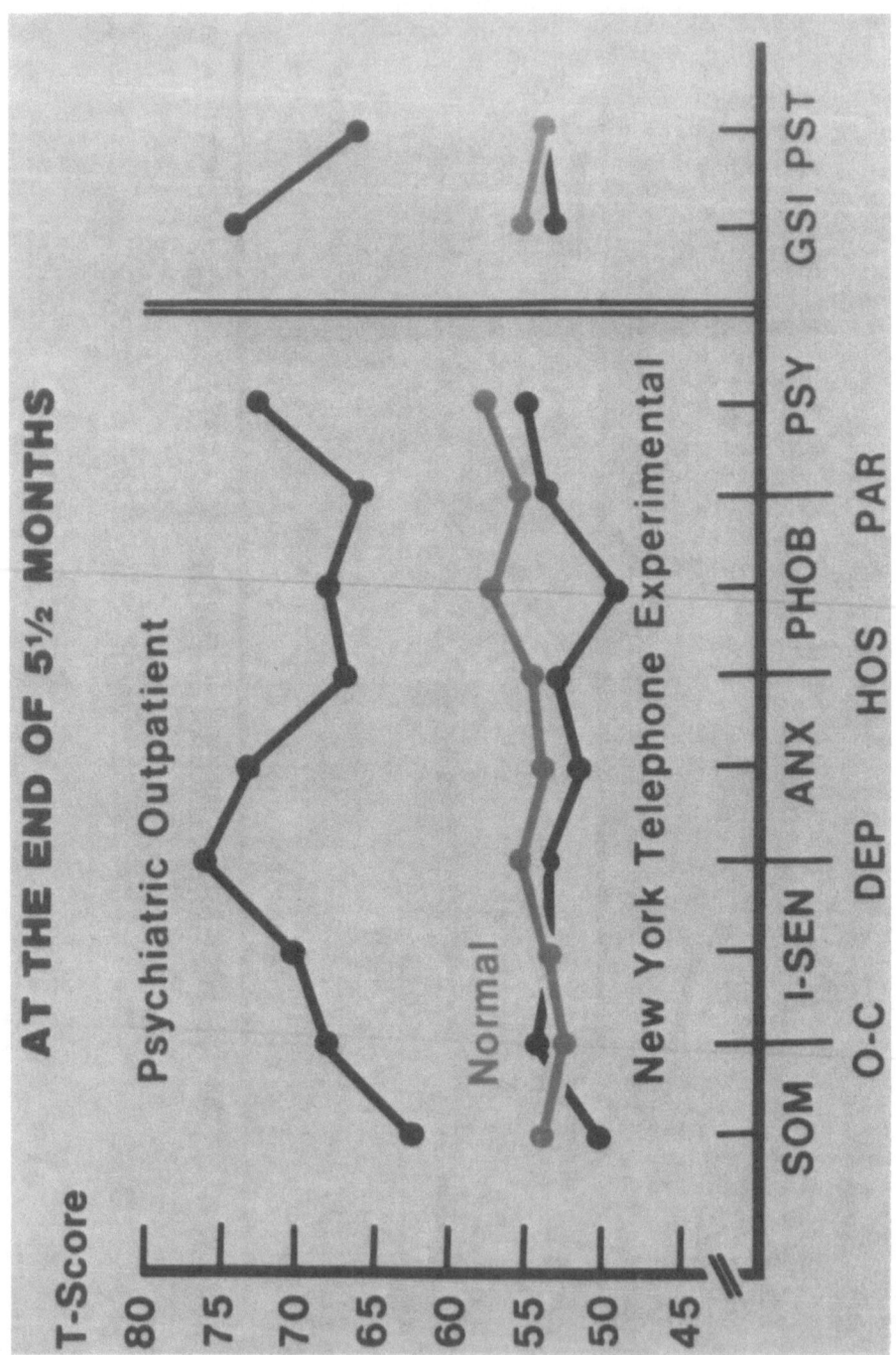

Figure 6.

SCL-90-R. In these general categories, the most frequently reported benefits were improvement in ability to think clearly, increased objectivity, greater alertness, better social functioning and enhanced enjoyment of life. These findings suggest that had appropriate additional objective measurements been applied, benefits of meditation training other than stress reduction might have been identified (e.g., improved efficiency, increased coping ability and greater satisfaction with life). These benefits may be particularly relevant for programs involving preventive health measures.

Of special interest from the point of view of employee health was the observation that physiological complaints related to psychosomatic disorders showed highly significant reductions with the use of the meditation-relaxation techniques. Also, those practicing these techniques showed there was also markedly lowered hostility, as well as a sharp decrease in moderate symptoms of depression. This lessened irritability appears especially relevant for the use of meditation in the workplace as well as for the management of such personality disorders as alcoholism where hostility scores on the SCL-90-R have frequently been found to be elevated.

I have already referred to the high compliance rates in the 70% - 80% range. It was interesting to note that, with but a single exception, all those subjects who did stop practicing did so within the first 3 months. Thereafter, while subjects might switch from frequent to occasional practicing, and back again, they did not discontinue their practice. This suggests that meditation-relaxation practice may stabilize within the first three months.

## 4  CONCLUSIONS FROM THE STUDY

The study demonstrated that semi-automated instruction in meditation could be used in an organizational setting with no loss of effectiveness over personal instruction in the technique. In addition, the timetable of attrition suggested that once it had been successfully adopted and practiced for a period of several months, meditation might become a permanent coping strategy which could then be called upon by the trainee when he or she has need of it, i.e., the strategic use of meditation is not likely to be abandoned. Semi-automated meditation training thus appeared to have considerable value for health maintenance programs in organizational settings, a value which is enhanced when the relative safety and inexpensiveness of this training is taken into account.

The study also showed that meditation could be highly effective in reducing stress levels among individuals who started out as distressed people. This was in contrast to the relative ineffectiveness which we had initially experienced in our application of meditation randomly to unselected employee populations. Therefore, it became significantly important to find out what the prevalence of distress was in our total employee population. In other words, how many distressed people we had at any particular time. To shed light on this subject, we conducted a survey of 4,000 randomly selected employees at all levels of the company from blue-collar craft workers to top executives. The survey instrument was the SCL-90-R which was completed and returned by 2,363 employees in a survey sample, for an overall response rate of 59%.

The findings from this survey were as follows:

1. A significant proportion (25%) of employees revealed stress levels in the clinical range, i.e., <u>distress</u>. This observation was true for every one of the stress categories on the SCL-90-R.

2. Level in the company was significantly related to stress, with higher and middle management revealing the lowest percentage of distressed persons (less than 20% in the clinical range) followed by lower management who had significantly higher scores (23% distressed) and then by non-management employees who revealed the highest stress levels (27% distressed). These distinctions were evident for both sexes but were particularly dramatic among female employees.

3. Male employees revealed higher proportions of stressed people than female employees when comparisons were made with the gender-keyed norms. 10% of male managers vs. 3% of female managers had scores greater than 2 standard deviations above the normative mean, with these proportions going to 12% for males vs. 4% for females among lower management and to 14% vs. 5% among non-management employees.

4. Male and female employees manifested different characteristic patterns of symptomatic stress. Males had a tendency to show higher levels of obsessive compulsive and hostility symptoms while females tended to reveal greater symptoms of phobic anxiety.

5. There was no evidence of substantial alteration in the above observations as a function of age.

We were able to use the data in this survey to calculate specific local SCL-90-R norms for each different employee sub-segment, i.e., upper management, lower management, and non-management by age, and sex groups. These norms now serve as effective reference values in the interpretation of the SCL-90-R scores obtained from individual

employee patients. Capitalizing on this ability to identify individuals with significantly elevated stress levels and drawing on
the conclusions from the aforementioned study and other experience
with health-promotion program implementation in the work setting,
an on-going program of meditation training was developed and is
now being implemented.

Since in our study the muscle-relaxing technique (PMR) did
not outperform controls, PMR was not included in the final program.
The two meditation techniques, CSM and ROM, were combined so that
they could be offered as parts of a single instructional system.
Trainees in the New York Telephone meditation program are thus
given the opportunity to move freely from one meditational approach
to the other. This is done to increase the probability that a
suitable technique will be adopted by the trainee.

The following summarizes the essential elements of the program:

A. Long-range goals

To provide an additional resource to employees which will
assist them in coping with stress. Secondarily, the goals
are to improve the productivity of employees and to reduce
the adverse personal effects of stress such as anxiety,
ineffectiveness, morbidity, and disability.

B. Strategy

Identify employees who are at a stressful period in their
lives and utilize that situation as a timely place to introduce them to meditation. Under these conditions based
on the findings from our prior studies, we anticipate
maximum acceptance and very little dropout losses.

C. Operations

The program is structured as part of the Company Medical
Department's preventive and health-maintenance effort.
Actual implementation is in the hands of specifically
qualified trainers.

The trainers initially learn meditation by means of cassette recordings and a programmed instruction workbook.
They are then trained in supervising the training process
by Company consultant(s) and the Company program coordinator.
The trainers work in close collaboration with clinicians
in the Medical Department who have responsibility for
individual case management.

Trainers periodically conduct meetins with the medical staff at various branch medical offices to introduce new staff members to meditation and to reinforce or upgrade the subject for old staff members. At these meetings a videotape describing the use of meditation in clinical practice is shown and discussion of its contents follows. The videotape presents indications for the use of meditation within an employee health maintenance program and outlines indications and contraindications for its use. The trainer then acquaints the medical staff with the mechanics of referring employees to the mediation training program and discusses any questions raised.

At the present time, to be eligible for the New York Telephone meditation training an employee must be referred by a member of the medical staff who considers him/her to be at risk with respect to developing stress-related symptoms. Program participants come from all management and non-management levels, the only criteria for admission being their medical status with respect to stress.

In the future we anticipate screening general employee groups (using the SCL-90-R or some other device) to pick out distressed people not currently under care in our Medical Department. Such people would also be eligible to enter the meditation training.

Once employees are referred to the program, the trainer contacts them by telephone and informs them of the next orientation meeting where they can learn about the meditation program and have an opportunity to decide whether they wish to sign up for it. The program is offered free of charge.

Orientation meetings are held in small groups of 10 to 20 persons at the Medical Department. Here employees referred to the program are shown a 25-minute videotape, "Relaxing With Meditation," which depicts Dr. Patricia Carrington (an authority on meditation) being interviewed on the subject. On the videotape, Dr. Carrington presents some of the research which has established meditation as a noncultic "no-nonsense" procedure and provides answers to most of the questions which those unfamiliar with the technique are likely to ask. When shown to groups of prospective trainees, this videotape has proven highly effective in encouraging enrollment in the meditation program. To date, over 95% of the employees who have viewed the videotape have signed up for the program.

At the orientation meeting the trainer answers questions about the method, describes the procedures for meditation training and works out schedules for home instruction and follow-up meetings. Participating employees are administered pretreatment psychological evaluations (SCL-90-R) on the spot and leave the orientation meeting taking with them the basic training materials which they will use (in their homes) to learn the meditation technique.

During the first week post-instruction, each participant is contacted by the trainer by telephone and the latter checks to see that the trainee is following the methods correctly, answers questions about the procedure, and helps the trainee to adjust to the technique to suit personal needs.

Two weeks into instruction, trainees assigned to a given group (maximum size 20 persons) assemble for their first follow-up training session. Here they learn to handle any problems encountered and to extend the process of meditation beyond the formal 10- to 20-minute sessions by using "mini meditations", short meditation sessions lasting 2 to 3 minutes which can be used strategically throughout the day, in addition to regularly scheduled longer sessions. This meeting affords trainees an opportunity to share their experiences and to help each other solve mutual problems, and serves as an excellent motivator for continued practice.

The trainer holds four additional follow-up meetings over the course of the first year. These are scheduled for six weeks, three months, and six months post-instruction, and at the end of one year. SCL-90-Rs are readministered at the three-month and one-year meetings respectively, for purposes of program evaluation.

At all of the follow-up meetings, the trainer checks on correctness of the practice, takes up problems of scheduling, interruptions, or resistances, encourages group members to share information on benefits derived from the practice, gives instruction in auxiliary techniques which can be combined with CSM or ROM, and encourages participant's continued meditation practice.

D.  Experience to Date

Implementation of this meditation training program was begun over a year ago. It is now operating in six of the eight branch company medical offices and so far has enrolled a total of 273 participants. These 273 participants have been in 19 different groups. To date there have been only 24 (8.8%) dropouts.

Three of the above groups have now been in existence over a year. There were 35 original participants in these three groups. After one year 6 (17%) had dropped out. The rest (83%) are actively practicing meditation regularly or on an intermittent basis as needed.

Observation of SCL-90-R scores on employees in the program has shown the same marked improvement that was found in our initial study, and individual anecdotal feedback has been very interesting. It reassures us that there is no question but that many of these employees have profited substantially in meaningful ways. Moreover, it is not an exaggeration to say that some lives have been literally transformed.   Objective measurement of the success of the program in terms of reduced absenteeism, disability, morbidity, and in terms of productivity increases is being carried out but it is too soon, unfortunately, to have results from these measures.

REFERENCES

1.   Carrington, P. et al. The Use of Meditation-Relaxation Techniques for the Management of Stress in a Working Population. Journal of Occupational Medicine 22 (1980) 221-231.

2.   Derogatis, L.R. SCL-90 Manual-L. (Baltimore, Johns Hopkins University School of Medicine, 1977).

A BEHAVIORAL APPROACH TO PREVENTION OF CORONARY HEART DISEASE

Chandra Patel

London School of Hygiene and Tropical Medicine
University of London
London, England

1   INTRODUCTION

Coronary heart disease (CHD) is the most common of all causes of death.  In men aged 45-64 years, up to 37% of deaths are attributed to CHD (207).  In the U.S.A., the epidemic of CHD has been on the wane since the mid-60's and on the balance of evidence, it seems unlikely that this could be due to changes in reporting. There has been a sharp decline in cigarette smoking, a shift in diet from animal to vegetable fats, an increased interest in exercise and more frequent treatment of hypertension in the U.S.A. However, the relationship between the decline in cardiovascular mortality and change in life styles are far from clear (63).  The largest decline occurred in black women and it is unlikely that they are the greatest beneficiaries of health education or hypertension treatment.  Neither are they likely to be the most  avid joggers!  In England and Wales, despite an early hint of a decline in the incidence, the mortality figures have remained disappointingly constant (199).

The highest incidence is found in Finland which is closely followed by Scotland and other English-speaking countries - Northern Ireland, New Zealand, Australia, United States, Eire, England and Wales and Canada.  Mediterranean countries like Greece, France and Spain have a much lower incidence, while Japan - inspite of industrialization, has the lower incidence.  In order to save men in the prime of their lives at a stage of development when they are of obvious economic importance to the communities and their families, we must mobilize all our resources.  It is, therefore, justifiable to explore any new ideas or theories on this subject. It is my aim to put forward a hypothesis and support it with the

results of studies carried out so far.   There is a lot of work to
be done before the hypothesis can be proven, but at least a start
has been made.

## 2   PATHOGENESIS OF CORONARY HEART DISEASE

Coronary heart disease or ischemic heart disease is often
due to atheroma in the coronary arteries.   It is now increasingly
being recognized that CHD is a spectrum of conditions ranging from
disease caused solely by atherosclerosis with or without thrombosis
to that in which coronary spasm plays a major role.

### 2.1   Coronary Spasm

A hundred years ago, angina pectoris was attributed to coronary
artery spasm but this theory was pushed aside as evidence accumulated
about the role of fatty deposits in the coronary arteries.   Forty
years ago, Friedberg & Horn (48) reported myocardial infarction
without the evidence of thrombotic occlusion of coronary arteries.
There is now angiographic evidence that coronary spasm does indeed
occur which not only explains angina occurring at rest (35, 95), but
also incidents of myocardial infarction with enzyme proof and ECG
changes in patients whose coronary arteries show no evidence of
organic occlusion (8, 23, 93, 108).   Coronary artery spasm in
patients with Prinzmetal angina has been well documented (128).   It
has also been suggested that in the vast number of patients with
CHD, both atheroma and spasm play a role.   The mechanism of coronary
spasm is not certain.   In 1910, William Osler speculated on
"Perverted internal secretion which favours spasm of the arteries".
Exposure to cold, emotion or other factors which disturbs autonomic
control, seem possible.   In favour of the spasm theory is also the
fact that drugs like Nifedipine and Verapamil are effective in
controlling angina, in as many as three-quarters or patients (3,
42, 132, 208).   Both drugs work by inhibiting the slow calcium
flow responsible for the contraction of the smooth muscles in the
arteries (182).

### 2.2   Atherosclerosis

There are several conflicting theories about the pathogenesis
of atherosclerosis.   The filtration theory postulates the inability
of the vessel wall to cope with lipid passing out of the lumen while
the accretion theory suggests that atheroma develops at the sites
of recurrent thrombus formation.   Fatty streaks are present in the
arterial walls of young children, while simple uncomplicated
atheromatous plaques make their appearance during early adult life.
The eventual fate of the plaque varies from patient to patient.   As
they enlarge and extend, the plaques can cause stenosis and eventually

occlusion of the involved vessel. A plaque full of lipid may behave as a miniature abscess, ulcerating and discharging its contents in to the arterial lumen to give lipid embolism and leaving a raw surface which provides a base for a thrombus to form. A thrombus may completely occlude the vessel or throw off platelet embolism. The occluded vessel may recanalize. Frequently, the plaques become calcified.

## 3  CONSEQUENCES OF CORONARY ARTERY DISEASE

The most common effect of atheroma in the coronary circulation or coronary spasm or the combination of both, are angina pectoris and myocardial infarction. A chest pain syndrome which is more severe than angina pectoris but falls short of myocardial infarction and occurs during rest has been variously called unstable angina, crescendo angina or coronary insufficiency. A variety of cardiac arrhythmia and heart failure also occur with or without previous history of chest pain. Sudden death was linked to angina pectoris by William Haberden in his 18th century description, but received little attention until recently. Community studies (4, 29) have shown that about two-thirds of coronary deaths occur rapidly, frequently outside hospital, only half of which have a history of previous heart attack or angina. For the remaining, sudden death while going about their everyday affairs is the first appearance of CHD. Some, of course, die in their sleep. The mortality amongst the group of patients who are admitted to hospital remains about 18-20%.

## 4  CONTRIBUTION OF CORONARY CARE UNITS

Modern treatment of CHD, such as Coronary Care Units (CCU) are expensive and have provided a limited beneficial effect on total mortality. In fact, serious doubts have been raised on the early high hopes about the contribution or coronary care units by two studies. In the first study, Mather and his colleagues (109) allocated selected cases of myocardial infarction to home care or CCU and found no difference in mortality. Many criticisms were made against the design of this study in the West Country, but a better planned and executed study in Nottingham has shown similar results (67).

It is beginning to be realized, particularly from animal experiments, that acute myocardial ischemia during the early part of a heart attack can cause self-perpetuating, re-entrant fatal arrythmia before the occurrence of myocardial infarction. Coronary care units are equipped to deal with these lethal ventricular arrythmia provided that patients are in CCU when they occur. Unfortunately, the majority of these early deaths occur within two hours of the onset of chest pain and often before the patient accepts the fact that there is something seriously wrong with him and seeks medical advice.

Following the pioneering work by the Belfast workers (131) it was claimed in Seattle (27) that sending a mobile coronary care unit (MCCU) to bring patients with suspected myocardial infarction to hospital saved a large number of lives. Most of the patients were resuscitated before the acute infarction developed. However, doctor-manned MCCU Studies from Nottingham (61, 62) have raised doubts about allocating resources to such projects..

## 5  AORTO-CORONARY BY-PASS SURGERY

Great advances have been made in the surgical treatment of severe angina with the use of a leg vein to by-pass coronary stenosis. Patients with chronic angina who fail to respond to medical treatment and who have only localized stenosis without any evidence of generalized myocardial fibrosis, seem to get symptomatic relief of angina, sometimes lasting several years. However, there is no evidence that it reduces long-term mortality. The risk attached to the operation is acceptably low in specialized units within a high level of expertise. Unfortunately, this highly expensive technique, although valuable in increasing the quality of life in selected individuals, cannot be expected to reduce the great burden of mortality from CHD in our communities (44, 122, 198).

## 6  SCOPE FOR PREVENTION

A series of WHO coordinated community studies have shown that 40% of the first attacks of myocardial infarction prove fatal. Of these, up to 60% occur within one hour of the onset of attack, without the presence of a doctor. Thus, even the most effective treatment can do nothing to reduce a large proportion of deaths (159). Besides, the patients who survive the first year after an infarct continue to have greater mortality than the average for their age and sex (147). The cry is not against CCU or new technological invention. They, indeed, play major roles in individual cases with specific complications as well as increasing our understanding of the whole subject. However, it is clear that major decrease in the burden of CHD can only occur as a result of an effective prevention program. If nothing is done to prevent CHD, it has been projected that one man in six can expect to get a heart attack before the age of retirement and half of these will be fatal (160). However, before we can do anything to prevent CHD, we need to know what causes it.

7 ETIOLOGY OF CORONARY HEART DISEASE

The cause of CHD is not known. Many studies conducted over
the last 35 years have demonstrated an association between certain
personal characteristics and the development of premature CHD (74).
These associated factors are known as risk factors. Numerous
risk factors have been identified, such as high blood pressure,
raised serum cholesterol, cigarette-smoking, diabetes or impaired
glucose tolerance, Type A behavior, sedentary living, obesity, age,
sex, and a positive family history. The first three are known as
the major risk factors because of the stronger and more consistent
association.


8 CAN REDUCTION IN RISK FACTORS REDUCE CHD?

There is a widespread view that reduction of the associated
risk factors will be effective in preventing CHD. As a result,
large scale complex multicentre intervention trials have assumed
massive commitment. Such enthusiasm is hardly justifiable when
one faces the fact that large number of CHD cases do not have
recognizable risk factors and significant proportion of subjects
with risk factors do not develop CHD. For example, Marmot and
Winklestein (107) reexamined the data of the report of the Intersociety Commission for Heart Disease Resourses (74), based on the
National Pooling Project which combines the results of eight major
prospective studies of CHD in the United States. Table I shows
the classification of 7,342 white men aged 30-59 in the Pooling
Project data by risk factor status at entry and gives the number
of cases that occurred in each group in the 10-year followup.

In the highest risk group with the presence of three risk
factors, 14% of the individuals developed CHD in ten years. In
other words, 86% of the high risk group would not develop CHD
in 10 years without any intervention. Alternatively, it can be
seen that 83% of CHD cases could not be predicted by the presence
of all three risk factors, as only 17% of the cases came from the
high risk group. If the high risk group is enlarged by including
population with two or more risk factors, we can predict 58% of
the cases but this increase in sensitivity is gained at the expense
of specificity. Thus, of this enlarged high risk group, approximately
91% will not develop CHD (100 - 10 year incidence rate). If there
were 100 successful pharmacological measure, they have to be applied
to 100 people to save nine lives and if the compliance rate, and
degree of success expected are say only 50% each, then the whole
exercise is likely to save only 2-3 lives. Against that, one must
also take into consideration the possible hazards of the treatment
as well as the total cost.

Thus, it is reasonable to conclude that although the ability to predict CHD from the presence of risk factors is very impressive, substantial proportion of CHD must occur for reasons other than the conventional risk factors. Maybe it is because of these facts that a number of intervention trials have consistently shown poor results. It is my intention to review literature and point out some gaps and then suggest a hypothesis which might fill those gaps.

## 8.1. Lipid Hypothesis

In the numerous national and interantional epidemiological studies, the topic most discussed is the link between coronary heart disease and cholesterol and other lipids present in diet, blood and the walls of coronary arteries. The hypothesis was based on a chain of evidence which began with an observation by 18th century pathologists that patients with angina pectoris had lesions in the coronary arteries. Later it was revealed that atherosclerotic lesions contained deposits of cholesterol and other fats (195). Theories were put forward to suggest that lipids from circulating blood were imbibed in the intima of the coronary arteries. This was supported by the observation of association between high serum cholesterol and coronary heart disease (16). Animal experiments showed that rabbits and chicken fed on high cholesterol diet developed lesions of atherosclerosis (2).

Keys and coworkers made an important contribution to this hypothesis. Their Seven Countries Study is internationally known (88). However, no significant part of the marked international variability among 16 cohorts could be explained by age, relative body weight, body fatness (skinfold thickness), smoking habits or physical activity. Although a number of studies had shown a strong association between cigarette smoking and CHD incidence, this study clearly failed to show the association. Similarly, there was no correlation between systolic hypertension and the CHD mortality, although in the Framingham Study this was considered to be a strong predictor of CHD, as well as other cardiovascular disease. They observed some correlation between diastolic blood pressure and CHD mortality, but even here, there was clearly no correlation between the levelof diastolic blood pressure and CHD mortality in the three countries with the highest incidence rates of CHD - Netherland, United States and Finland. Between population, there was a strong correlation between levels of serum cholesterol and CHD incidence, but there was no evidence that in any single population group high fat consumers were the ones who developed CHD. The Diet Heart Report (124) finally concluded that "the evidence that coronary heart disease migh be reduced through dietary means is most suggestive but not convincing".

McMichael (123) suggested that a high correlation ( =0.81) between the level of blood cholesterol, and the incidence of

coronary heart disease in the Seven Countries Study was largely due
to the inclusion of a population from East Finland, which has double
the incidence of CHD compared to the population from West Finland
at the same level of serum cholesterol. Exclusion of this population
from East Finland, which is not representative of any average
population, would leave a much less convincing evidence and the
correlation between the fat in the diet, serum cholesterol and
coronary incidence would drop to a statistically insignificant
level ( = 0.38). The relationship between fat in the diet,
serum cholesterol and CHD is so weak that Mann (101) has even gone
to the extent of pronouncing "diet-heart: end of an era". The
evidence to support his contentions comes from various epidemiological
observations.

The first line of evidence comes from examining human dietary
habits. Dietary habit was examined by Kannel & Gordon (81) in about
1,000 persons in the Framingham Study and found no relationship
between dietary habits and cholesterolaemia. Similarly, there was
no relationship between the levels of serum cholesterol and the
dietary habits of 2,000 persons in the Tecumseh Study (125).

The next line of evidence comes from clinical trials with
diet therapy. In primary prevention trial people who are intially
free from coronary heart are involved. The Finnish trial (114)
based on 29,217 person-years in two mental hospitals showed some
reduction in the CHD incidence in low fat diet group but overall
mortality remained unchanged. This has been criticized by Mann as
"only an apparent influence on what the attending physician thought
the cause of death to be". The Primary Prevention Trial in Los
Angeles (36) again gave no improvement in total mortality, although
the coronary component was signficantly reduced. Bassler commented
that this difference might be due to difference in any number of
heavy smokers in two groups (6). There were 70 heavy smokers
(over a pack a day) in the control group and 70 CHD deaths. In
the diet group, there were 48 CHD deaths and only 45 heavy smokers.
There were more deaths due to cancer in the treated (diet) group.
This rather disquieting hazard has been shown in another trial
also (41).

The dietary treatment in a secondary prevention trial in
Oslo (92) showed reduction in angina pectoris and non-fatal myocardial
infarction, but the incidence of sudden death was increased. Two
trials in England involving over 600 survivors of myocardial
infarct did not show any evidence of reduced recurrence (156, 157).

The cholesterol reducing drugs Clofibrate and Niacin were
used in the Coronary Drug Project (31) in 8,141 patients who had
either recovered from myocardial infarction or had angina symptoms.
Although the level of serum cholesterol was reduced by 15-20%, this
did not make any difference to the death rate in patients with

established CHD.  One of the disturbing side  effects of cholesterol lowering regimen had been the doubling of the incidence of gall stones (32).  In a study from Scotland (158), survival of patients with angina  was  reported to be prolonged with no benefit to patients who had already had myocardial infarction.

A large WHO coordinated primary prevention study of cholesterol-lowering Clofibrate drug was recently reported  from Europe (30). In a double-blind study, 15,000 men aged between 30-59 years in Edinburgh, Prague, and Budapest were divided into three groups of 5,000 men each.  Group A with high initial serum  cholesterol were treated with 1.6G of Clofibrate daily, while the  control Group B with high initial level of serum cholesterol  and another control Group C with normal level  of serum cholesterol, were treated with capsules filling with olive oil.  At a 5-year followup, serum cholesterol level in the treated group was  reduced by 9.7% (15% reduction was expected).  Although there  was significant reduction in incidence of non-fatal myocardial infarction in the treated group, there was no significant difference in  the incidence of angina or fatal heart attacks.  The total mortality in  the Clofibrate group was actually higher (162) than in  either of the control groups (127 and 93  respectively).  The  causes of this excess death rate were due to increase in neoplasia as well as diseases of the liver,  gall bladder and intestines.   The Lancet editorial commented on the outcome of the study  "The treatment was successful but unfortunately the patient died" (25).  On the balance of evidence, Clofibrate  can no longer be recommended as a lipid-lowering agent for general use.

## 8.2  Other Discrepancies in Lipid Hypothesis

Groen et al  (58) sutdied Benedictine and Trappist Monks, both living in rural areas away from social and economic problems.  The Benedictine monks ate a mixed diet substantially high in saturated fat, while the Trappist monks ate  a vegetarian diet devoid of butter, eggs, and meat.  Despite the high mean level of serum cholesterol in the Benedictine monks, no significant difference was found in coronary heart disease prevalence between them, while both groups showed prevalence much lower than that of the general population.

Medale and  his colleagues studied various ethnic groups in Israel (112, 113) and found a substantial range of fat  intake varying from 1-5% calories from saturated fat intake in the lowest decile to 15-49% in the highest decile.  However, there was no relationship between saturated fat intake and incidence of myo-cardial infarction.  Prior and his colleagues (146) from New Zealand showed  that Maories in the Island  of Pukapuka had a greater intake of saturated fat in the form  of  coconut oil than Maories in Rarotonga, who are more Europeanized, and yet the Rarotongans had

higher serum cholesterol and a greater prevalence of ischemic
heart disease.  Similarly, an inverse relationship between fat
intake and serum cholesterol was found on the Island of Palau by
Laberthe and coworkers (91).  The last authors, on the other hand,
found consistent correlation between the degree of modernization
and levels of blood pressure, serum cholesterol, obesity, ECG
abnormality and cardiovascular symptoms.

Shaper et al (179, 180) reported a  much lower incidence of
atherosclerosis and serum cholesterol levels in the Samburu tribe
of Kenya and the milk and meat eating Masai of Tanganyika than those
of Americans, although the  fat  contents of their diet was at least
as high and probably higher than that of most Americans.  This
was confirmed by other workers (102).

Malhotra showed, among Indian railway workers, a very low
incidence of CHD in North India where the average fat intake
was 10-20 times higher,  mostly in the form of saturated fat, compared
with a very high incidence in South India where the fat intake was
much lower (3.5% calories from fat) and contained a large proportion
from fat) and contained a large proportion  of polyunsaturated fat.
Mean cholesterol levels in the North and South Indian groups did
not show difference (99).

## 8.3  Stress and Serum Cholesterol

In all the lipid intervention studies, emphasis is placed on
dietary  fat only, completely disregarding the fact that diet only
plays a minor role and that there are other important contributory
factors.  Friedman, Rosenman and Carrol (52) observed in a group
of accountants a gradual rise in the level of serum cholesterol
associated with an increase in occupational stress before the tax
deadline.  Once the deadline was met, the serum cholesterol began
to fall.  High peaks of serum cholesterol were also found in new
cadets in the Air Force Academy during the early weeks considered
to be the highest in environmental stress (24).  Following this
stressful phase of training, however, the cholesterol level decreased.
Rahe et al (152) found in underwater demolition team trainees
that cholesterol levels increased under the stress of learning
new skills or when the subjects felt fearful, angry or depressed.

## 8.4  Essential Hypertension and Coronary Heart  Disease

The fact that hypertension is a strong predictor of cardiovascular disease is undenied, although its etiology remains unknown.
It is generally agreed that essential hypertension results from
the interaction between hereditary predisposition and environmental
factors.  Since genetic factors cannot be removed, the therapeutic
efforts must be concentrated  upon counteracting environmental
factors in the hope of mitigating genetic influence.  Sir George

Pickering (144) stated that environmental factors working through the mind are important. The environment can affect us in two different ways:

1. the noxious effects of the environments themselves, and
2. the physiological response of the individual to his environment.

Scotch & Geiger (176) reviewed the literature on essential hypertension and concluded that hypertension results from a failure of the individual to adapt to a changing environment. Cruz-Coke (33, 34) introduced the concept of an "ecological niche" to explain the consistently low pressures found in groups living in isolated regions and enjoying an unchanging and unchallenged tradition. When people from these groups migrate to areas of "western", urban civilization, their blood pressures begin to rise.

Henry & Cassel (66) arranged data from 18 epidemiological studies from various parts of the world into three groups according to the social and psycholgoical environment of the groups. They showed that where the population did not show a rise in blood pressure with age, the culture had remained stable, traditional forms were honored and group members were secure in their roles and had adapted to them from an early age. With the onset of industrialization, urbanization and migration, social, cultural and economic values change and the individual is required to make continuous behavioral adjustments. As people become older, this process of adaptation becomes more and more stressful and is reflected in rising blood pressures with age. Beaglehold et al (7) followed up a population of a south sea island, Tokelau, during their migration to New Zealand. It was revealed that the rise in blood pressure was proportional to the interaction with an integration into New Zealand society as judged by the ethnicity of workmates and friends, club membership, participation in the Tokelauan community and religious activities, language fluency and so on.

Nearly 25 centuries ago, Hippocrates told his contemporaries that (203) those things which one has been accustomed to for a long time, although worse than the things which one is not accustomed to, usually give less disturbance. Those who advocate environment of essential hypertension are constantly criticized by those who cannot conceive that there can be more stress today with so much material comfort around. Strange as it may seem, the more we get, the more we strive, the more responsibility we are prepared to take and the longer we work. The rich feel just as insecure and worried about the future as the poor. It has been said "hypertension is a new disease and stress disease, the price a millionaire pays for his directorship and a clerk for his failure" (127).

Cobb & Rose (28) found in air traffic controllers requiring constant vigilance and extreme responsibility, a higher mean arterial pressure, higher prevalence and increased annual incidence of hypertension occurring at a younger age, compared with second class airmen. Even amongst the controllers, those working at high traffic density towers had a higher incidence than those working at low traffic density towers. Kasl & Cobb (84) followed a number of blue collar workers after a plant shutdown and found their blood pressure rose and remained high during the period of unemployment. Among those who were fortunate enough to find permanent re-employment, the blood pressure began to come down.

## 8.5 Drug Treatment of Hypertension

Earlier studies of drug treatment of hypertension were shown to reduce the incidence of uraemia, strokes, and heart failure, but not of myocardial infarction (15). Such benefit was evident in men with an initial diastolic blood pressure between 125-129mm of Hg in the Veterans Administration Study published in 1967. In the second study, the benefit with the exception of myocardial infarction was also evident in men with an initial diastolic blood pressure between 90-114mm Hg(193). In a subsequent analysis it was revealed that a significant reduction in morbid events had occurred only in the subgroup with a diastolic pressure between 105-114mm Hg, but not in the group with an initial diastolic pressure of 90-104mm Hg. (194).

The value of therapy, it was suggested, might be related to the onset and type of treatment since hypotensive therapy may be ineffective, it started too late (10). In secondary prevention trials, beta adrenoreceptor blocking drugs were shown to be partially cardo-protective and reduced the incidence of sudden death, although it is not known that this was contributed by its specific action on risk factors (1, 200, 201). In one such large scale trial with one of the initial beta blocking drug Practolol, severe side effects were reported (121). Practolol was later withdrawn from the market. A number of studies are under way to evaluate the benefit of lowering mildly elevated blood pressure with diastolic pressure between 90-109mm Hg. (120). A study from Australia (100) was recently published showing that drug treatment of mild hypertension is beneficial in reducing strokes and other complications, but reduction in CHD mortality was not significant.

A community-based Hypertension Detection and Followup Program (73) from the United States reported a significant reduction in mortality from all causes, including 20% difference in mortality from CHD in patients with mild hypertension (DBP 90-104mm Hg.) allocated to the "stepped care" therapy with systematic approach to strict control of blood pressure in comparison with the "Referred Care" group patients who were allocated to

their usual source of medical care. The deaths from hypertensive
disease were the same in both groups. The greater decrease in
mortality in the "Stepped Care" group was not due to greater
reductions in other risk factors like cigarette smoking, body
weight, or serum cholesterol. By the fifth years, 75% of the
"Stepped Care" patients and 54% of the "Referred Care" patients
were on anti-hypertensive drugs and 64% and 43% respectively were
at or below the goal blood pressure status. The difference in
mean systolic pressure between the groups was less than 5mm Hg.
which makes one wonder whether cheaper non-drug behavioral approaches
might not be better alternatives to putting a large part of the
population on a life-long antihypertensive drug therapy with
associated hazards and a substantial cost.

## 8.6 Cigarette Smoking

The striking importance of cigarette smoking as a risk factor
for coronary heart disease has been established both in the U.K.
(154, 170) and the United States (60, 80). Yet in many countries
with both low and high incidence of CHD, smoking has been found
to be unrelated or unimportant. The Seven Countries Studies (88)
is a striking example. The same was true in Puerto Rico (56).
Even if the harmful effects are established, this does not
necessarily mean that they are reversible if smoking is abandoned
after many years. However, Doll and Hill (40) observed encouraging
results in a 10-year followup of British doctors. This low
mortality in ex-smokers was confirmed in other observational
studies (60, 80). It is difficult to interpret that the reduction
in mortality was due to smoking cessation from these observational
studies, since people who stop smoking on their own often come
from higher social classes and probably also change other behaviors
at the same time. Therefore, the benefit of smoking cessation can
only be proved by a radomized controlled trial.

In such a trial involving middle-aged men, Rose and Hamilton
(161) showed that an active intervention program, consisting of
a series of personal interviews with a doctor, was highly
successful in helping smokers to reduce or stop smoking, compared
with the normal care group program in which the decision to advise
on the smoking habit was left to their own general practitioners.
However, over a period of eight year followup, there was no
evidence at all of reduction in overall mortality in the active
intervention group. It is possible that the followup period was
not long enough for the benefit to be obvious. Alternatively,
it is possible that we are missing out an important link. If
smoking is, at least partially, a sign of stress, then in a
randomized controlled trial like this one would probably increase
stress in people who give up cigarettes on medical advice and
this may counteract the benefits of giving up smoking. When
people give up smoking on their own, it may be that they have

learned to cope with their stress and it is not necessary for them to be dependent on cigarette smoking. In these ex-smokers one would see not only the advantages of stopping smoking but also the benefits of stress reduction. Russeks (171) reported lower prevalence of CHD in ex-smokers compared with the group which never smoked.

## 8.7 Diabetes Mellitus

The evidence that diabetes or impaired glucose tolerance is a risk factor for CHD is very confused. Population study in Bedford (86) showed an increased frequency of ECG abnormality and of arterial disease in persons with impaired glucose tolerance. A study from Tecumseh (130) in the United States, similarly showed increased association of arterial disease. However, in neither of these studies, was the association independent of other risk factors such as hypertension and hyperlipaemia. The Whitehall Study (53) showed increased prevalence of ECG abnormalities in upper decile of glucose distribution with no evidence of trend below the 90th centile. Both Bedford (85) and Busselton (197) studies indicated that diabetes may be relevant as a risk factor for CHD in women but not possibly in men. Diabetes is relatively common in Japan, in spite of the low incidence of CHD (12). A study in Israel showed that although the Asian born subjects had the lowest incidence of myocardial infarction but they had higher prevalence rate and the highest incidence rate for diabetes mellitus (112, 113). A long-term prospective study showed that diabetes is a risk factor when combined with hypertension (143). It is also becoming apparent that part of the cardiac mortality in diabetics is not due to CHD but to several pathological entities grouped together as diabetic cardiopathy (94). Unfortunately, a large scale trial revealed that treatment of diabetes with Phenformin or Tolbutamide may increase the number of ischemic cardiac events (189). There have been arguments regarding the proper management of diabetes, but many believe that it should be controlled on diet alone whenever possible. There is some evidence that stress may be responsible for poor control of diabetes if not actually a precipitating factor (76).

## 8.8 Obesity

Obesity has often been found to be associated with the increased incidence of CHD. However, it was argued that this might be due to its association with other risk factors; for example, high blood pressure and elevated serum cholesterol and that if the major risk factors are excluded, obesity is not an independent risk factors are excluded, obesity is not an independent risk factor. The Pooling Project Research Group (145) showed high relative weight was associated with increased risk of CHD only in men under the age of 50; between 50-55 years there was no extra risk;

while over the age of  55 there was slight reduction in the risk.
On the other hand, cross sectional study in Finland failed to show
any association (78).

This may be considered an academic argument only because, in
practice, reduction in weight is frequently  associated with decrease
in blood pressure and also lowering of serum cholesterol within
days of dieting and before any significant weight loss.  This
was explained by a concommitant reduction in salt intake (153),
but reduction in blood pressure in obese patients on reducing diet
have been demonstrated, even when sodium intake was kept constant
(155).  Recent evidence suggests that the underlying mechanisms
may be reduction in catecholamine metabolism  (77) as well as
plasma renin activity (188), thus implicating sympathetic over
activity associated with both obesity, as well as high blood pressure.
No prospective study, however, has shown that reducing weight reduces
the incidence of CHD.  Another important point is that theoretically
it may sound a simple therapeutic measure, but clinical experience
of many is that in practice it is quite difficult to maintain
reduction in body weight in the obese population generally.

## 8.9  Coronary-Prone Behavior

Many astute physicians in the past have observed relevant and
often profound details of behavior characteristics of coronary-
prone men suggesting a link between self-generated psycho-social
stress and symptoms of angina pectoris or myocardial infarction.
Osler (129) described a coronary-prone man as a "keen and ambitious
man, the indicator of whose engine is set full speed ahead."  Wolf
(204) described a coronary-prone person as one who not only meets a
challenge by putting out extra effort, but who takes little
satisfaction from his accomplishment.  Kemple (87) described him as
an aggressive, ambitious individual with an intense emotional
drive, unable to delegate authority or responsibility with ease,
possessing no hobbies and concentrating all his thoughts and
energy in the narrow groove of his career.

Friedman and Rosenman (50) described Type A coronary-prone
behavior as an overt pattern characterized by intense ambition,
competitive drive, constant preoccupation with occupational deadlines
and a keen sense of time urgency.  A typical Type A person, Rosenman
says (163) is an individual engaged in a relatively chronic excessive
struggle to obtain unlimited number of things from his environment
in the shortest period of time against the opposing effects of other
things or persons in the same environment.  Type A individual speaks
louder and faster than non-coronary prone Type B person (175).  He
is less satisfied with his job (72) and although working closer to
his endurance limits on a treadmill, he is rarely likely to express
fatigue (21).  Russek and Zohman (172) failed to recognize such
overt behavior pattern in their group of young coronary patients,

but remarked at their striking degree of self-control, dignified reserve and outward complacency. They found that long hours of work, job responsibility and severe emotional stress of occupational origin were more signficantly correlated than positive family history or a high fat diet.

Friedman and Rosenman developed an interview technique which utilized standardized 15-minute challenging questioning. By carefully attending to the style as well as to the content of the responses, they were able to distinguish coronary-prone Type A persons from non-coronary prone Type B. In a prospective study known as the Western Collaborative Group Study (WCGS) they classified 3,524 initially CHD-free, middle-aged, middle-class men according to, their behavior pattern and followed them for 8.5 years (164). Through the followup period, Type A showed greater propansity to get CHD, compared with only 79 out of 1,565 Type B men. Even when all the confounding factors like age, blood pressure, serum cholesterol and cigarette smoking were statistically controlled, Type A still proved to be an important risk factor (165). Type A individuals who survived myocardial infarction also showed greater risk of having a recurrence (75). These observations have recently been confirmed in another large propsective study based on the Framingham sample, even though the investigators used much simpler measure of Type A behavior known as the Framingham Type A Questionnaire (64).

Type A individuals have more angiographic evidence of coronary artery occlusion compared with Type B (14) and faster progression of this occlusion (90). They also respond to stressful and challenging stimuli with greater increase in systolic blood pressure, heart rate, epinephrine and norepinephrine (37-39, 55). Correlation between systolic and diastolic pressures and Type A behavior has been reported only by Howard et al (71). It has also been suggested that Type A may interact with other risk factors such as diastolic blood pressure and enhance CHD risk in a manner which is multiplicative rather than additive (167). Although the recognition that competitive, aggressive, time-pressured Type A behavior as a contributing factor to CHD is now more widespread, intervention programs to reduce risk associated with this Type A behavior have been very scanty (166, 168, 185) and it is far too early to know if current approaches will eventually prove effective. Any primary prevention program in Type A men who are not considered sick by themselves, their families or companies and who are active, energetic, highly productive, fulfilling their family obligation and social roles, pose special problems. Even if the mass of evidence in favor of Type A behavior as a health risk qualifies it for therapeutic intervention, the issues still remain debatable as to what in the Type A behavior we are seeking to intervene and how to validate the success of intervention. To be competitive, ambitious and hard-working may increase chances of CHD on one hand, but it also increases the chances of social, economic and occupation success. Thus, there are conceptual, methodological and ethical problems (169).

## 8.10  Regional and Social Class Difference

Just as there is a discrepancy between CHD mortality in East Finland and West Finland at a similar level of risk factor, there are pronounced differences in CHD mortality within different groups in Scotland.  Thus, West-Central Scotland has a considerably greater mortality, probably the highest in the world, compared with either East-Central or North-East Scotland.  Serum cholesterol concentrations do not seem to be greater in Scotland than in Southern England and it has been speculated that excess mortality might be partially due to excess sudden death (177).  It is possible that in the areas of higher unemployment and poor socio-economic background, a traditional desire to gain more education and technical skills to compete for the dearth of jobs might be important.

Once upon a time, CHD was considered to be a disease of affluence, being much more common in rich industrialized countries and upper social classes (117).  Yet, contrary to this opinion, CHD is now more common among the working class men and women in England and Wales (104).  Women in social classes IV and V always had higher mortality compared with the women of social classes I and II, while in men a similar trend seemed to have started between 1951 and 1961.  This national trend was confirmed in a longitudinal study of 17,530  Civil Servants working in London over a period of 7.5 years (105).  Men in the lowest grade (messengers) had 3.6 times the CHD mortality of men in the highest employment grade (administrators).  Men in the low employment grades were  slightly shorter, heavier, had slightly higher blood pressure, higher plasma glucose, smoked more, reported less leisure time physical activity and, curiously enough, lower serum cholesterol compared with men  in the higher grade.  Even when allowances were made for the influence on mortality of all the risk factors, this could only partially explain the differences in mortality between the groups.  Indeed, employment grade was a stronger predictor of risk of dying from CHD than any of the familiar risk factors.

It is possible that unfit men tend to have been  selected into the lowest grade, but it could also be that  high expectations of the working class, increased competition and job responsibilities, breakdowns in the social hierarchy,  aggressive  behavior overtly manifest in militant union activities, insecurities associated with less skilled jobs (which are first to go with mechanization, especially in times of economic recession), rising unemployment and inflation, are particularly stressful to low socio-economic classes of men in a changing social structure.

This association between the high rate of CHD and the low position at work has been observed  by other workers as well

(181, 187). Syme and Berkman (186) proposed an increase in the generalized susceptibility of becoming ill in lower socio-economic groups by pointing out that not only the increased incidence of CHD, but virtually every disease or cause of death, including such diverse conditions like lung cancer, gastric ulcers, difficulties in pregnancy, sarcoidosis and depression. In 270,000 employees of telecommunication industry, the incidence of heart disease over a three year period was greatest among workers than executives (68). This was thought to be due to differences in education rather than occupation.

In the Western Collaborative Study of middle-aged men in California over 8.5 years, CHD was inversely linked to educational achievement but unrelated to income (164). For men aged 50-59 at entry, the average annual rate per 1,000 was 9.1 in college graduates and 16.8 for those without higher education. Similar pattern was also found in women by Kitagawa and Hauser (89).

## 8.11  Physical Activity

Urbanization, industrialization and mechanization of transport have all led to a great decrease in the amount of physical activity in the last few decades, so it is not surprising that it has become a suspect associated factor. It was explained that increased physical activity of the working class occupation was responsible for lower mortality (118, 119), but mechanization has now made their job physically less demanding. On the other hand, increase leisure time activity in the upper class administrators might be protective and may partially explain the apparently inverse relationship between the employment grade and CHD mortality (104, 105, 115, 116). However, the lack of physical activity concept does not explain the continuous higher rate in working class women. Besides, CHD mortality in East Finns is the highest in the world and yet most of them are lumber jacks and farmers engaged in most strenuous activity and despite consuming over 4,000 calories a day, they are lean and tall.

It may be impossible to establish beyond scientific doubt whether or not exercise is beneficial because for such proof one would have to randomly allocate a large group of people into two groups, one of whom took regular exercise and the other none and both the groups would have to be identical with respect to age, sex, mean blood pressure, serum cholesterol levels, smoking habits and so on , and the trial would have to continue for several years before an effect of exercise can be evaluated. The evidence so far has been summed up in a report by the working group of the Scottish Home and Health Department (178) by saying that it was unconvinced that physical activity had a protective effect.

## 8.12  Alcohol and Associated Factors

St. Leger et al (183) reported detailed analyses of factors associated with cardiac mortality in 18 developed countries in Western Europe, North America, Australia, and New Zealand.  A surprising revelation was a strong  and negative association between CHD and wine consumption.  Countries  with hard drinking habits of beer and spirits, such as Finland, Scotland, U.S.A., Canada, Australia and New Zealand, have 3-5 times the mortality from CHD, especially in men aged 35-64, contrary to countries where alcohol is chiefly taken in the form  of wine, such as France and Switzerland.  The association does not automatically mean that we can reduce CHD  incidence simply by increasing our wine con-sumption.  Prospective studies which are just beginning might shed some light on  this new factor.  A positive association between higher blood pressure and alcohol consumption was shown by Beevers (9).

## 8.13 Social Mobility, Immigration and Acculturation

Social scientists and epidemiologists have, in recent years, pointed out the unfavorable effects of difficulties of adjustment to new environments and unfamiliar cultures which the people must face following immigration, moving to new location within the same country or following changes in personal environment.  In North Dakota, CHD rates were twice as high in men who had several job changes and geographic moves; the rates were three times as high in men who moved to the city or moved up in the social class (186).  Berkman and Syme (11) followed up 6,928 adults for nine years in Alameda County, California, and showed that those who lacked social and community ties were more likely to die prematurely from various diseases compared with those who have more extensive social contacts.  In a followup study in Evans County, Georgia, between 1960 and 1969, Kaplan and his associates (83) found twice the prevalence of  CHD  among lower status persons who had moved upwards in social status during the period compared with those who remained at the same level.  Social inconsistency, such as discrepancies between the class of origin and adult status or educational standard and income, are thought to promote conflicting cultural expectations, disruption of interpersonal relationships and confusion about social roles (13).  People displaying such status inconsistency are exposed to stress of moving into social circumstances with which they are not familiar or have not been previously prepared for.  Such stress is thought to make them extra vulnerable to CHD.

Israel, having a large population of immigrants, has naturally been a subject to study the effect on health of moving into a new unfamiliar culture.  Although the relative mortality rates followed the patterns of the country from which these immigrants originally came, a rise in the rate of myocardial infarction was common in most groups followed by a sharper rise in all first-born Israelis, no matter where their fathers were born. However, the incidence rate began to fall in the second generation (112, 113). It is possible that their fathers, despite having to make adjustments, had no great difficulties in accepting themselves as foreigners while the first generation face the problems of identity. Coming from a different home background, they could not identify themselves with the true natives of Israel, at the same time having nothing in common with the countries of their fathers' origin. By the second generation, identity with Israel is gradually established with a decline in CHD mortality.

There is some evidence that social and cultural factors may interact with the conventional biological factors in an important manner which influence the incidence rate of CHD. Japan has the lowest rate of CHD in any industrialized nation, while the United States has one of the highest incidence. Gordon (56, 57) found an increasing gradient in mortality from CHD in Japanese living in Japan, Hawaii, and California respectively. It is possible that the low incidence of CHD in Japan is due to the increased social and emotional support people derive from each other due to strong family bonds and group cohesiveness. It has been explained that the Japanese institutions encourage free expression of emotion and group support (110). On the other hand, the stress of adjusting to a new society which is highly anonymous, might increase the susceptibility.

Marmot and Syme (106) suggested that if that was the case, the Japanese-Americans who have remained traditional, maintaining contact with Japanese language and habits, would have lower rate of CHD than the Japanese-Americans who had adopted Western American culture. In a very elegant study, they showed that the prevalence of definite CHD and, indeed, each characteristic, angina pectoris, the pain of myocardial infarction, and major ECG abnormality for each age group were greater in the Westernized group compared with the traditional Japanese living in California. This difference could not wholly be explained by the age standardized differences in the conventional risk factors: dietary preference, serum cholesterol, cigarette smoking, blood pressure, triglycerides, body weight or serum glucose. Those who were brought up in the Japanese culture, but who later adopted western lifestyles had intermediate incidence rate. It is an interesting concept to think that the high expected susceptibility due to special incongruity described earlier may, in fact, be counteracted to some extent by the protective effect of the Japanese culture in early life.

There are other examples of traditional social network buffering the harmful effects of highly individualized western culture. Bruhn et al (17) examined a close-knit community consisting of predominantly

German Protestant stock in the town of Nazareth, Pennsylvania.
People with CHD were more likely to be non-German minority than
controls and had lived in Nazareth for a comparatively shorter
time.  Striking differences were also found between Catholic-
Americans of Italian origin in Rosetto, Pennsylvania and  neighboring
communities (184).  Despite high levels of animal fat in the diet,
the inhabitants of the close knit and highly supportive Rosetto
community had significantly lower rate of CHD.  Following quote
from Ecclesiastes seems appropriate (82):

> "9.   Two are better than one because they have good
>       reward for their labour.
> 10.   For if they fall, the one will lift up his fellow;
>       but woe to him that is alone when he falleth, and
>       hath not another to lift him up.
> 11.   Again if two lie together, then they have warmth,
>       but how can one be warm alone?
> 12.   And if a man prevail against him that is alone,
>       two shall withstand him; and a three-fold cord
>       is not quickly broken."

                    Ecclesiastes 4: 9-12

Religious belief too can be a source of social support in
time of stress.  Caplan (20) points out that it can help the
faithful to proceed calmly with their routine, leaving it to the
deity and to the expectable social safeguards of society to ensure
their wellbeing.  In a study of 10,000 Israeli Civil Servants,
Medalie and Goldbourt (111) found that incidence of angina
pectoris in men who perceived their wives as loving and supportive,
was only half to those whose wives were seen as non-supportive.
Sachar (174) suggests that a man well-related to a supportive
and healthy society is adept at finding ways to cope with stress.
On the other hand, as Henry (65) suggests if he feels rejected,
inferior  in some way, unloved and uncared for, if he lacks status
in his social group and is a stranger to their ways and cannot
call on anyone for assistance with goods or services, he becomes
vulnerable.

We are constantly trying to discover factors which cause
illness.  Maybe we should try and elucidate factors which keep
people healthy.  House (70) has gone farthest in developing  an
instrument to measure social support, the concept which has been
amply reviewed by Caplan and Killilea (19) and Cobb (26).  Kobasa
(79) put forward a rather interesting concept of "hardy personality",
a characteristic which keeps persons healthy who ought to be ill by
all the measure of social, occupational and personal environments.

8.14 Life Events

Death from a "broken heart" may be a figure of speech from a
bygone age, but Parkes et al (133) showed in a longitudinal study of
4,486 widowers of 55 years and over that grief can indeed kill
through the heart. The mortality was report to be 40% higher than
expected in married men of the same age in the first six months
after bereavement, after which the mortality rate gradually began
to fall. By far, the commonest cause of death was CHD, which was
67% higher than expected.

Rahe and associates (149, 150, 151) developed a schedule of
Recent Experience (SRE) life change questionnaire to measure stress
due to changes in life events like death of a loved one, a change
in job or residence, illness in the family, a marriage, a financial
crisis, the birth of a child and so on. Each event was assigned a
life change unit (LCU) to represent a score of the relative stress.
They found a positive relationship between LCU and intensity build
up in the year or two prior to illness and the severity of illness.
A lot of work in this area has been retrospective and it is possible
that those who already have a disease are more likely to recall such
life events to account for their illness.

8.15 Multiple Risk Factor Intervention

When single risk factor intervention proved disappointing
it was pointed out that to have an appreciable effect, as many
risk factors as possible must be controlled together. Accordingly,
a comprehensive community program was started in North Karelia
County of Finland with the highest CHD mortality in the world.
It was relatively successful in reducing risk factor levels compared
with those of the control county of Kuopio (148). However, this
did not result in greater reduction in mortality in North Karalia
over a 5-year followup (173). It is possible that followup period
was not long enough. Another explanation could be the general
decline in CHD mortality in all counties of Finland (190).

In the Stanford Study (45), three towns were selected from
Northern California. The town of Tracey served as a control
while Gilmore and Watsonville received multimedia campaign via
newspaper, radio and television, supplemented by an intensive
personal instruction program for high risk subjects in Watsonville.
After two years of intervention, there were modest decreases in the
levels of risk factors in the intervention towns while the risk
slightly increased in the control group. The net estimated
reduction in coronary risk was calculated to be 23-28%. No data
on morbidity or mortality were published.

In the United Kingdom which is one of the countries participating
in the European multifactorial intervention trial (206), the

heart disease prevention project team randomly allocated 24 factories
or occupational groups, comprising 18,210 men aged 45-59 years, into
intervention or control groups.  Men in the intervention groups
received advice on dietary reduction of fat and cholesterol, stopping
or reducing  cigarette smoking, regular exercise and reducing
weight in the overweight, while people with hypertension were
treated by antihypertensive drugs.  In addition to the group campaign,
the top 10-15% of the higher risk group  received personal counselling
and personal letters of advice and followup.  At  the end of 5-year
followup, there were no clear differences between the intervention
and control groups in  the total risk estimates (162).  In a
subanalysis of men in the higher risk group, the estimated reduction
in risk, calculated from the changes in risk factor levels using
multiple  logistic function, was 9% at the end of 5 years or an
average of 11% over the last 3 years of followup.

It was pointed out that the above trial does not have the
statistical power to detect such small difference and thus it is
possible that when the trial  is finally concluded, it may not show
significant reduction in CHD mortality and miss a difference  as
important  as 10-15% (103).  It is of crucial importance that every
effort should be  made to elucidate other important etiological
factors so that the  future intervention  trials  not  only  show
large enough differences in morbidity and mortality to be  detected
by  the available statistical means but also make an impressive
contribution in eradicating  the  great burden of mortality from
CHD.


9  STRESS HYPOTHESIS

From the critical review of the literature, it is apparent
that the conventional major risk factors only account for part of
the  occurence of CHD.  On the other hand, in a constitutionally
susceptible person, psychological factors, personality, or behavior
characteristics  of the individual his social, ecological and
cultural environments and the way he copes  with  rapidly changing
increasing hostile environments with dwindling social support of
fragmentary nuclear family and highly  indifferent urban society,
are also important.  In spite of such  evidence, most intervention
trials have confined their attention to reducing three major risk
factors by conventional methods:  drug treatment of hypertension,
dietary or drug treatment of high serum cholesterol and advice to
stop smoking, with occasional mention of weight reduction or
increased physical activity.  It is not surprising, therefore,
that as yet there are no signs of major decline in mortality from
CHD or even clear-cut answers to the problem.  To plan further
trials on lines similar  to the ones in progress and some in
pipelines (Minnesota, Oslo, Stanford, Pawtacket) would
be pointless.

On the other hand, to look at the entire problem from a different angle would not only throw light on new facets but also probably help generate different treatment approaches. With this in mind, I suggest that psychosocial stress may be a causative factor (Figure 1). Working through appropriate neuro-endocrine stimulation and biochemical disturbances, it can lead to sudden death, probably through fatal arrhythmia (97). It may also lead to myocardial infarction (CHD) through gradual development of atherosclerosis, thrombosis or prolonged vasospasm of the coronary arteries. The disease can occur directly or indirectly through various risk factors. It is well-recognized that emotional stress can be one of the factors which lead to over-eating, cigarette smoking or alcohol consumption. Need to continue working in our highly pressurized, industrial environments, in spite of fatigue turns individuals to coffee, nicotine, and food, all of which sustain stimulation (65), while alcohol can calm one down when social situations get uncomfortable. Need to control and compete leads to aggressive, hostile behavior (51) and physical inactivity possibly by promoting early fatigue (126).

Overwhelming stress can result in the production of stress hormones leading to decrease in insulin and increase in blood glucose and free fatty acids (43). Its contribution to hypertension (59, 66) and raised serum cholesterol (24, 50, 152) is gradually being revealed. If the hypothesis is right and if effective intervention procedures can be found to counteract psycho-social-occupational stress, then we cannot only expect to see reduction in CHD but also see some reduction in the conventional risk factors in process.

One of the attractions of this hypothesis is that it can explain cases of CHD in individuals without the presence of conventional risk factors. It can also explain why some people who get myocardial infarction are overweight, while others have high blood pressure or high serum cholesterol, depending upon their genetic susceptibility.


10 POSSIBLE INTERVENTION STRATEGIES

The idea behind a broad and fairly simple stress hypothesis I put forward is to generate a treatment approach which is prac-tically feasible, ethically responsible, scientifically sound and which leads to clinically meaningful therapeutic changes. Assuming that underlying physiological response to recurrent internal and external environmental demands is the hypothalamic defense alarm reaction or the sympathetic fight or flight response (18) in varying intensity reflected in the behavioral and emotional correlates ranging from aggression, anger, frustration, frantic activity to fearful alertness, one can understand various mechanisms

292

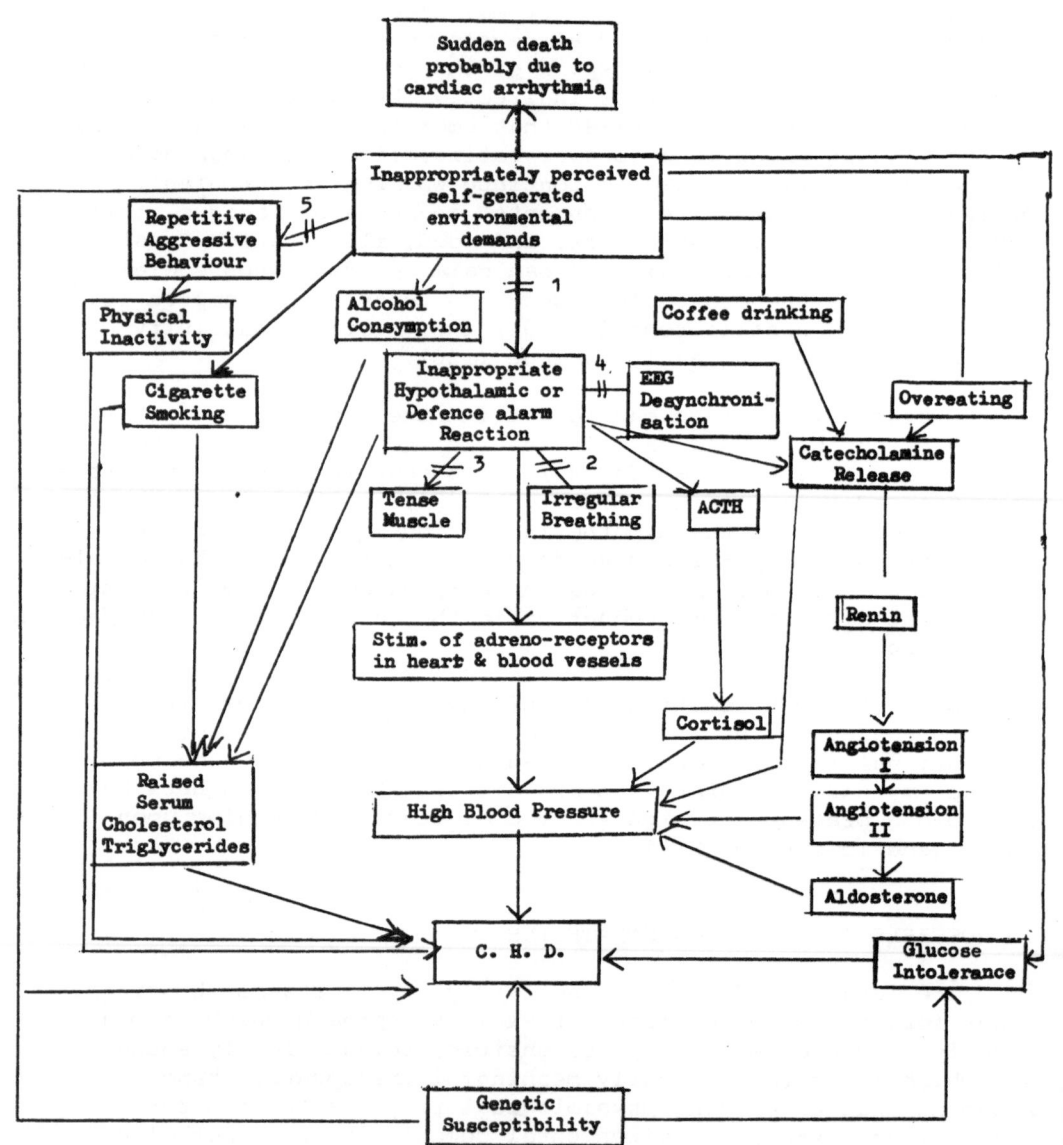

Figure 1

which can lead to high blood pressure (138), raised serum cholesterol
and other lipids, abnormal glucose intolerance and eventually CHD
(Figure 1). By directing intervention strategies to various pathways
(1-5 in Figure 1), one could modulate the entire response and by
repeated practice of these strategies, hope to prevent CHD. I
started to work on this concept in its primitive form, in 1973, and
though it has been refined and further strategies have been added
through experience, it has turned out to be more robust than I
expected from the start as it will become clear through the results
of the studies to be described. In the main, five strategies
are used (1-5 in Figure 1).

## 10.1 Cognitive Restructuring

It is understood that the intensity of the response depends
upon individuals' appraisal of the situation. Faulty interpretation
leads to inappropriate emotional response, maladaptive behavior and
damaging physiological reactions. Through an audio-visual health
education program, individuals are helped in shaping their emotional
response to everyday life situations as well as in working out
coping strategies. It is not easy to change longstanding habitual
response but through trial and error and diligent perseverance,
persons' usual pattern of cognition can be modestly changed.

## 10.2 Breathing Exercise

He is taught simple breathing exercise at first. It known that
breathing is erratic when a person is excited, yet low  and regular
when he is calm and composed. By a simple, rhythmic diaphragmatic
breathing exercise, a certain amount of physical calmness is induced.
This exercise can be performed anywhere and in any position without
anyone even noticing it. This is followed by:

## 10.3 Deep Muscle Relaxation

Increase in muscle tension is part and parcel of the fight
or flight response. An effective intervention strategy would,
therefore, be to relax. The person is asked to lie down, close the
eyes and systematically relax each part of the body. He is told
that for full benefit he should do this exercise with an empty stomach
and bladder. The fact that deep muscle relaxation reduces the
intensity of the hypothalamic response is evident from animal
experiments. For example, increase in proprioception through passive
movements increases the intensity and a greater rise in blood pressure,
while a decrease in proprioception through curarization decreases
the intensity and causes a small rise in blood pressure when the
hypothalamus is electrically stimulated (54, 69). It is thought
that the intensity of the response is directly proportional to
the amount of sensory input to the brain. In this context, it is
also interesting to note that an increase in isometric contraction,

294

such as a tight hand grip or the carrying of a heavy suitcase, a
considerable rise in blood pressure has been observed (96). Maybe
we live in a world with far too much sensory stimulation. It is
assumed that a reduction in sensory input due to mental and physical
relaxation would reduce the sympathetic responsiveness of the hypothalamus, and eventually lower blood pressure and other risk factors.

10.4 Meditation

After a few sessions in breathing exercise and deep muscle
relaxation, a type of mental relaxation is introduced in the form
of passive concentration and eventually meditation. One definite
advantage of meditation is that it at least prevents sleep.
Relaxation is very conducive to sleep in accordance with the
mechanisms of sleep (98). But if the patient is allowed to sleep
then the whole concept of voluntary control is nullified. Meditation
is also known to change the ECG pattern into a more synchronized
one with high amplitude, slow wave pattern of the relaxed brain not
passing into sleep (196). It is also known to increase coherence
between two hemispheres as well as between the anterior and posterior
parts of each hemisphere (5).

10.5 Biofeedback

In short, the points so far discussed in the program are aimed
at reducing the levels of arousal. The biofeedback instruments are
used to train patients more efficiently to shift into a low arousal
state. One of the two very simple instruments are used. A
Galvanic Skin Resistance (GSR) which by and large informs the
patient about his level of skin resistance and indirectly of the
level of his arousal or an Electromyographic Feedback Machine (EMG)
which continuously measures and displays his level of muscular
tension. As the patient relaxes, the sound becomes fainter and
the clicks become fewer until they stop. The sensitivity is then
turned up to give further signals and the patient has to relax
further to stop the signal and so on. The idea behind this procedure
is that the knowledge of results reinforces the learning. In
addition to this relaxation feedback, the patient is also given an
overall feedback of his blood pressure level at the end of each
session. Every success the patient has is taken as an opportunity
to raise his self esteem and his motivation to continue the program
on a long-term basis. Each session is about 30 minutes long.
Originally, the patients had three training sessions per week,
but experience as well as more comprehensive educational program
have shown that on average one training session per week for eight
weeks may be adequate. In addition, the patient is asked to
practice twice a day on his own for 15 to 20 minutes. Recent
studies have included loaning the patient an instruction cassette
tape for home practice.

## 10.6 Stress Management

The sixth point in the plan is integrating relaxation response
into daily activities. It would be useful to know what situations
in an individual's life contribute to hypertension or atherosclerosis
- so that one could desensitize that individual against those
situations. In practice, it is not possible to identify these
situations in every individual. However, we know that environments
of urbanized industrialized society are important, possibly through
repeated aggressive behavior with concomittant neurohormonal changes.
Therefore, we can assume that desensitization against situations
of modern civilizations would be beneficial. A counter-conditioning
or the method of reciprocal inhibition is used in which fear or
aggression, inducing stimulus is paired with another neutral stimulus,
such as relaxation, which inhibits fear or aggression (205). For
example, car driving is one of the modern activities which raises
blood pressure in some individuals and causes aggression. What the
patient is asked to do is to take one deep breath, relax and "let
go" at every red traffic light or intersection. He uses the same
method before answering a telephone, speaking in public, during an
interview, while waiting for a bus or in a dentist's surgery, and
so on. This list is inexhaustive and can be made up by an individual
to suit his requirement. A tiny, colored paper disc is stuck to his
wrist watch dial, so every time he looks at the watch he is reminded
to relax, and we know how time pressure is considered to be one of
the important risk factors (51).

Another way of integrating meditation in everyday life is
through what is known as meditation in action. It is seen when a
meditator becomes one with whatever he is doing at that point.
For example, when an artist is painting or a sculpturist is sculpting
or a dancer is dancing; when his mind is so concentrated on the
thing he is doing that he becomes completely engrossed. It is a
way of releasing or channelling emotional energy. We do not have
to pursue higher arts for this. We can practice meditation in
action during our everyday work or leisure activity, whether
interviewing, washing up or jogging, provided we could learn to
concentrate on the activity at hand with our body and mind shut
out irrelevant ideas and associated anxieties.


## 11 EVALUATION OF INTERVENTION STRATEGIES

The aim of intervention is prevention of CHD. However, to
prove that the proposed intervention package was actually effective,
we would require very large and expensive long-term study where
morbidity and mortality were accepted end points. It is not possible
to plan such a study merely on theoretical reasoning. A series of
steps have to be taken before one can reach the ultimate goal.
What I am about to describe is efforts to climb some of those initial
steps.

11.1 Hypertension

At first I chose to study the effect of the intervention package on blood pressure in hypertensive patients because it was likely to be relatively easier to evaluate and if found effective, the behavioral intervention would establish itself as one of the treatment approaches for a single most potent contributing factor to morbidity and mortality. In a pilot study (134), 20 hypertensive patients controlled on antihypertensive drugs were recruited. Twenty similar hypertensive controls were age and sex matched. The treatment group was offered intervention strategies described, over a study period or three months. The control group was given attention placebo. If during the study period blood pressure became normal, drugs were gradually reduced or eliminated.

At the end of three months, five patients in the treatment group stopped antihypertensive medication altogether; a further seven patients had reductions made in their drug dosage ranging from 33-66%; another four patients had a better control of blood pressure at the same dosage, while the remaining four patients did not show significant benefit as far are blood pressure is concerned, although one of them stopped having almost daily migraine attacks. In addition to this reduction in antihypertensive drug requirement, average drops in systolic and diastolic pressures in the treated group were 20 and 14mm Hg., respectively. In the control group of hypertensive patients who were already familiar to me and my nursing staff as well as the procedure of blood pressure measurement, increased attention and repeated measurements did not cause significant change in blood pressure or antihypertensive medication.

The groups were followed up up to 12 months (135) and with continued practice of cognitive and behavioral strategies, reductions in blood pressure and antihypertensive medications were maintained in the treated group, while those in the control group did not change significantly.

In order to produce a better evidence of efficacy, a randomized controlled trial was carried out (140). Thirty-four hypertensive patients of at least six months duration, controlled on antihypertensive medications were randomly allocated after the baseline blood pressure was established. The patient in each group attended twice a week for six weeks. The treatment group patient was given training in biofeedback-aided relaxation and meditation as well as learning to appraise everyday life situations more appropriately and better stress management. The control group patient was asked to lie down and relax in his own manner. After the trial period of six weeks, patients in both the groups were followed up once a fortnight for three months. An average of all measurements made during followup was taken as the final pressure. The drugs were kept constant.

The results showed small but significant reductions in systolic
and diastolic pressures in the control group (8 and 4mm Hg.
respectively) and differences between the groups were highly
significant (P =    .001) for systolic and P =    .005 for diastolic
changes).  Two months after the last followup examination, the
patients were recalled.  The results at this visit showed that blood
pressure in the control group had gone back to at least its original
levels while most of the reduction in the treatment group was
maintained, thus demonstrating a typical placebo effect in the
control group, meaning that it lasts as long as the placebo factors
are operating, whatever they may be.  On the other hand, the treated
group patients had learned a skill which maintained blood pressures
at a lower level.

By chance, random allocation had not divided patients into
two equal groups.  The study was extended in phase 2 during which
the intervention package was offered to the control group over
the next six weeks.  The results showed lowering in both systolic
and diastolic pressures in an almost identical pattern shown by
the previous treated group.

## 11.2 Reduction in Blood Pressure Reactivity

Although hypertension is one of the major risk factors and
mechanisms exist by which it  can damage the intima of the blood
vessels and render them more liable to the process of atherosclerosis,
there are a number of coronary-prone persons in whom resting blood
pressure is within normal limits.  Individuals with Type A behavior
is a case in point.  Apart from one study (71) most investigators
report that resting pressures in Type A individuals do not differ
from those in Type B persons.  It is more than likely that the
mechanisms through which Type A behavior exerts its harmful effects
are their physiological and biochemical hyperactivity to challenging
stimuli.  Type A individuals create their own stress not only by
perceiving challenge where Type B do not; but also by showing a
sharper rise in blood pressure and other biochemical changes which
are slower to return to baseline (37, 47, 49, 202).

A number of studies have shown that compared with normotensives,
hypertensive patients respond to physical, emotional or painful
stimuli with more intensive and prolonged pressor response.  The
pressure load on the left ventricle and the vessel walls is neither
a resting pressure, nor an occasional peak of pressure, but an
integrated average pressure over long periods.  If frequency,
intensity and duration of these pressor responses could be  reduced,
the cumulative benefit over a number of years could be very
substantial.

Thirty-two hypertensive patients were randomly allocated into treatment and control groups (136, 138). All of the patients were subjected to two experimental stressors - a standardized exercise test and a cold pressor test. These tests were repeated after six weeks, during which the treated group received behavioral intervention program while the control group received attention placebo similar to previous studies. The results showed significant reduction in the magnitude as well as duration of pressure rises in the treatment group compared with the control group in all measures except for systolic rise following the exercise test (two-tailed between group differences). Although the measurements were made intermittently using an ordinary mercury sphygmomanometer, this study demonstrates the possibility of potentially profound benefits which could be obtained by behavioral methods.

12 MULTIPLE RISK FACTOR INTERVENTION BY BEHAVIORAL MODIFICATION

Having seen fairly convincing evidence that behavioral strategies outlined above can reduce hypertension and blood pressure reactivity and some indications from two pilot studies (137, 139) that it may also reduce serum cholesterol and cigarette smoking, a randomized controlled trial was set up to see if all of the major risk factors can be reduced at once in unselected group of people engaged in full-time jobs (142). One thousand thirty-two employees of a large manufacturing industry between 35-64 years of age were screened. Those with two or more risk factors were reexamined. The risk factors were defined as an average of two measurements of B.P. to be 140/90 or more; serum cholesterol of 6.3mmol/l or more and current cigarette smoking of 10 or more cigarettes per day. If the person still qualified on the grounds of two or more risk factors at the second examination, he was invited to participate in the study. In a sub-group, a further sample of blood was withdrawn for plasma renin activity (PRA) and plasma aldosterone assays. Two hundred four or 89% of those qualified consented and were randomly allocated to treatment and control groups. The treatment consisted of training in relaxation-meditation and other behavioral methods one hour a week for eight weeks. Additionally, both groups were given health education literature including low cholesterol diet.

The results (Table 1) showed significantly greater reduction in systolic and diastolic pressures in the treatment group, whether the analysis included the whole group or was confined to the high risk subgroups with initial pressure of 140/90 or more. These reductions were maintained at eight-month followed up (P = .001). Serum cholesterol was significantly lower in both groups at eight weeks as well as at eight months (P = .001) within group by paired to test. However, the greater drop in the treatment

| Risk factor group | Men in each group | Cumulative % of CHD Cases | Ten year incidence % |
|---|---|---|---|
| All three | 595 | 17 | 14 |
| Any two | 2178 | 58 | 9 |
| Any one | 3320 | 94 | 5 |
| None | 1249 | 100 | 2 |
| TOTAL | 7342 | 100 | 7 |

Table 1. Ten Year Incidence of CHD According to Risk Factor Status at Entry in White Men Aged 30-59; adapted from (107).

group was only significant at eight weeks and was confined to the high risk subgroup (P = .025).

Our dietary analysis showed that groups were similar at entry in their intake of total calories and animal fats and that both groups had reduced their intake of saturated fats and increased polyunsaturated fats. However, control group had made slightly greater changes. Body weight also remained unchanged, suggesting that blood pressure and cholesterol difference between the groups were unrelated to dietary or weight changes. More people reduced smoking in the treatment group compared with the control group (68% vs. 39%) and these changes were largely maintained up to eight month followup. Although these differences were statistically significant, one might have hoped for a greater effect judging from the result of our pilot study (139).

Plasma renin activity and aldosterone were analysed in a sub-sample of 54 subjects. There were significantly greater reductions in both the parameters in the treatment group at eight weeks, but not at eight months (P = .05). There were no correlations between the changes in blood pressure and changes in PRA in either group, but there were signficant correlations between changes in aldosterone and changes in both systolic and diastolic blood pressure at eight weeks. Plasma renin activity is mediated through beta-adrenoreceptors, while it is possible that blood pressure was reduced by a central mechanism involving both alpha and beta adrenoreceptors as well as hormonal changes.


13   IMPLICATIONS

Although the hypothesis that psychosocial stress is a causative factor is not yet proven, there is enough evidence from the studies carried out so far that it is at least an important  risk factor. Assuming that the greater reductions in blood pressure, cigarette smoking and cholesterol achieved in this study would reduce  the mortality from CHD, we can calculate the potential reduction in mortality using the multiple logistic function from the London Whitehall Study (104). The figure at eight weeks is 21% reduction in the predicted risk of CHD death while at eight  months the figure is 18% which can be attributed to relaxation only.

This may not sound very impressive, but when one considers the fact that subjects in this study had elevations of risk factors too mild to warrant  the hazards of  pharmacological intervention and yet serious enough to increase their risk of dying  from CHD, the results obtained may not  be a mean achievement. It is possible that  reduction in risk may occur  through paths other than through the conventional risk factors, although it is not possible to estimate its magnitude from the present study.  In fact, the results are quite encouraging when comparisons are made with other multiple  risk factors intervention studies using conventional methods (148, 162).  The predicted reductions in mortality from CHD in these studies followed up to a 5-year  period have been estimated from 9-17.4%.  Followup period in our study has been comparatively short.  Therefore, one must remain cautious in making claims.  However, there is no reason why relaxation therapy cannot be combined with conventional therapies so that the future intervention trials not only show large enough differences in morbidity and mortality to be detected by the available statistical means, but also make an impressive contribution in eradicating the great burden of mortality  from CHD in our communities.

REFERENCES

1.   Anderson, M.P., P. Bechsgaard, J. Frederikson et al.  Effect of Alprenolol on Mortality Among Patients with Definite or Suspect Acute Myocardial Infarction.  Lancet II (1979) 865-867.

2.   Anitschkow, N.  Arterosclerosis.  In E.V. Cowdry (Ed.) Arterosclerosis (New York, Macmillan, 1933).

3.   Antman, E., J. Muller, S. Goldberg et al.  Nifedipine Therapy for Coronary Spasm:  Collective Clinical Experience in the United States.  Presentation, American Heart Association Meeting 1979 (Abstract  Circulation, Suppl. II to 59 & 60, II 76).

4.   Armstrong, A., B. Duncan, M.F. Oliver et al.  Natural History of Acute Coronary Heart Attacks:  A Community Study. Brit. Heart J. 34 (1972) 67-80.

5.   Banquet, J.P., Spectral Analysis of the EEG in Meditation. Electroenceph. Clin. Neurophysiol. 35 (1973) 143-151.

6.   Bassler, T.J., Smoking and Coronary Heart Disease, Lancet, II (1979) 1211.

7.   Beaglehole, R., C.E. Salmond, A. Hooper et al.  Blood Pressure and Social Interaction in Tokelauan Migrants in New Zealand.  J. Chron. Dis.  30 (1977) 803-812.

8.   Bemiller, C.R., C.J. Pepine, A.K. Rogers.  Long Term Observation in Patients with Angina and Normal Coronary Arteriogram.

9.   Beevers, D.G.  Alcohol and Hypertension.  Lancet, II (1977) 114-115.

10.  Berglund, G., L. Wilhemsen, R. Sannerstedt et al.  Coronary Heart Disease After Treatment of Hypertension.  Lancet I (1978) 1.

11.  Berkman, L.F. and L. Syme.  Social Networks, Lost Resistance and Mortality:  A Nine Year Followup Study of Alameda County Residents.  Amer. J. Epid.  189 (2) (1979) 186-204.

12.  Blackard, W.G., Y. Omor and L.R. Freedman. The Epidemiology of Diabetes Mellitus in Japan. J. Chron. Dis. 18 (1965) 415-427.

13.  Blalock, H.M. Status Inconsistency, Social Mobility: Status Integration and Structural Efects. Amer. Soc. Rev. 32 (1967) 790-800.

14.  Blumenthal, J.A., R.B. Williams, Y. Kong et al. Coronary Prone Behavior and Angiographically Documented Coronary Disease Circulation. 58 (1978) 634-639.

15.  Breckenridge, A., C.T. Dollery, E.H.O. Parry. Prognosis of Treated Hypertension. Quart. J. Med. 39 (1970) 411-429.

16.  Bronte-Stewart, B., A. Key, and J.F. Brook. Serum Cholesterol Diet and Coronary Heart Disease. Lancet II (1955) 1103.

17.  Bruhn, J.C., S. Wolf, T. Lynn et al. Social Aspects of Coronary Heart Disease in Pennsylvannia German Comunity. Soc. Sci. Med. 2 (1968) 201,212.

18.  Cannon, W.R. The Emergency Function of the Adrenal Medulla in Pain and Major Emotions. Amer. J. Physiol. 33 (1941) 356-372

19.  Caplan,G. and M. Killilea. Support Systems and Mutual Help. (New York, Greene and Straton, 1976)

20.  Caplan,G. Mastery of Stress: Psychosocial Aspects. Am. J. Psychiatry. 138 (1981) 413-420.

21.  Carver, C.S., A.E. Coleman and D.C. Glass. The Coronary-Prone Behaviour Pattern and Suppression of Fatigue on a Treadmill Test. Journal of Personality and Social Psychology 33 (1976) 460-466.

22.  Cassel, J. The Contribution of the Social Environment to Host Resistance. American Journal of Epidemiology. 102(2) (1976) 107-123.

23.  Cheng, T.O., T. Bashour, B.K. Singh, and G.A. Kelser. Myocardial Infarction in the Absence of Arteriosclerosis: Result of Coronary Spasm. Am. J. Cardiol. 30 (1972) 680-682

24.  Clark, D.A., E.L. Arnorld, J. Foulds et al. Serum Urate and Cholesterol Level in Air Force Academy Cadets. Aviat. Space Environ. Med. 46 (1975) 1044.

25.  Clofibrate: A Final Verdict. The Lancet II (1978) 1131-1132

26.  Cobb,S. Social Support as a Moderator of Life Stress. Psychosomatic Medicine. 38(5) (1976) 300-314.

27.  Cobb, L.A., H. Alvarez, M.K. Compass. A Rapid Response System for out of Hospital Cardiac Emergencies. Med. Clin. North Am. 60 (1976) 283-290.

28.  Cobb, S., and E.M. Rose. Hypertension, Peptic Ulcer and Diabetes in Air Traffic Controllers. J.A.M.A. 224 (1973) 489-492.

29.  Colling, A., A.W. Dellipiani, R.J. Donaldson, and P. MacCormack. Teeside Coronary Survey: An Epidemiological Study of Acute Attacks of Myocardial Infarction. Brit. Med. J. 2 (1976) 1169-1172.

30.  Committee of Principal Investigators.  A Cooperative Trial
     in the Primary Prevention of Ischaemic Heart Disease Using
     Clofibrate.  Brit. Heart J. 40 (1978) 1069-1118.
31.  Coronary Drug Project Research Group.  Clofibrate and Niacin
     in Coronary Heart Disease.  JAMA 231 (1975) 360.
32.  Coronary Drug Project Research Group.  Gall Bladder Disease
     as a Side  Effect of Drugs Influencing Lipid Metabolism.
     N. Engl. J. Med. 296 (1977) 1185-1190.
33.  Cruz-Coke, R. Environmental Influences and Arterial Blood
     Pressure.  Lancet II (1960) 885-886.
34.  Cruz-Coke, R., R. Etcheverry, and R. Nagel.  Influence of
     Migration on Blood Pressure of Eastern Islanders.  Lancet
     I (1964) 697-699.
35.  Day, L.J. and E. Sowton.  Clinical Features and Follow Up
     of Patients with Angina and Normal Coronary Arteries.
     Lancet II (1976) 334-337.
36.  Dayten, S., M.L. Pearce, S. Hasimoto, et al.  A Controlled
     Clinical Trial of a Diet High in Unsaturated Fat in Preventing
     Complication of Artherosclerosis.  Circulation 40 (Suppl. II)
     1969.
37.  Debroski, T., J. MacDougall and J. Shields.  Physiologic
     Reactions to Social Challenge in Persons Evidencing the
     Type A Coronary-Prone Behaviour Pattern.  J. Human Stress
     3(3) (1977) 2-9.
38.  Debroski, T. and J. MacDougall.  Stress Effects on Affiliation
     Preference Among Subjects Possessing the Type A Coronary-
     Prone Behaviour Pattern.  J. Personality & Social Psychology
     36 (1978) 23-33.
39.  Dembroski, T.M., J.M. MacDougall, J.A. Herd, and J.L. Shields.
     Effect of Level of Challenge on Pressor and Heart Rate Responses
     in Type A and B. Subjects.  J. Applied Soc. Psychology 9 (1979)
     209-228.
40.  Doll, R. and A.B. Hill.  Mortality in Relation to Smoking:
     Ten Years' Observation of British Doctors.  Brit. Med. J.
     I (1964) 1339-1410.
41.  Ederer, F., P. Laren, O. Turpeinen, et al.  Cancer Among
     Men on Cholesterol-Lowering Diets:  Experiments from Five
     Clinical Trials.  Lancet II (1971) 203-206.
42.  Endo, M., I. Kanda, S. Hosoda et al.  Prinzmetal's Variant
     Form of Angina Pectoris:  Reevaluation of Mechanisms.
     Circulation 52 (1975) 33-37.
43.  Efendic, S., E. Cerasi, and R. Luft.  Trauma:  Hormonal
     Factors with Special Reference to Diabetes Mellitus.  Acta
     Anaesthesiol. Scand. Suppl. 55, 107-119.
44.  European Coronary Surgery Study Group.  Coronary-Artery
     By-Pass Surgery in Stable Angina Pectoris:  Survival of
     Two Years.  Lancet I (1979) 889.
45.  Farquhar, J.W., N. MacCoby, P.D. Wood, et al.  Community
     Education for Cardiovascular Health.  Lancet I (1977)
     1192-1195.

304

46. Folklow, B., M. Hallback, Y. Lundgren, et al. Importance of Adaptive Changes in Vascular Design for Establishment of Primary Hypertension. Studied in Man and in Spontaneously Hypertensive Rats. Circulation 32-33(Suppl. 1) (1973) 2-16.

47. Frankenhaeuser, M. Sympathetic Adrenomedullary Activity, Behavior and the Psychosical Environment. In P. Venables and M.J. Christi (Eds.) Research in Psychophysiology. Chichester, Wiley, 1975).

48. Friedberg, C.K., and H. Horn. Acute Myocardial Infarction not Due to Coronary Artery Occlusion. JAMA 112 (1939) 1675-1679.

49. Friedman, M., S. Byers, J. Diamant, and R.H. Rosenman. Plasma Catecholamine Response of Coronary Prone Subjects (Type A) to a Specific Challenge. Metabolism 24 (1975) 205-210.

50. Friedman, M. and R.H. Rosenman. Association of Specific Overt Behaviour Pattern with Blood and Cardiovascular Findings. JAMA 169 (1959) 1286-1296.

51. Friedman,M. and R. Rosenman. Type A Behaviour and Your Heart. (New York, Alfred A. Knopf, 1974).

52. Friedman, M. R.H. Rosenman, and V. Carrol. Changes in the Serum Cholesterol and Blood Clotting Time in Men Subjected to Cyclic Variation of Occupational Stress. Circulation 17 (1959) 852-861.

53. Fuller, J.H., P. McCartney, R.J. Jarrett et al. Hyperglycaemia and Coronary Heart Disease: The Whitehall Study. J. Chron. Dis. 32 (1979) 721-728.

54. Gellhorn, E. and W.F. Kiely. Mystical States of Consciousness: Neurological and Clinical Aspects. J. Nerv. Men. Dis. 154 (1972) 399-405.

55. Glass, D.C., L.R. Krakoff, R. Contrada, et al. Effects of Harrassment and Competition Upon Cardiovascular Catecholamines Responses in Type A and Type B Individuals. Psychophysiology 17 (1980) 453-463.

56. Gordon, T. Mortality Experience Among the Japanese in the United States, Hawaii and Japan. Public Health Reports 72 (1957) 543-553.

57. Gordon, T. Further Mortality Experience Among Japanese-Americans. Public Health Reports 82 (1967) 973-984.

58. Groen, J.J., B.K. Tijong, A.F. Willebrandt, and C.J. Kamminga. Influence of Nutrition, Individual and Different Forms of Stress on Blood Cholesterol: Results Experiment of 9-Months Duration in 60 Normal Volunteers. Proceedings of the First International Congress on Dietetics (Voeding 10, 1959).

59. Guttman, M.C. and H.F. Benson. Interaction of Environmental Factors and Systemic Arterial Blood Pressure. Medicine 50 (1971) 543-553.

60. Hammond, E.C. Smoking in Relation to the Death Rate of One Million Men and Women. National Cancer Institute Monograph 19 (1966) 127-204.

61. Hampton, J.R., M. Dowling, and C. Nicholas. Comparison of Results from a Cardiac Ambulance Manned by Medical and Non-Medical Personnel. Lancet I (1977) 526-529.

62. Hampton, J.R. and C. Nicholas. Randomized Trial of a Mobile Coronary Care Unit for Emergency Calls. Brit. Med. J. 1 (1978) 1118-1121.

63. Havlik, R.J. and M. Feinleib (Eds.) Procedings of the Conference on the Decline in Coronary Heart Disease Mortality. NIH Publication No. 79-1610, May 1979.

64. Haynes, S.G., M. Feinleib, and W.B. Kannel. The Relationship of Psychosocial Factors to Coronary Heart Disease in the Framingham Study: III. Eight Years Incidence of CHD. American Journal of Epidemiology III (1980) 37-58.

65. Henry, J.P. Social and Biological Processes in Disease. Social Science and Medicine, 1981.

66. Henry, J.P. and J.C. Cassel. Psychosocial Factors in Essential Hypertension. Recent Epidemiological and Animal Experiemental Evidence. Amer. J. Epidemiology 90(3) (1969) 171-200.

67. Hill, J.D., J.R. Hampton, J.R.A. Mitchell. A Randomized Trial of Home vs. Hospital Management for Patients with Suspected Myocardial Infarction. Brit. Med. J. II (1976) 1035.

68. Hinkle, L.E., L.H. Whitney, E.W. Lehman, et al. Occupation, Education, and Coronary Heart Disease. Science 161 (1968) 238-246.

69. Hoes, R. Electroencephalographic Synchronization Resulting from Reduced Proprioceptive Drive Caused by Enruomuscular Blocking Agents. Electroenceph. Clin. Neurophysiol. 14 (1962) 220-232.

70. House, J. Barriers to Work Stress I: Social Support. Presented at the NATO Advanced Study Institute: Behavioral Medicine: Work, Stress, and Health. Castle Bonas, Castera-Verduzan, France, August 1981.

71. Howard, J.H. D.A. Cunningham, P.A. Rechnitzer. Health Patterns Associated With Type A Behavior: A Managerial Population. J. Human Stress 2(1) (1976) 24-33.

72. Howard, J.H., D.A. Cunningham, P.A. Rechnitzer. Work Patterns Associated with Type A Behavior: A Managerial Population. Human Relations 30 (1977) 825-836.

73. Hypertension Detection and Follow Up Program: Cooperative Group. Five-Year Findings of the Hypertension Detection and Follow Up Program. 1. Reduction in Mortality of Persons with High Blood Pressure, Including Mild Hypertension. JAMA 242 (1979) 2562-2571.

74. Intersociety Commission for Heart Disease Resources. Primary Prevention of the Atherosclerotic Diseases. Circulation 42 (1970) A55-A95.

75. Jenkins, C.D., S.J. Zyzanski, and R.H. Rosenman. Risk of New Myocardial Infarction in Middle-Aged Men with manifest Coronary Heart Disease, Circulation 53 (1976) 342-347.

76.   Johnson, J.B.   Psychological Factors in Juvenile Diabetes:
      A Review.  Journal of  Behavioral Medicine 3 (1979) 95-116.
77.   Jung, R.T., P.S. Shetty, M. Barrard, et al.  Role of Cate-
      cholamines in Hypertensive Response to Dieting.  Brit. Med.
      J. I  (1979)  12-13.
78.   Juustilia, H.  Overweight and Ischaemic Heart  Disease.
      Amer. J. Cardiol. 41 (1978) 622.
79.   Kobasa, S.  Hardy Personality.  Presented at the NATO
      Advanced Study Institute, Behavioral Medicine:   Work, Stress
      and  Health.  Castle  Bonas, Catera-Verduzan, France, August
      1981.
80.   Kahn, H.A.  The Corn Study of Smoking and Mortality Among
      U.S. Veterans:   Report on 8.5 Years Observation.   National
      Cancer Institute Monograph No. 19  (1966) 1-125.
81.   Kannel, W.B., Gordon, T.  The Framingham Diet Study.  Diet
      and Regulation of Serum Cholesterol (Sect. 24), Department
      of Health, Education and Welfare, Washington, DC, 1970.
82.   Kaplan, B.H.  A Note on Religious Beliefs  and Coronary
      Heart Disease.  J. South Carolina Med. Assoc. (February,
      1976, Suppl.) 60-64.
83.   Kaplan, B.H., J.C. Cassel, H.A. Tyroler, et al.  Occupational
      Mobility and Coronary Heart Disease.  Arch. Int. Medicine
      128 (1971) 936-942.
84.   Kasl, S.V. and S. Cobb.  Blood Pressure Changes in Men
      Undergoing Job Loss:  A  Preliminary Report.  Psychosom.
      Med. 32 (1970) 19-38.
85.   Keen, H., R.J. Jarrett, K.G.M.M. Alberti.  Diabetes Mellitus:
      A New Look at Diagnostic Criteria.  16 (1979) 283-285.
86.   Keen, H., G.A. Rose, D.A. Puke et al.  Blood Sugar and
      Arterial Disease.  Lancet II (1965) 505-508.
87.   Kemple, C.  Rorschach Method and Psychosomatic Diagnosis.
      Psychosom. Med. 7 (1975) 85-89,
88.   Keys, A.  Coronary Heart Disease in Seven Countries.
      Circulation 41 (Suppl) (1970) 1-199.
89.   Kitagawa, E.M. and P.M.Hauser.  Differential Mortality in
      the U.S.:  A Study in Socioeconimic Epidemiology. (Cambridge,
      Massachusetts, Harvard University Press, 1973).
90.   Krantz, D.S., M.I. Sanmorco, R.H. Selvester, and K.A. Matthews.
      Psychological Correlates of Progression of Atherosclerosis
      in Men.  Psychosom. Med. 41 (1979) 467-476.
91.   Labarthe, D., D. Reed, J. Brody, R.A. Stallones.  Health
      Effects of Modernization in Palau.  Amer. J. Epidemiol. 98
      (1973) 161-174.
92.   Laren, P.  The Effect of Plasma Cholesterol Lowering Diet in
      Male Survivor of Myocardial Infarction.  Acata. Med. Scand.
      466 Suppl. (1962) 5-92.
93.   Lavey, E.B., R.A. Winkle  Continuing Disability of Patients
      with Chest Pain and Normal Coronary Arteriograms.  J. Chron.
      Dis. 32 (1979) 191-196.

94. Leder, T., B. Neubauer, N.J. Christensen, and K. Lundback. Diabetic Cardiopathy. Diabetologia 1 (1979) 207-209.

95. Kikoff, W., B.L. Segal, and H. Kasparian. Paradox of Normal Selective Coronary Angiogram in Patients Considered to Have Unmistakable Coronary Heart Disease. New Eng. J. Med. 276 (1967) 1063-1066.

96. Lind, A.R., S.H. Taylor, P.W. Humphreys. The Circulatory Effects of Sustained Voluntary Muscle Contraction. Clin. Sci. 27 (1964) 229-244.

97. Lown, B. and R.L. Verrier. Neural Activity and Ventricular Fibrillation. New England Journal of Medicine 294 (1976) 1165-1170.

98. Mogoun, H.W. The Waking Brain. (Springfield, Illinois, Charles Thomas, 1963).

99. Malhotra S.L. Georgraphical Aspects of Acute Myocardial Infarction in India with Special Reference to Patterns of Diet and Eating. Brit. Heart J. 29 (1967) 337-344.

100. Management Committee. The Australian Therapeutic Trial in Mild Hypertension. Lancet I (1980) 1261-1267.

101. Mann, G.V. Diet Heart: End of an Era. New England Journal of Medicine 297 (1977) 644-650.

102. Mann, G.V., R.D. Shaffer, R.S. Andersson, and H.H. Sandstead. Cardiovascular Disease in the Masai. Atheroscler. Res. 4 (1964) 289-312.

103. Marmot, M.G. Epidemiological Basis for the Prevention of Coronary Heart Disease. Bull. W.H.O. 57(3) (1979) 331-347.

104. Marmot, M.G., A.M. Aldelstein, N. Robinson and G.A. Rose. Changing Social Class Districution of Heart Disease. Brit. Med. J. II (1978) 1109-1112.

105. Marmot, M.G., G. Rose, M. Shipley, and P.J.S. Hamilton. Employment Grade and Coronary Heart Disease in British Civil Servants. J. Epidem. Comm. Health 32 (1978B) 244-249.

106. Marmot, M.G. and S.L. Syme. Acculturation and Coronary Heart Disease in Japanese-Americans. Amer. J. Epidemiol. 104 (1976) 225-246.

107. Marmot, M. and W. Winkelstein. Epidemiologic Observation on Intervention Trials for Prevention of Coronary Heart Disease. Amer. J. Epidem. 101 (1975) 177-181.

108. Maser, A., A. L'Abbote, G. Baroldi, et al. Coronary Spasm as a Possible Cause of Myocardial Infarction. New Eng. J. Med. 299 (1978) 1271-1277.

109. Mather, H.G., N.G. Pearson, K.L.Q. Read, et al. Acute Myocardial Infarction: Home and Hospital Treatment. Brit. Med. J. 3 (1971) 334.

110. Matsumoto, Y.S. Social Stress and Coronary Heart Disease in Japan: A Hypothesis. In Hans Peter Dreitzel (Ed.) Social Organization of Health (London, Collier-Macmillan Ltd., 1971.

308

111. Medalie, J.H. and U. Goldbourt. Angina Pectoris Among 10,000 Men. II. Psychosocial and Other Risk Factors as Evidence by a Multivariate Analysis of a 5-Year Incidence Study. Amer. J. Med. 60 (1976) 910-921.

112. Medalie, J.H., H.A. Kahn, H.N. Neufeld et al. Myocardial Infarction Over a 5-Year Period. I. Prevalence Incidence and Mortality Experience. J. Chron. Dis. 26 (1973) 63-83.

113. Medalie, J.H., H.A. Kahn, H.N. Neufeld, et al. Five-year Myocardial Infarction Incidence. I. Association of Single Variables to Age and Birth Place. J. Chron. Dis. 26 (1973) 329-349.

114. Miettinen, M., O. Turpeinen, M.J. Karvonen. Effect of Cholesterol Lowering Diet on Mortality from Coronary Heart Disease and Other Causes: A 12-Year Clinical Trial in Men and Women. Lancet II (1972) 835-838.

115. Morris, J.N., S.P.W. Chava, C. Adam, et al. Vigorous Exercise in Leisure Time and the Incidence of Coronary Heart Disease. Lancet I (1973) 333-339.

116. Morris, J.N., M.G. Everitt, R. Pollard, et al. Vigorous Exercise in Leisure Time: Protection Against Coronary Heart Disease. Lancet (1980) 1207-1210.

117. Morris, J.N., J.A. Heady, and R.G. Barley. Coronary Heart Disease in Medical Practitioners. Brit. Med. J. I (1952) 503-520.

118. Morris, J.N., J.A. Heady, P.A.B. Raffle, et al. Coronary Heart Disease and Physical Activity of Work. Lancet II (1953) 1053-1057.

119. Morris, J.N., A. Kagan, D.C. Pattison, et al. Incidence and Prediction of Ischaemic Heart Disease in London Busmen. Lancet II (1966) 553-559.

120. M.R.C. Working Party on Mild to Moderate Hypertension. Brit. Med. J. I (1977) 1437.

121. Multicenture International Study. Improvement in Prognosis of Myocardial Infarction by Long-Term Beta-Adrenoreceptor Blockade Using Practolol. Brit. Med. J. 3 (1975) 735-740.

122. McIntosh, H.D. and G.A. Garcia. The First Decade of Aorto Coronary By-Pass Grafting, 1967-77: A Review. Circulation 57 (1978) 405-431.

123. McMichael, I. Diet and Exercise in Coronary Heart Disease. Lancet I (1974) 1340-1341.

124. National Diet Heart Study Research Group. The National Diet Heart Study: Final Report. American Heart Assoc. Monograph No. 18, 1968.

125. Nichols, A.B., C. Ravenscroft, D.E. Lamphiear, et al. Daily Nutritional Intake and Serum Lipid Levels: The Tecumseh Study. Am. J. Clin. Nutri. 29 (1976) 1384-1392.

126. Nixon, P. Human Function Curve with Special Reference to Cardiovascular Disorders. Part I. Practitioner 217 (1976) 765-770.

127. Ogilvie, H.   In Praise of Idleness.   Brit. Med. J. 1 (1949) 645-651.

128. Oliva, B., D.E. Potts, and R.G. Pluss.   Coronary Artery Spasm in Prinzmetal Angina.   New Eng. J. Med. 288 (1973) 745-751.

129. Osler, W.   Lumlein Lectures on Angina Pectoris.   Lancet I (1910) 839-844.

130. Ostrander, L.D. Jr., T. Francis Jr., N.S. Hayner et al. The Relationship of Cardiovascular Disease to Hyperglycaemia. Ann. Intern. Med. 62 (1965) 1188-1198.

131. Pantridge, J.F. and J.S. Geddes.   A Mobile Intensive Care Unit in the Management of Myocardial Infarction.   Lancet II (1967) 271-273.

132. Parodi, O., A. Masseri, and I. Simonetti.   Management of Unstable Angina at Rest by Verapamil:   A Double-Blind Cross-Over Study in the Coronary Care Unit.   Brit. Heart J. 41 (1979) 167-174.

133. Parkes, C.M., B. Benjamin and R.G. Fitzgerald.   Broken Heart: A Statistical Study of Increased Mortality Among Widowers. Brit. Med. J. 1 (1969) 740-743.

134. Patel, C.H.   Yoga and Biofeedback in the Management of Hypertension.   Lancet II (1973) 1053-1055.

135. Patel, C.   Twelve-Month Follow Up of Yoga and Biofeedback in the Management of Hypertension.   Lancet I (1975A) 62-65.

136. Patel, C.   Yoga and Biofeedback in the Management of "Stress" in Hypertensive Patients.   Clin. Sci. Mol. Med. Vol. 48, $171_s$, $174_s$ Suppl.   Proceedings of Third Symposium of the International Society of Hypertension.   Milan, September 1974.   (Oxford, Blackwell Scient. Publ, 1975).

137. Patel, C.   Reduction of Serum Cholesterol and Blood Pressure in Hypertensive Patients by Behaviour Modification.   J. Roy. Coll. General Practitioners 26 (1976) 211-215.

138. Patel, C.H.   Biofeedback-Aided Relaxation and Meditation in the Management of Hypertension.   Biofeedback and Self-Regulation.   2 (1977) 1-41.

139. Patel, C. and M. Carruthers.   Coronary Risk Factor Reduction Through Biofeedback-Aided Relaxation and Meditation.   J. Roy. Coll. General Practitioners 27 (1977) 401-405.

140. Patel, C.H. and W.R.S. North.   Randomized Controlled Trial of Yoga and Biofeedback in the Management of Hypertension. Lancet II (1975) 93-95.

141. Patel, C. M.M. Marmot, and D.J. Terry.   Controlled Trial of Biofeedback-Aided Behavioural Methods in Reducing Mild Hypertension.   Brit. Med. J. 282 (1981) 2005-2008.

142. Patel, C.H., M. Marmot, D.J. Terry, et al.   Coronary Risk Factor Reduction Through Biofeedback Aided Relaxation and Meditation.   Paper presented at the 52nd Annual Scientific Meeting, Anaheim, California, November 1979.   Circulation 60(2) Abstraction 882 (1979) II-226.

143. Pell, S., and C.A. D'Alonzo.   Some Aspects of Hypertension in Diabetes Mellitus.   JAMA 202 (1967) 10.

144. Pickering, G.W.  High Blood Pressure.  2nd Edition (London,
     J. & A. Churchill, 1968).
145. The Pooling Project Research Group.  Relationship of Blood
     Pressure, Serum Cholesterol, Smoking Habits, Relative Weight
     and ECG Abnormalities to Incidence of Major Coronary Events:
     A Final Report of the Pooling Project.  J. Chron. Dis. 3
     (1978) 201-306.
146. Prior, I.M.,  H.P.B. Harvey, M.I. Neave, and F. Davidson.
     The  Health of Two Groups of Cook Island Maorios.  Medical
     Research  Council of New Zealand.  Department of Health.
     Special Report  Series, No. 26,  1966.
147. Prognosis  After Myocardial Infarction.  Leading  Article.
     Brit. Med. J. 2 (1979) 1311-1312.
148. Puska, P., J. Tuomilehto, J. Salonen et al.  Changes in
     Coronary Risk Factors During Comprehensive 5-Year Community
     Programme to Control Cardiovascular Disease (North Karelia
     Project) Brit. Med. J. ii (1979) 1173-1178.
149. Rahe, R.H.  Subjects Recent Life Changes and Their Near
     Future Illness Susceptibility.  Advances in Psychosom.
     Med. 18 (1972) 2-19.
150. Rahe, R.H.  Subjects Recent Life Changes and Their Near
     Future Illness Reports.  Ann. Clin. Res. 4  (1972) 250-265.
151. Rahe, R.H. and J. Paasikivi.  Psychosocial Factors and Myo-
     cardial Infarction.  II. An Out-Patient Study in Sweden.
     J. Psychosom. Res. 15 (1971) 33-39.
152. Rahe, R.H., R.T. Rubin, E.K.E. Gunderson and R.J. Arthur.
     Psychologic Correlates of Serum Cholesterol Level in Man:
     A Longitudinal Study.  Psychosom. Med. 33 (1971) 399-410.
153. Ramsey, L.E., M.H. Ramsey, J. Hettarachchi et al.  Weight
     Reduction  in  a Blood Pressure Clinic.  Brit. Med. J. 2
     (1978) 244-245.
154. Reid, D.D., P.J.S. Hamilton,  P. McCartney et al.  Smoking
     and Other Risk Factors for Coronary Heart Disease in British
     Civil Servants.  Lancet II (1976) 979-984.
155. Reisin, E., R. Abel, M. Modan et al.  Effect of Weight Loss
     Without Salt Restriction on the Reduction of Blood Pressure.
     New Eng. J. Med. 298 (1978)  1-6.
156. Research Committee.  Controlled Trial of  Soya Bean Oil  in
     Myocardial Infarction.  Lancet II (1968) 693-700.
157. Research Committee.  Low Fat Diet in Myocardial Infarction:
     A Controlled Trial.  Lancet III (1965) 501-504.
158. Research Committee of the Scottish Society of Physicians.
     Ischaemic Heart Disease:  A Second Prevention Trial Using
     Clofibrate.  Brit. Med. J. 4 (1971) 775-784.
159. Rose, G.A.  The Contribution of Intensive Coronary Care.
     Brit. J. Prev. Soc. Med. 29 (1975) 147-150.
160. Rose, G.  Coronary Heart Disease:  Check the Healthy Patient.
     Modern Medicine 21 (4) (1976) 6-11.
161. Rose, G. and P.J.S. Hamilton.  A Randomized Control Trial
     of the Effect on Middle-Aged Men of Advice to Stop Smoking.

J. Epidem.Comm. Health 32 (1978) 275-281.

162. Rose, G., R.F. Heller, H.T. Pedoe and D.G.S. Christie.
Heart Disease Prevention Project: A Randomized Controlled
Trial in Industry. Brit. Med. J. i (1980) 747-751.

163. Rosenman, R.H. The Role of Behaviour Patterns and Neuro-
genic Factors in the Pathogenesis of Coronary Heart Disease.
In R.S. Elliott (Ed.) Stress and the Heart (New York, Futura
Publishing Company, 1974).

164. Rosenman, R.H., R.J. Brand, C.D. Jenkins et al. Coronary
Heart Disease in Western Collaborative Group Study: Final
Follow Up of 8½ Years. JAMA 233 (1975) 872.

165. Rosenman, R.H., R.J. Brand, R.I. Sholtz, and M. Friedman.
Multivariate Prediction of Coronary Heart Disease During
8.5 Year Follow Up in the Western Collaborative Group Study.
Am. J. of Cardiology 37 (1976) 902-910.

166. Rosenman, R.H. and M. Friedman. Modifying Type A Behaviour
Pattern. J. Psychosom. Res. 21 (1977) 323-333.

167. Rosenman, R.H., M. Friedman, R. Straus et al. Coronary
Heart Disease in the Western Collaborative Group Study:
A Follow Up Experience of Two Years. JAMA 195 (1966)
130-134.

168. Roskies, E., H. Kearney, M. Spevack et al. Generalizability
and Durability of Treatment Effects in an Intervention
Program for Coronary-Prone (Type A) Managers. J. Behav.
Med. 2 (1979) 195-207.

169. Roskies, E. Considerations in Developing a Treatment
Program for the Coronary-Prone (Type A) Behaviour Pattern.
In P. Davidson and S.M. Davidson (Eds.) Behavioural Medicine:
Changing Health Life Styles. (New York, Brunner/Mazel, 1980).

170. Royal College of Physicians. Smoking or Health. (London,
Pitman Medical, 1977).

171. Russek, H.I. and L.G. Russek. Behaviour Patterns and
Emotional Stress in the Etiology of Coronary Heart Disease:
Sociological and Occupational Aspects. In D. Wheatly (Ed.)
Stress and the Heart (New York, Raven Press, 1977).

172. Russek, H.I. and B.L. Zohman. Relative Significance of Heredity,
Diet and Occupational Stress in Coronary Heart Disease of
Young Adults. Amer. J. Med. Sci. 235 (1958) 266-277.

173. Salonen, J.T., P. Puska, and H. Mustaniemi. Changes in Morbidity and Mortality During Comprehensive Community Programme
to Control Cardiovascular Diseases During 1972-77 in North
Karelia. Brit. Med. J. ii (1979) 1178-1183.

174. Sachar, .EJ. Hormonal Changes in Stress and Mental Illness.
In D.T. Kriger and J.C. Hughes (Eds.) Neuroendocrinology:
The Interrelationships of Body's Two Major Integrative
Systems in Normal Physiology and in Clinical Disease.
Sunderland, Massachusetts, Sinauer Associates).

175. Schucker, T. and D.R. Jacobs. Assessment of Behavioural
Risk for Coronary Heart Disease by Voice Characteristics.
Psychosomatic Medicine 39 (1977) 219-228.

176. Scotch, N.A. and J.H. Geiger. The Epidemiology of Essential Hypertension. A Review with Special Attention to Psychologic and Sociocultural Factors. Psychologic and Sociocultural Factors in Etiology. J. Chron. Dis., 16 (1963) 1183-1213.
177. Scottish Hearts Editorial. Lancet II (1979) 726,727.
178. Scottish Home and Health Department. Research into Coronary Heart Disease in Scotland. Report to the Chief Scientist by a Working Group. Edinburgh, (1979).
179. Shaper, A.G. Cardiovascular Studies in the Sambaru Tribe of Northern Kenya. Am. Heart J., 63 (1962) 437.
180. Saper, A.G., M. Jones, and J. Kyobe. Plasma Lipids in an African Tribe Living on a Diet of Milk and Meat. Lancet II (1961) 1324-1327.
181. Shekelle,R.B., A.M. Ostfeld, and O. Paul. Social Status and Incidence of Coronary Heart Disease. J. Chron. Dis. 22 (1969) 381-394.
182. Singh, B., G. Ellardt, and C.T. Peter. Verapamil: A Review of its Pharmacological Properties and Therapeutic Use. Drugs, 15 (1978) 169-197.
183. St. Leger, A.S., A.L. Cochrane, and F. Moore. Factors Associated with Cardiac Mortality in Developed Countries with Particular Refernce to the Consumption of Wine. Lancet I (1979) 1017-1020.
184. Stout, C., J.Marrow, E. Brandt, and S. Wolf. Unusually Low Incidence of Death from Myocardial Infraction in an Italian-American Community in Pennsylvania. J. Am. Med. Ass. 188 (1964) 845-849.
185. Suinn, R.M. The Cardiac Stress: Management Program for Type A Patients. Cardiac Rehabilitation, 5 (1975) 13-15.
186. Syme, S.L. and L.F. Berkman. Social Class, Susceptibility and Sickness. Amer. J. Epidem., 104 (1976) 1-8.
187. Syme, S.L., M.N. Hyman, and P.E. Enterline. Some Social and Cultural Factors Associated with the Occurrence of Coronary Heart Disease. J. Chron. Dis., 17 (1964) 277-289.
188. Tuck, M.L., J. Sowers, L. Dornfeld et al. The Effect of Weight Reduction, Blood Pressure, Plasm Renin Activity and Aldoster Levels in Obese Patients. New Eng. J. Med. 304 (1981) 930-933.
189. University Group Diabetes Program. A Study of the Efect of Hypoglycaemic Agents on Vascular Complications in Patients with Adult- Onset Diabetes.VI. Supplementary Report on non-fatal Events in Patients Treated with Tolbutamide. Diabetes, 25 (1976) 1129-1153.
190. Valkonen, T. and M.L. Niemi. Decline of Mortality from Cardiovascular Disease in North Karelia. Brit. Med. J. I (1980) 46.
191. Vaughan Williams, E.M., N.O. Hassan, J.S. Floras et. al. Adaption of Hypertensives to Treatment with Cardioselective and Non-selective Beta-blockers. Absence of Correlation between Bradycardia and Blood Pressure Control and Reduction

in Slope of QT/RR Relation. Brit. Heart J., 44 (1980) 437-487.

192. Veterans Administration Co-operative Study Group on Anti-hypertensive Agents. Effects of Treatment on Morbidity in Hypertension: Results in Patients with Diastolic Blood Pressures Averaging 115 Through 129 mm.Hg. J. Am. Med. Ass., 202 (1967) 1028-1034.

193. Veterans Administration Co-operative Study Group on Anti-hypertensive agents. Effects of Treatment on Morbidity in Hypertension. II. Results in Patients with Diastolic Blood Pressures Averaging 90 Through 114 mm.Hg. J. Am. Med. Ass. 213 (1970) 1143-1152.

194. Veterans Administration Co-operative Study Group on Anti-hypertensive Agents. Effects of Treatment on Morbidity in Hypertenion. III. Influence of Age, Diastolic Pressure and Cardiovascular disease. Circulation, 45 (1972) 991-1004.

195. Virchow, R. Cellular Pathology as Based upon Physiological and Pathological Histology. Translated from the Second German Edition Originally Published by J.P. Lippincott and Co. 1863. New York, Dover Publications, 1971.

196. Wallace, R.K. and H. Benson. The Physiology of Meditation. Scientific American., 226 (1972) 84-90.

197. Welborn, T.A. and K. Wearne. Coronary Heart Disease Incidence and Cardiovascular Mortality in Busselton with Reference to Glucose and Insulin Concentration. Diabetes Care., 2 (1979) 154-160.

198. Westaby, S., R.N. Sapsford, and H.H. Bentall. Return to Work and Quality of Life after Surgery for Coronary Artery Disease. Brit. Med. J., II (1979) 1028-1931.

199. Why the American Decline in Coronary Heart Disease? Editorial, Lancet I (1980) 183,184.

200. Wilcox, R.G., J.M. Roland, D. Banks et.al. Randomised Trial Comparing Prppanolol with Atenol in Immediate Treatment of Suspected Myocardial Infarct. Brit. Med. I (1980) 885-888.

201. Wilhelmsson, C., J.A. Vedin, L. Wilhelmsson et. al. Reduction of Sudden Deaths after Myocardial Infarction by Treatment with Alprenolol. Lancet II 1157-1160.

202. Williams, R.B., M. Friedman, D.C. Glass et. al. Summary Statement. Mechanisms Linking Behavioural and Pathophysio-logical Processes. In T. Dembroski (Ed.) Proceedings of the Forum on Coronary Prone Behaviour. Washington, D.C. Dept. of Health, Education and Welfare. Publication No. (NIH) 199 78-1451, 157-169.

203. Wolf, S. In Society, Stress and Disease. Vol. I, L. Levi (Ed.) Oxford University Press. (1971) 5

204. Wolf, S.G. Cardiovascular Reactions to Symbolic Stimuli. Circulation, 18 (1958) 187-292.

205. Wolpe, J. Psychotherapy by Reciprocal Inhibition. Stanford University Press, (1958).

206. World Health Organisation European Collaborative Group. An International Controled Trial in the Multifactorial Prevention of Coronary Heart Disease. Internat. J. Epidem., 3 (1974) 219-224.
207. World Health Statistics Annuals 1968-79. Geneva World Health Organisation, 1979.
208. Yasue, H., M. Touyama, H. Kato et. al. Prinzmetal Variant Form of Angina as a Manisfestation of Alpha- Adrenergic Receptor Mediated Coronary Artery Spasm Documented by Angiography. Am. Heart J., 91 (1976) 148-155.

THE BROADER ISSUE - HEALTH-CARE MANAGEMENT AT THE INDIVIDUAL AND
SYSTEMS LEVEL

Gilbeart H. Collings, Jr.

Corporate Medical Director
The New York Telephone Company
New York, New York

In our sessions here at the Chateau de Bonas, we have been
exploring what is known about the effects of stress, its causes,
and the interplay between stress, health, and work, i.e., how
stress relates to health and therefore to productivity and function
and how its effects can be mitigated or modified.  We have thus
been directing our attention to the body of knowledge about stress.
A different issue is how does one apply that body of knowledge in
a fruitful way.  In other words, how can it be incorporated into
practical action programs which can intervene in the real world
with reasonable hope of success commensurate with the effort
expended.  This question brings up new considerations and opens
up a whole spectrum of additional subjects for discussion.  Many
of these are important, indeed essential, to evolving a workable
stress intervention.  But, as you know, stress is only one factor
in health.  Among others are heredity, nutrition, quality of medical
care, aging, the physical environment, etc.  The broader issue then
commands a look at stress not as a stand-alone factor but as one
piece in a multifactorial complex.

We have extensive experience with single-factor intervention
programs other than stress and somewhat less experience with integrated interventions aimed more broadly at the multifactorial
health complex.  But stress, whether approached independently as
a single factor or jointly as a part of the broader complex, has
only recently received attention in action-oriented programs.
Limited though it is, our experience so far with stress management
leads us to believe it will not present fundamentally different
challenges from other health factors which have previously pursued.
We will, therefore, draw from our prior experience with other health

interventions as we plan to incorporate stress reduction into our
health-promotion programs. I would like to explore with you some
of the considerations which we may expect to encounter as we set
out to do something about stress.

First, however, it would be appropriate for me to diverge
briefly and tell you a bit about the background of my own particular
experience with regard to these matters. Our company is a large
company, having 80,000 employees working in 1,237 locations
throughout the state of New York. Our main concentration of
47,000 employees is in the New York City metropolitan area. The
population is 47% women and mean age is 41 years with a gradual
trend upward. Total company costs for health impairment in this
population, as projected for 1981, are on the order of $200 million,
an amount equal to 10% of total wage payments and more than 10%
greater than last year. Our medical department of about 225
employees includes 40 full-time physicians, 40 nurses, 3 rehabilitation counselors and 4 health counselors. Health policy is guided
by a medical cabinet of senior medical directors in the headquarters
group, chaired by the Corporate Medical Director. Such policy is
implemented through 8 area medical offices of varying sizes
throughout the state. Each of these offices has a professional
staff headed by an Area Medical Director. We have a partial medical
information system (MIS) operating in all areas and a complete
prototype MIS in one area serving about 9,000 employees. Our
medical department staffs work hard to develop and maintain sound
relationships with upper management supervisors, union leaders and
employees in general. In this environment, we provide many
standard intervention programs, some not-so-standard intervention
programs, and we do applied research in the development of new
intervention programs.

Let us now consider the stress management problem. How can
we best make use of the knowledge we currently have about stress?
How can we minimize the negative effects stress has on the target
population? How can we capitalize on its positive effects? And,
how can we improve the resultant wellness and coping ability of
the population we serve?

As one considers these questions in relationship to a specific
target population, the first solution that pops into mind is
education of the population so that they will understand stress
and its relationships well enough to take action. Usually, the
decision to educate assumes that if people only knew enough about
a problem to understand it they would automatically be prompted
to do something about it. Unfortunately, of course, this is not
the case often enough. Furthermore, such logic depends on the
presumed wisdom of people to be able to make their action appropriate and effective. Moreover, the educational approach assumes

that people have the capability of making the necessary crucial
decisions and devising the appropriate strategies to adapt general
knowledge to meet their own specific needs as individuals. A bit
of reflection on this will probably bring us to the conclusion -
which is the correct conclusion, by the way - that left to their
own devices very few people are likely to work out effective
answers. Which in turn leads us to the second conclusion: that
we will probably have to provide additional amounts of education
beyond an academic understanding of stress, to try to help
people with the "how to" part of coping with stress. In other
words, we are prompted to provide additional education and training
to supplement the individual employee's limited ability to manage
his or her own program.

This may come as an unwelcome revelation to you but our experience with health interventions generally has been that the
simple education of participants either in regard to the facts of
a subject itself or in regard to the ways to achieve practical
goals with that subject has been unsuccessful in producing more
than marginal results.

On the other hand, our experience has been that generally
people respond better to a leader who possesses special knowledge
and capability in a particular subject area than they do to the
opportunity to acquire sufficient depth of understanding of that
subject area to be self-sufficient. While people need to participate freely and actively and not be coerced, they also need
guidance and suggestions as to how to proceed and finally they need
ongoing encouragement and a place to resolve the problems and
frustrations that arise.

As a result of all this we have concluded that if one really
wants to change the state of affairs for a group of people, a
different approach from the standard garden variety of health
education is required. An approach which we find successful is a
partnership between the participant employee and the professional
within the system with mutual respect and cooperation on both
sides, aimed not at making the employee a self-sufficient expert
fully competent in his/her own right and totally responsible for
the eventual outcome, but aimed at a joint approach with the
sharing of as much information as is necessary to accomplish the
desired ends. Not only does such an approach work better than
education alone, it turns out to require less total effort than
education alone because it is not wasteful of education and it is
not necessary to bring all participants up to a high level of
expertise on all subjects relevant to their health status. An
example may make this point clear. It is simply more efficient
for me to go to a qualified auto-mechanic who tells me that the
bearing in my car is burned out, replaces the bearing, and then
gives me enough education so that I will keep the bearing lubricated,

than it is for me to learn enough about auto mechanics to be able
to identify and understand about bearings and then work out the
repair and continuing maintenance details for myself.

Now, let us talk a bit about what our experience has shown us
with regard to the requirements for an effective health partnership.  The following are the fundamentals:

1.  It must appeal to and obtain the full voluntary partici-
    pation of each individual.

2.  It must provide a minimum of education for the participating
    individual consisting only of the facts necessary for
    success.

3.  It must present to the participating individual practical
    strategies for action at appropriate times.

4.  And, it must follow-up, support, reinforce, and evaluate
    its success on a continuing basis.

Let us probe a bit deeper into number three above, "The
strategies for action...":

Consider the following for a moment:  Suppose your responsibility was to deal with all the pneumonia and all the diabetes in
a population.  Would you give the whole population an antibiotic
and give the whole population insulin?  Of course not.  It could
be argued, however, that such action would in fact take care of
most of the pneumonia and the diabetes.  But, you would immediately
point out that such an approach is wasteful, almost certainly not
cost-effective and moreover would be attended by substantial side
effects on the people that had no pneumonia or diabetes.  To say
nothing of being hard to administer in such a way as to achieve
the proper therapeutic dosages in each case of disease.  While we
recognize the absurdity of the foregoing approach to the medical
treatment of disease, we seem to assume that when it comes to
other forms of intervention such as stress-management or to preventive interventions, different ground rules pertain and we set
out to apply our interventions on a wholesale basis.  The truth
of the matter is that this approach is no more viable in the latter
circumstances than it is in the medical therapeutic interventions.
Should everyone who is fat have his/her weight reduced to normal?
I don't think so.  The fat man who is going to survive in relatively
good health to a ripe old age doesn't need his weight reduced.
Should eveyone stop smoking?  I doubt it.  Most smokers are not
going to die of smoke-related illnesses.  Should everyone be trained
in stress reduction?  If so, should everyone have the same kind of
training?  Should everyone have the same action plans?

What we are facing into is a common dilemma in prevention, the disparity between the large diffuse target population and the small number of effective hits from any particular intervention. Obviously, we must find ways to reduce this disparity and some attempts to do so are already evident (so-called health hazard appraisal, and other forms of risk or need assessment have come to the fore in an attempt to reduce the targeted population to those with a statistically higher need). But, this is only the beginning and we must go much further. We must not only increase the precision of "need identification," we must prognosticate the yield from that intervention as well, since all high-need individuals do not respond in the same degree relative to the yield from any given intervention. We can thus postulate high-need, high-yield equations for more effective preventive intervention. Due to the present lack of hard data, filling in the controlling variables in these equations is something we can only partially do today. However, the direction in which we must move is clear. We need to work toward an armamentarium which is less of a shotgun and more a rifle.

Having looked at the single intervention of stress management and remembering what we said earlier, that in the real world single-factor interventions must often coexist and interrelate with multiple numbers of other factors, some of which may also have interventions, what can we learn from experience with multiple interventions in the same population?

We have found that individual programs such as hypertension control, exercise programs, weight reduction, or what have you, are often only marginally cost-effective or ineffective at first but can sometimes be brought into the black by dilligent management and adaptation. At best, however, such stand-alone programs are inefficient since they address very wide target populations and by their very nature generate high overheads. As a consequence, as experience with such stand-alone programs has accumulated, the natural tendency has been to combine several of these interventions into a single, coordinated, hopefully more efficient format. This led, a number of years ago, to the emergence of so-called multiphasic approaches where individual elements or interventions share in a common overhead and can be directed by common medical management to a common target population. Although much improved in efficiency as compared to the older single-element programs, these multi-element programs have not provided the ultimate answer. They did, however, serve to bring into clearer focus the nature of the real problems facing intervention professionals and to stimulate the development of improved methods of administration. And, experience with them clarified the important basic principles of integrated intervention management, which are:

1. Standardized interventions although superficially attractive because they are easy to apply to large numbers of people, seldom work out well. Health interventions need to be individualized to fit the specific situation of each participant if real efficiency and effective results are to be obtained.

2. Although individualization is the key to the successful intervention, the collective administration of such interventions needs to be conceptualized and carried out on an integrated basis as a whole and not in separate isolated programs.

3. The delivery system must be managed in such a way as to optimize its opportunities to achieve the most productive overall cost-benefit ratios.

For a number of years we have been developing such a system at New York Telephone and are vigorously pursuing its maturation. We call it Health Care Management (HCM). I would like to briefly describe this system, not because it is the best in the world but because I am most familiar with it and it can serve as a basis for discussion which may be stimulated by this presentation.

Briefly, our concept of HCM is oriented to the whole spectrum of health itself wherein those services nearer to the good-health end of the spectrum (specifically health education, preventive measures, early diagnosis, and presymptomatic ambulatory care) provide relatively low-cost leverage to control the high-cost services closer to the poor-health end. These latter include symptomatic ambulatory care, crisis care, and rehabilitative and domiciliary care. Such control is exerted only in proportion to the quality and extent of the leverage services. We view these services as best provided through application of management by objectives which is so well known in the business world but almost unknown among medical professionals except for the traditional mandated objective to alleviate the patient's disease.

We have somewhat arbitrarily divided HCM into three levels of management. All depend on an information base able to define the health "norm" for individuals and for groups (requiring a detailed health profile for each individual on a voluntary and confidential basis and periodically updated).

We define Level I management as what we do about acute departures from the norm of an individual. This is a disease-oriented, crisis-type care for which physicians are trained and its objective is the restoral of the norm, either the old one or a new one and as early and as cost-effectively as possible. This type of care we sometimes deliver ourselves but more often work in conjunction with community health-care providers since we are not in the business of acute-care delivery. It is this level of HCM that has caused us to extensively involve ourselves in a number of business groups on health, health maintenance organizations, and the like, and to hire and train a director of health resources management. Although we may work through a community practitioner who delivers the actual care, we do not relinquish our management role during Level I care process; our professionals are committed to follow a case through to the achievement of the objective.

Level II management in our view is uniquely suited to in-house delivery. It too is oriented to the individual employee and is essentially the dividing of an individual's health profile (his norm) into pieces to be managed over a long term. Each management unit which we call a "monad" is characterized and assigned long-term objectives. And, strategies are developed to achieve those object-ives. The processing of all such monads results in what we call the lifetime health strategy. This includes the scheduling of periodic encounters to measure progress toward objectives and to modify those objectives as appropriate. The basic premise for Level II management is the promotion of wellness.

Finally, Level III management is designed to manage the pop-ulation and is based on the idea of the high-need, high-yield module. In this system, the sub-populations of our employees at high risk for a variety of high-cost and treatable or preventable diseases such as hypertension or low-back syndrome, or stress are identified. Individuals falling into such a group are presented to our health professionals along with options for interventions "prioritized" according to yield. The professional may or may not select one of these options but he must take some action and docu-ment it, thus adding to our information base for future decision-making. In addition, Level III management is intended to facilitate the management of the system itself for better operating efficiency, maximum resource utilization, more productive strategy planning, and finally for evaluation.

In summary, HCM is an integrated manageable system through which an individual employee's total health can be addressed with efficiency. It permits the simultaneous and flexible application of a variety of interventions (such as stress-control) with some expectation that each will not be wasted on low-need people while being effectively brought to bear where they can be expected to do the greatest good.

Although this or some other system is a necessary basis for optimum health management, it is not the entire solution. For there is also the matter of _practice_ which we may call the practice of health-care management.   This, like clinical practice, is both an art and a science.   And, although it is a new form of practice for most of us, it is one which will respond to experience and capability and common sense and one which offers substantial opportunities for growth and achievement of professionals engaged in helping others to improve the quality of life.

# SUBJECT INDEX